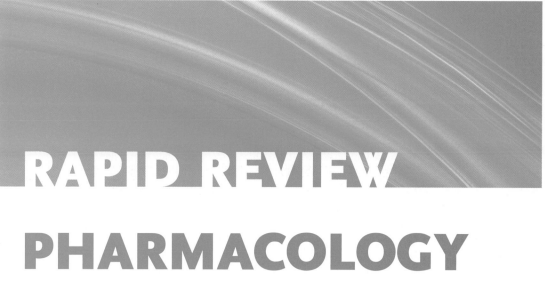

RAPID REVIEW

PHARMACOLOGY

THIRD EDITION

Thomas L. Pazdernik, PhD
Chancellor's Club Teaching Professor
Department of Pharmacology, Toxicology, and Therapeutics
University of Kansas Medical Center
Kansas City, Kansas

Laszlo Kerecsen, MD
Professor
Department of Pharmacology
Arizona College of Osteopathic Medicine
Midwestern University
Glendale, Arizona

D1439238

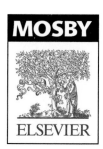

MOSBY

ELSEVIER

MOSBY
ELSEVIER

3251 Riverport Lane
Maryland Heights, Missouri 63043

RAPID REVIEW PHARMACOLOGY, Second Edition
Copyright © 2010, 2007, 2003 by Mosby, Inc., an affiliate of Elsevier Inc.

ISBN: 978-0-323-06812-3

Notice

Knowledge and best practice in this field are constantly changing. As new research and experience broaden our knowledge, changes in practice, treatment and drug therapy may become necessary or appropriate. Readers are advised to check the most current information provided (i) on procedures featured or (ii) by the manufacturer of each product to be administered, to verify the recommended dose or formula, the method and duration of administration, and contraindications. It is the responsibility of the practitioner, relying on their own experience and knowledge of the patient, to make diagnoses, to determine dosages and the best treatment for each individual patient, and to take all appropriate safety precautions. To the fullest extent of the law, neither the Publisher nor the Authors assume any liability for any injury and/or damage to persons or property arising out or related to any use of the material contained in this book.

Library of Congress Cataloging-in-Publication Data
Pazdernik, Thomas.
   Rapid review pharmacology / Thomas L. Pazdernik, Laszlo Kerecsen. — 3rd ed.
     p. ; cm. — (Rapid review series)
   Includes index.
   Rev. ed. of: Pharmacology. 2nd ed. c2007.
   ISBN 978-0-323-06812-3
  I. Pharmacology—Examinations, questions, etc. I. Kerecsen, Laszlo. II. Title.
   III. Series: Rapid review series.
    [DNLM: 1. Pharmaceutical Preparations—Examination Questions. 2. Pharmaceutical Preparations—Outlines. 3. Drug Therapy—Examination Questions. 4. Drug Therapy—Outlines. QV 18.2 P348r 2011]
  RM105.P39 2011
  615'.1—dc22

2009045661

Acquisitions Editor: James Merritt
Developmental Editor: Christine Abshire
Publishing Services Manager: Hemamalini Rajendrababu
Project Manager: Nayagi Athmanathan
Design Direction: Steven Stave

To my wife, Betty; my daughter Nancy and my granddaughter Rebecca Irene; my daughter Lisa and her husband, Chris; and my triplet grandchildren, Cassidy Rae, Thomas Pazdernik, and Isabel Mari

TLP

To Gabor and Tamas, my sons

LK

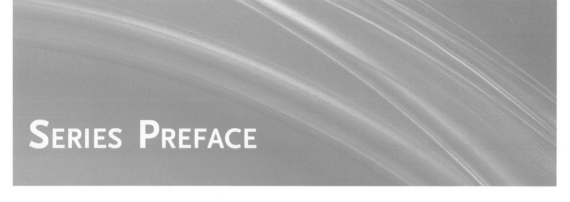

SERIES PREFACE

The First and Second Editions of the *Rapid Review Series* have received high critical acclaim from students studying for the United States Medical Licensing Examination (USMLE) Step 1 and consistently high ratings in *First Aid for the USMLE Step 1*. The new editions will continue to be invaluable resources for time-pressed students. As a result of reader feedback, we have improved upon an already successful formula. We have created a learning system, including a print and electronic package, that is easier to use and more concise than other review products on the market.

SPECIAL FEATURES

Book

- **Outline format:** Concise, high-yield subject matter is presented in a study-friendly format.
- **High-yield margin notes:** Key content that is most likely to appear on the exam is reinforced in the margin notes.
- **Visual elements:** Full-color photographs are utilized to enhance your study and recognition of key pathology images. Abundant two-color schematics and summary tables enhance your study experience.
- **Two-color design:** Colored text and headings make studying more efficient and pleasing.

New! Online Study and Testing Tool

- A minimum of **350 USMLE Step 1–type MCQs:** Clinically oriented, multiple-choice questions that mimic the current USMLE format, including high-yield images and complete rationales for all answer options.
- **Online benefits:** New review and testing tool delivered via the USMLE Consult platform, the most realistic USMLE review product on the market. Online feedback includes results analyzed to the subtopic level (discipline and organ system).
- **Test mode:** Create a test from a random mix of questions or by subject or keyword using the timed **test mode**. USMLE Consult simulates the actual test-taking experience using NBME's FRED interface, including style and level of difficulty of the questions and timing information. Detailed feedback and analysis shows your strengths and weaknesses and allows for more focused study.
- **Practice mode:** Create a test from randomized question sets or by subject or keyword for a dynamic study session. The **practice mode** features unlimited attempts at each question, instant feedback, complete rationales for all answer options, and a detailed progress report.
- **Online access:** Online access allows you to study from an internet-enabled computer wherever and whenever it is convenient. This access is activated through registration on www.studentconsult.com with the pin code printed inside the front cover.

Student Consult

- **Full online access:** You can access the complete text and illustrations of this book on www. studentconsult.com.
- **Save content to your PDA:** Through our unique Pocket Consult platform, you can clip selected text and illustrations and save them to your PDA for study on the fly!
- **Free content:** An interactive community center with a wealth of additional valuable resources is available.

ACKNOWLEDGMENT OF REVIEWERS

The publisher expresses sincere thanks to the medical students and faculty who provided many useful comments and suggestions for improving both the text and the questions. Our publishing program will continue to benefit from the combined insight and experience provided by your reviews. For always encouraging us to focus on our target, the USMLE Step 1, we thank the following:

Patricia C. Daniel, PhD, Kansas University Medical Center

Steven J. Engman, Loyola University Chicago Stritch School of Medicine

Omar A. Khan, University of Vermont College of Medicine

Michael W. Lawlor, Loyola University Chicago Stritch School of Medicine

Lillian Liang, Jefferson Medical College

Erica L. Magers, Michigan State University College of Human Medicine

ACKNOWLEDGMENTS

The authors wish to acknowledge Jim Merritt, Senior Acquisitions Editor, Christine Abshire, Developmental Editor, and Nayagi Athmanathan, Project Manager, at Elsevier. We also thank Eloise DeHann for editing the text and Matt Chansky for his excellent illustrations. A very special thanks to Dr. Edward F. Goljan, Series Editor, who read each chapter quickly after it was sent to him and provided both valuable editing and suggestions for marked improvements to each chapter. We give thanks to Tibor Rozman, MD, for his contributions to the development of clinically relevant questions and to Tamas Kerecsen for processing the questions. We also thank the faculty of the Department of Pharmacology, Toxicology, and Therapeutics at the University of Kansas Medical Center and the faculty of the Department of Pharmacology at Arizona College of Osteopathic Medicine, Midwestern University, for their superb contributions to the development of materials for our teaching programs. Dr. Lisa Pazdernik, Ob/Gyn provided valuable input into Chapter 26 (Drugs used in Reproductive Endocrinology). Finally, we thank the numerous medical students who, over the years, have been our inspiration for developing teaching materials.

—Thomas L. Pazdernik, PhD
Laszlo Kerecsen, MD

CONTENTS

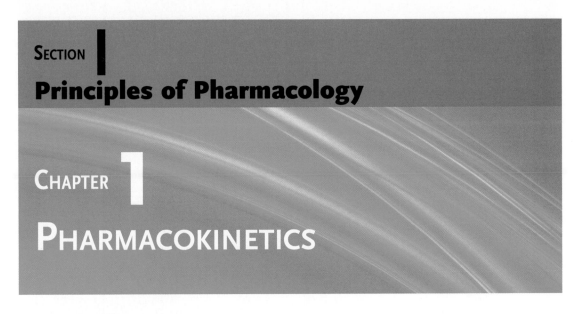

CHAPTER **1**

PHARMACOKINETICS

I. **General** (Fig. 1-1)
   A. **Pharmacokinetics is the fate of drugs within the body.**
   B. **It involves drug:**
      1. Absorption
      2. Distribution
      3. Metabolism
      4. Excretion

ADME— Absorption, Distribution, Metabolism, Excretion

II. **Drug Permeation**
   • Passage of drug molecules across biological membranes
   • Important for pharmacokinetic and pharmacodynamic features of drugs
   A. **Processes of permeation** (Fig. 1-2)
      1. Passive diffusion
         a. Characteristics
            (1) Does *not* make use of a carrier
            (2) *Not* saturable since it doesn't bind to a specific carrier protein
            (3) Low structural specificity since it doesn't require a carrier protein
            (4) Driven by concentration gradient

Passive diffusion driven by concentration gradient.

         b. Aqueous diffusion
            (1) Passage through central pores in cell membranes
            (2) Possible for low-molecular-weight substances (e.g., lithium, ethanol)

Aqueous diffusion via pores in cell membranes.

         c. Lipid diffusion
            (1) Direct passage through the lipid bilayer
               • Facilitated by increased degree of lipid solubility
            (2) Driven by a concentration gradient (nonionized forms move most easily)
            (3) Lipid solubility is the most important limiting factor for drug permeation
               • A large number of lipid barriers separate body compartments.
            (4) Lipid to aqueous partition coefficient (PC) determines how readily a drug molecule moves between lipid and aqueous media.

High lipid-to-oil PC favors lipid diffusion.

      2. Carrier-mediated transport

Most drugs are absorbed by passive diffusion.

         a. Transporters are being identified and characterized that function in movement of molecules into (influx) or out (efflux) of tissues
            • See Tables 3-1; and 3-2 of Biochemistry Rapid Review for further details on the movement of molecules and ions across membranes.
         b. Numerous transporters such as the ABC (ATP-binding cassette) family including P-glycoprotein or multidrug resistant-associated protein type 1 (MDR1) in the brain, testes, and other tissues play a role in excretion as well as in drug-resistant tumors.

Carrier-mediated transport is mediated by influx and efflux transporters.

         c. Characteristics of carrier-mediated transport
            (1) Structural selectivity
            (2) Competition by similar molecules
            (3) Saturable

Drug competition at transporters is a site of drug-drug interactions.

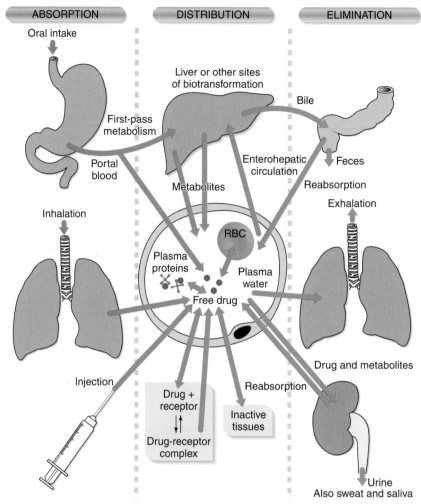

| ABSORPTION | DISTRIBUTION | ELIMINATION |

1-1: Schematic representation of the fate of a drug in the body (pharmacokinetics). Orange arrows indicate passage of drug through the body (intake to output). Orange circles represent drug molecules. RBC, red blood cell.

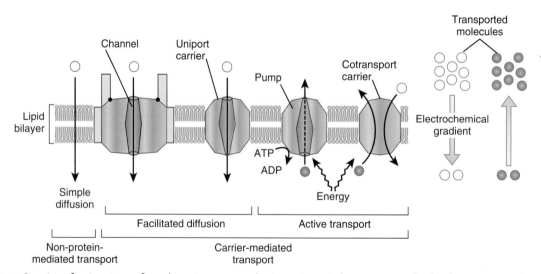

1-2: Overview of various types of membrane-transport mechanisms. Open circles represent molecules that are moving down their electrochemical gradient by simple or facilitated diffusion. Shaded circles represent molecules that are moving against their electrochemical gradient, which requires an input of cellular energy by transport. Primary active transport is unidirectional and utilizes pumps, while secondary active transport takes place by cotransport proteins. *(From Pelley JW and Goljan EF. Rapid Review Biochemistry, 2nd ed. Philadelphia, Mosby, 2007, Figure 3-1.)*

     d. Active transport
       (1) Energy-dependent transporters coupled to ATP hydrolysis (primary active transport); others take place by cotransport proteins (secondary active transport)
       (2) Movement occurs against a concentration or electrochemical gradient
       (3) Most rapid mode of membrane permeation
       (4) Sites of active transport
         (a) Neuronal membranes
         (b) Choroid plexus
         (c) Renal tubular cells
         (d) Hepatocytes

> Active transport requires energy to move molecules against concentration gradient.

     e. Facilitated diffusion
       (1) Does *not* require energy from ATP hydrolysis
       (2) Involves movement along a concentration or electrochemical gradient
       (3) Examples include: movement of water soluble nutrients into cells
         (a) Sugars
         (b) Amino acids
         (c) Purines
         (d) Pyrimidines

> Sugars, amino acids, purines, pyrimidines and L-dopa by facilitated diffusion

   3. Pinocytosis/endocytosis/transcytosis
     a. Process in which a cell engulfs extracellular material within membrane vesicles
     b. Used by exceptionally large molecules (molecular weight >1000), such as:
       (1) Iron-transferrin complex
       (2) Vitamin B_{12}-intrinsic factor complex

III. Absorption

- Absorption involves the process by which drugs enter into the body.

A. Factors that affect absorption

   1. Solubility in fluids bathing absorptive sites
     a. Drugs in aqueous solutions mix more readily with the aqueous phase at absorptive sites, so they are absorbed more rapidly than those in oily solutions.
     b. Drugs in suspension or solid form are dependent on the rate of dissolution before they can mix with the aqueous phase at absorptive sites.
   2. Concentration
     - Drugs in highly concentrated solutions are absorbed more readily than those in dilute concentrations
   3. Blood flow
     a. Greater blood flow means higher rates of drug absorption
     b. Example—absorption is greater in muscle than in subcutaneous tissues.
   4. Absorbing surface
     a. Organs with large surface areas, such as the lungs and intestines, have more rapid drug absorption
     b. Example—absorption is greater in the intestine than in the stomach.

> Blood flow to site of absorption important for speed of absorption.
>
> Drugs given intramuscularly are absorbed much faster than those given subcutaneously.
>
> Absorbing surface of intestine is much greater than stomach.

   5. Contact time
     - The greater the time, the greater the amount of drug absorbed.
   6. pH
     a. For weak acids and weak bases, the pH determines the relative amount of drug in ionized or nonionized form, which in turn affects solubility.
     b. Weak organic acids donate a proton to form anions (Fig. 1-3), as shown in the following equation:

$$HA \leftrightarrow H^+ + A^-$$

     where HA = weak acid; H^+ = proton; A^- = anion
     c. Weak organic bases accept a proton to form cations (see Fig. 1-3), as shown in the following equation:

$$HB^+ \leftrightarrow B + H^+$$

     where B = weak base; H^+ = proton; HB^+ = cation
     d. Only the nonionized form of a drug can readily cross cell membranes.
     e. The ratio of ionized versus nonionized forms is a function of pK_a (measure of drug acidity) and the pH of the environment.
       (1) When pH = pK_a, a compound is 50% ionized and 50% nonionized
       (2) Protonated form dominates at pH less than pK_a
       (3) Unprotonated form dominates at pH greater than pK_a.

> Weak organic acids are un-ionized (lipid soluble form) when protonated.
>
> Weak organic bases are ionized (water soluble form) when protonated.

1-3: Examples of the ionization of a weak organic acid (salicylate, top) and a weak organic base (amphetamine, bottom).

(4) The Henderson-Hasselbalch equation can be used to determine the ratio of the nonionized form to the ionized form.

$$\log \frac{[\text{protonated form}]}{[\text{unprotonated form}]} = pK_a - pH$$

   f. Problem: Aspirin is a weak organic acid with a pKa of 3.5. What percentage of aspirin will exist in the lipid soluble form in the duodenum (pH = 4.5)?
      • Solution:

$$HA \rightleftarrows A^- + H^+$$

$$|pKa - pH| = \Delta$$

$$|3.5 - 4.5| = 1$$

Antilog of $1 = 10$

pH 4.5 is more alkaline than pKa 3.5

Thus, $HA = 1; A^- = 10$

and

$$\%HA \ (\text{Lipid soluble form}) = [HA/(HA + A^-)] \times 100$$

or

$$\%HA = [1/(1 + 10)] \times 100$$

or

$$\%HA = \text{about } 9.1\%$$

Weak organic acids pass through membranes best in acidic environments.

Weak organic bases pass through membranes best in basic environments.

Bioavailability depends on the extent of an orally administered drug getting into the systemic circulation

Sublingual nitroglycerin avoids first-pass metabolism, promoting rapid absorption.

Slow release formulations are designed to extend the time it takes a drug to be absorbed so that the drug can be administered less frequently.

Bioequivalence depends on both rate and extent of absorption.

IV. Bioavailability
   • Bioavailability is the relative amount of the administered drug that reaches the systemic circulation.
   • Several factors influence bioavailability.
   ### A. First-pass metabolism
      • Enzymes in the intestinal flora, intestinal mucosa, and liver metabolize drugs *before* they reach the general circulation, significantly decreasing systemic bioavailability.
   ### B. Drug formulation
      • Bioavailability after oral administration is affected by the extent of disintegration of a particular drug formulation.
   ### C. Bioequivalence
      1. Two drug formulations with the same bioavailability (extent of absorption) as well as the same rate of absorption are bioequivalent.
      2. Must have identical:
         a. T_{max} (time to reach maximum concentration)
         b. C_{max} (maximal concentration)
         c. AUC (area-under-the-curve from concentration versus time graphs)
   ### D. Route of administration (Table 1-1)

TABLE 1-1. **Routes of Administration**

ROUTE	ADVANTAGES	DISADVANTAGES
Enteral		
Oral	Most convenient Produces slow, uniform absorption Relatively safe Economical	Destruction of drug by enzymes or low pH (e.g., peptides, proteins, penicillins) Poor absorption of large and charged particles Drugs bind or complex with gastrointestinal contents (e.g., calcium binds to tetracycline) Cannot be used for drugs that irritate the intestine
Rectal	Limited first-pass metabolism Useful when oral route precluded	Absorption often irregular and incomplete May cause irritation to rectal mucosa
Sublingual/ buccal	Rapid absorption Avoids first-pass metabolism	Absorption of only small amounts (e.g., nitroglycerin)
Parenteral		
Intravenous	Most direct route Bypasses barriers to absorption (immediate effect) Suitable for large volumes Dosage easily adjusted	Increased risk of adverse effects from high concentration immediately after injection Not suitable for oily substances or suspensions
Intramuscular	Quickly and easily administered Possible rapid absorption May use as depot Suitable for oily substances and suspensions	Painful Bleeding May lead to nerve injury
Subcutaneous	Quickly and easily administered Fairly rapid absorption Suitable for suspensions and pellets	Painful Large amounts cannot be given
Inhalation	Used for volatile compounds (e.g., halothane and amyl nitrite) and drugs that can be administered by aerosol (e.g., albuterol) Rapid absorption due to large surface area of alveolar membranes and high blood flow through lungs Aerosol delivers drug directly to site of action and may minimize systemic side effects	Variable systemic distribution
Topical	Application to specific surface (skin, eye, nose, vagina) allows local effects	May irritate surface
Transdermal	Allows controlled permeation through skin (e.g., nicotine, estrogen, testosterone, fentanyl, scopolamine, clonidine)	May irritate surface

V. Distribution

- Distribution is the delivery of a drug from systemic circulation to tissues.
- Drugs may distribute into certain body compartments (Table 1-2).

A. Apparent volume of distribution (V_d)

1. Refers to the space in the body into which the drug appears to disseminate
2. It is calculated according to the following equation:

$$V_d = \frac{\text{Amount of drug given by IV injection}}{C_0}$$

where C_0 = extrapolated concentration of drug in plasma at time 0 after equilibration (Fig. 1-4).

3. A large V_d means that a drug is concentrated in tissues.
4. A small V_d means that a drug is in the extracellular fluid or plasma; that is, the V_d is inversely related to plasma drug concentration.
5. Problem: 200 mg of drug X is given intravenously to a 70 kg experimental subject and plasma samples are attained at several times after injection. Plasma protein binding

Large V_d when drug concentrated in tissue.

Low V_d when drug remains in plasma.

TABLE 1-2. **Body Compartments in Which Drugs May Distribute**

COMPARTMENT	VOLUME (L/KG)	LITERS IN 70-KG HUMAN	DRUG TYPE
Plasma water	0.045	3	Strongly plasma–protein bound drugs and very large–molecule drugs (e.g., heparin)
Extracellular body water	0.20	14	Large water-soluble drugs (e.g., mannitol, aminoglycosides)
Total body water	0.60	42	Small water-soluble drugs (e.g., ethanol)
Tissue	>0.70	>49	Drugs that avidly bind to tissue (e.g., chloroquine; 115 L/kg)

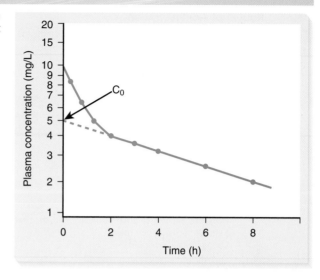

1-4: Semilogarithmic graph of drug concentration versus time; C_0 = extrapolated concentration of drug in plasma at time 0 after equilibration

was determined to be 70% and the extrapolated concentration at time zero was found to be 5.0 mg/L. Which of the following compartments does this drug appear to be primarily found in?

- Solution:

$$V_d = amt_{IV}/C_0$$

or

$$V_d = 200 \text{ mg}/5.0 \text{ mg/L}$$

or

$$V_d = 40L$$

Thus, this drug appears to distribute in a volume close to total body water (see Table 1-2)

B. Factors that affect distribution

- Plasma protein and tissue binding, gender, age, amount of body fat, relative blood flow, size, and lipid solubility
1. Plasma protein binding
   a. Drugs with high plasma protein binding remain in plasma; thus, they have a low V_d and a prolonged half-life.
      - Examples—warfarin, diazepam
   b. Binding acts as a drug reservoir, slowing onset and prolonging duration of action.
   c. Many drugs bind reversibly with one or more plasma proteins (mostly albumin) in the vascular compartment.
      Tissue protein binding favors larger V_d.
      - Examples—chlordiazepoxide, fluoxetine, tolbutamide, etc.
   d. Disease states (e.g., liver disease, which affects albumin concentration) or drugs that alter protein binding influence the concentration of other drugs.
      - Examples of drugs—Furosemide or valproate can displace warfarin from albumin
2. Sites of drug concentration (Table 1-3)
   a. Redistribution
      (1) Intravenous thiopental is initially distributed to areas of highest blood flow, such as the brain, liver, and kidneys.
      (2) The drug is then redistributed to and stored first in muscle, and then in adipose tissue.

Plasma protein binding favors smaller V_d.

Thiopental's anesthetic action is terminated by drug redistribution.

TABLE 1-3. **Sites of Drug Concentration**

SITE	CHARACTERISTICS
Fat	Stores lipid-soluble drugs
Tissue	May represent sizable reservoir, depending on mass, as with muscle Several drugs accumulate in liver
Bone	Tetracyclines are deposited in calcium-rich regions (bones, teeth)
Transcellular reservoirs	Gastrointestinal tract serves as transcellular reservoir for drugs that are slowly absorbed or that are undergoing enterohepatic circulation

b. Ion trapping
  (1) Weak organic acids are trapped in basic environments.
  (2) Weak organic bases are trapped in acidic environments.
3. Sites of drug exclusion (places where it is difficult for drugs to enter)
  a. Cerebrospinal, ocular, endolymph, pleural, and fetal fluids
  b. Components of blood-brain barrier (BBB)
    (1) Tight junctions compared to fenestrated junctions in capillaries of most tissues
    (2) Glia wrappings around capillaries
    (3) Low cerebral spinal fluid (CSF) drug binding proteins
    (4) Drug-metabolizing enzymes in endothelial cells
      • Examples of enzymes—monoamine oxidases, cytochrome P-450s
    (5) Efflux transporters

VI. Biotransformation: Metabolism
  • The primary site of biotransformation, or metabolism, is the liver, and the primary goal is drug inactivation.
  ### A. Products of drug metabolism
    1. Products are usually less active pharmacologically.
    2. Products may sometimes be active drugs where the prodrug form is inactive and the metabolite is the active drug.
  ### B. Phase I biotransformation (oxidation, reduction, hydrolysis)
    1. The products are usually more polar metabolites, resulting from introducing or unmasking a function group ($-OH$, $-NH_2$, $-SH$, $-COO^-$).
    2. The oxidative processes often involve enzymes located in the smooth endoplasmic reticulum (microsomal).
    3. Oxidation usually occurs via a cytochrome P-450 system.
    4. The estimated percentage of drugs metabolized by the major P-450 enzymes (Fig. 1-5)
    5. Non-microsomal enzymes include:
      a. Esterases
      b. Alcohol/aldehyde dehydrogenases
      c. Oxidative deaminases
      d. Decarboxylases
  ### C. Phase II biotransformation
    1. General
      a. Involves conjugation, in which an endogenous substance, such as glucuronic acid, combines with a drug or phase I metabolite to form a conjugate with high polarity
      b. Glucuronidation and sulfation make drugs much more water soluble and excretable.
      c. Acetylation and methylation make drugs less water soluble; acetylated products of sulfonamides tend to crystallize in the urine (i.e., drug crystals)

Weak organic acids are trapped in basic environments.

Weak organic bases are trapped in acidic environments.

L-Dopa is converted dopamine after transport across BBBB.

Diseases that affect the liver influence drug metabolism.

Valacyclovir (good oral bioavailability) is a prodrug to acyclovir (treats herpes).

Phase 1: oxidation, reduction, hydrolysis.

Many oxidations by microsomal cytochrome P-450 enzymes.

Phase II are synthesis reactions; something is added to the molecule.

Conjugation reactions (e.g., glucuronidation, sulfation) usually make drugs more water soluble and more excretable.

Methylation and acetylation reactions often make drugs less water soluble.

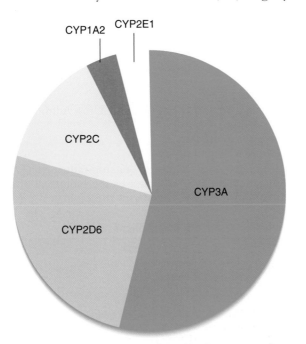

1-5: Diagram showing the estimated percentage of drugs metabolized by the major cytochrome P-450 enzymes.

2. Glucuronidation
   a. A major route of metabolism for drugs and endogenous compounds (steroids, bilirubin)
   b. Occurs in the endoplasmic reticulum; inducible
3. Sulfation
   a. A major route of drug metabolism
   b. Occurs in the cytoplasm
4. Methylation and acetylation reactions
   • Involve the conjugation of drugs (by transferases) with other substances (e.g., methyl, acetyl) to metabolites, thereby decreasing drug activity

D. Phase III disposition processes

Transporters responsible for influx and efflux of molecules involved in absorption, distribution, and elimination

E. Drug interactions

May occur as a result of changes to the cytochrome P-450 enzyme system

1. Inducers of cytochrome P-450
   a. Hasten metabolism of drugs; lowers therapeutic drug level
   b. Examples:
      (1) Chronic alcohol (especially CYP2E1)
      (2) Phenobarbital
      (3) Phenytoin
      (4) Rifampin
      (5) Carbamazepine
      (6) St. John's wort (herbal product)
2. Inhibitors of cytochrome P-450
   a. Decreases metabolism of drugs; raises therapeutic drug level (danger of toxicity)
   b. Examples:
      (1) Acute alcohol
      (2) Cimetidine
      (3) Ketoconazole
      (4) Erythromycin
3. Inhibitors of intestinal P-glycoprotein transporters
   a. Drugs that inhibit this transporter increase bioavailability, thus, resulting in potential toxicity.
   b. Example of inhibitors—grapefruit juice increases the bioavailability of verapamil
   c. Examples of drugs made more toxic—digoxin, cyclosporine, saquinavir

F. Genetic polymorphisms

1. Influence the metabolism of a drug, thereby altering its effects (Table 1-4)
2. Pharmacogenomics
   a. Deals with the influence of *genetic* variation on drug responses due to *gene expression* or *single-nucleotide polymorphisms* (SNPs)
   b. This impacts the drug's *efficacy* and/or *toxicity*
   c. Many are related to drug metabolism
3. Personalized medicine uses patient's *genotype* or *gene expression* profile to tailor medical care to an individual's needs
4. Drugs recommended by the U.S. Food and Drug Administration (FDA) for pharmacogenomic tests
   a. Warfarin for anticoagulation
      (1) Adverse effect—bleeding
      (2) Genes—*CYP2C9* and vitamin K epoxide reductase (*VKORC1*)
         (a) Deficiency of *CYP2D9* increases the biological effect of warfarin
         (b) Mutation in *VKORC1* decreases the biological effect of warfarin

TABLE 1-4. **Genetic Polymorphisms and Drug Metabolism**

PREDISPOSING FACTOR	DRUG	CLINICAL EFFECT
G6PD deficiency	Primaquine, sulfonamides	Acute hemolytic anemia
Slow *N*-acetylation	Isoniazid	Peripheral neuropathy
Slow *N*-acetylation	Hydralazine	Lupus syndrome
Slow ester hydrolysis	Succinylcholine	Prolonged apnea
Slow oxidation	Tolbutamide	Cardiotoxicity
Slow acetaldehyde oxidation	Ethanol	Facial flushing

G6PD, glucose-6-phosphate dehydrogenase.

Margin notes:

Newborn babies have very low enzyme glucuronysyltransferase activity, *cannot* eliminate chloramphenicol → "Gray baby" syndrome

Phase III of disposition; influx and efflux transporters.

Many anticonvulsants induce cytochrome P-450 enzymes but valproic acid inhibits these enzymes.

Inducers of drug metabolism: chronic alcohol, phenobarbital, phenytoin, rifampin, carbamazepine, St. John's wort

Inhibitors of drug metabolism: acute alcohol, cimetidine, ketoconazole, erythromycin.

Personalized medicine means adjusting dose according to individual's phenotype.

  b. Isoniazid for antituberculosis
     (1) Adverse effect—neurotoxicity
     (2) Gene—N-Acetyltransferase (*NAT2*)
  c. Mercaptopurine for chemotherapy of acute lymphoblastic leukemia
     (1) Adverse effect—hematological toxicity
     (2) Gene—thiopurine S-methyltransferase (*TPMT*)
  d. Irinotecan for chemotherapy of colon cancer
     (1) Adverse effects—diarrhea, neutropenia
     (2) Gene—UDP-glucuronosyltransferase (UGT1A1)
  e. Codeine as an analgesic
     (1) Response—lack of analgesic effect
     (2) Gene—*CYP2D6*

G. Reactive metabolite intermediates
  1. Are responsible for mutagenic, carcinogenic, and teratogenic effects, as well as specific organ-directed toxicity
  2. Examples of resulting conditions:
     a. Acetaminophen-induced hepatotoxicity
     b. Aflatoxin-induced tumors
     c. Cyclophosphamide-induced cystitis

VII. Excretion

• Excretion is the amount of drug and drug metabolites excreted by any process per unit time.

A. Excretion processes in kidney
  1. Glomerular filtration rate
     a. Depends on the size, charge, and protein binding of a particular drug
     b. Is lower for highly protein-bound drugs
     c. Drugs that are *not* protein bound and *not* reabsorbed are eliminated at a rate equal to the creatinine clearance rate (125 mL/minute).
  2. Tubular secretion
     a. Occurs in the middle segment of the proximal convoluted tubule
     b. Has a rate that approaches renal plasma flow (660 mL/min)
     c. Provides transporters for:
        (1) Anions (e.g., penicillins, cephalosporins, salicylates)
        (2) Cations (e.g., pyridostigmine)
     d. Can be used to increase drug concentration by use of another drug that competes for the transporter (e.g., probenecid inhibits penicillin secretion)
     e. Characteristics of tubular secretion
        (1) Competition for the transporter
        (2) Saturation of the transporter
        (3) High plasma protein binding favors increased tubular secretion because the affinity of the solute is greater for the transporter than for the plasma protein
     f. Examples of drugs that undergo tubular secretion:
        (1) Penicillins
        (2) Cephalosporins
        (3) Salicylates
        (4) Thiazide diuretics
        (5) Loop diuretics
        (6) Some endogenous substances such as uric acid
  3. Passive tubular reabsorption
     a. Uncharged drugs can be reabsorbed into the systemic circulation in the distal tubule.
     b. Ion trapping
        (1) Refers to trapping of the ionized form of drugs in the urine
        (2) With weak acids (phenobarbital, methotrexate, aspirin), alkalinization of urine (sodium bicarbonate, acetazolamide) increases renal excretion.
        (3) With weak bases (amphetamine, phencyclidine), acidification of urine (ammonium chloride) increases renal excretion.

B. Excretion processes in the liver
  1. Large polar compounds or their conjugates (molecular weight >325) may be actively secreted into bile.
     • Separate transporters for anions (e.g., glucuronide conjugates), neutral molecules (e.g., ouabain), and cations (e.g., tubocurarine)

Codeine has to be converted by *CYP2D6* to morphine in brain to be an active analgesic.

FDA recommends phenotyping for: warfarin, isoniazid, mercaptopurine, irinotecan, codeine.

Acetaminophen overdose common choice for suicide attempts.

A drug with a larger V_d is eliminated more slowly than one with a smaller V_d.

Probenecid inhibits the tubular secretion of most β-lactam antimicrobials.

Excretion by tubular secretion is rapid, but capacity limited.

Weak organic acids are excreted more readily when urine is alkaline.

Weak organic bases are excreted more readily when urine is acidic.

Size of molecule determines if a compound is more likely to be actively secreted in kidney (small molecular weights) or liver (larger molecular weights).

2. These large drugs often undergo enterohepatic recycling, in which drugs secreted in the bile are again reabsorbed in the small intestine.

    a. The enterohepatic cycle can be interrupted by agents that bind drugs in the intestine (e.g., charcoal, cholestyramine).

    b. Glucuronide conjugates secreted in the bile can be cleaved by glucuronidases produced by bacteria in the intestine and the released parent compound can be reabsorbed; antibiotics by destroying intestinal bacteria can disrupt this cycle.

C. Other sites of excretion

- Example—excretion of gaseous anesthetics by the lungs

VIII. Kinetic Processes

- The therapeutic utility of a drug depends on the rate and extent of input, distribution, and loss.

A. Clearance kinetics

1. Clearance

    a. Refers to the volume of plasma from which a substance is removed per unit time

    b. To calculate clearance, divide the rate of drug elimination by the plasma concentration of the drug.

2. Total body clearance

    a. It is calculated using the following equation:

$$Cl = V_d \times K_{el}$$

where V_d = volume of distribution, K_{el} = elimination rate

    b. Problem: Drug X has a volume of distribution of 100 L and a K_{el} of 0.1 hr^{-1}. What is its total body clearance (Cl)?

- Solution:

$$Cl = V_d \times K_{el}$$

or

$$Cl = 100 \text{ L} \times 0.1 \text{ hr}^{-1}$$

or

$$Cl = 10 \text{ L/hr or } 167 \text{ mL/min}$$

3. Renal clearance

    a. It is calculated using the following equation:

$$Cl_r = \frac{U \times C_{ur}}{C_p}$$

where U = urine flow (mL/min), C_{ur} = urine concentration of a drug, C_p = plasma concentration of a drug

    b. Problem: What is the renal clearance (Cl$_r$) of Drug X if 600 mL of urine was collected in one hour and the concentration of Drug X in the urine was 1 mg/mL and the mid-point plasma concentration was 0.1 mg/mL?

- Solution:
  $Cl_r = (60 \text{ mL/min} \times 1 \text{ mg/mL})/0.1 \text{ mg/min}$
  $Cl_r = 600 \text{ mL/min}$; this drug must be eliminated by tubular secretion since clearance approaches renal plasma flow

B. Elimination kinetics

1. Zero-order kinetics

    a. Refers to the elimination of a constant amount of drug per unit time

- Examples—ethanol, heparin, phenytoin (at high doses), salicylates (at high doses)

    b. Important characteristics of zero-order kinetics

      (1) Rate is independent of drug concentration.

      (2) Elimination pseudo-half-life is proportional to drug concentration.

      (3) Small increase in dose can produce larger increase in concentration.

      (4) Process only occurs when enzymes or transporters are saturated.

    c. Graphically, plasma drug concentration versus time yields a straight line (Fig. 1-6A).

2. First-order kinetics

    a. Refers to the elimination of a constant percentage of drug per unit time

- Examples—most drugs (unless given at very high concentrations)

    b. Important characteristics of first-order kinetics

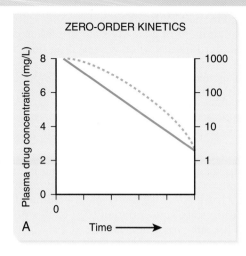

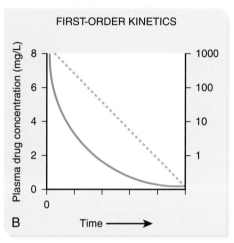

1-6: Kinetic order of drug disappearance from the plasma. Note that the scale on the left x-axis is arithmetic, yielding a relationship shown by the solid line, and the scale on the right x-axis is logarithmic, yielding a relationship shown by the dashed line.

(1) Rate of elimination is proportional to drug concentration.
(2) Drug concentration changes by some constant fraction per unit time (i.e., 0.1/hr).
(3) Half-life ($t_{1/2}$) is constant (i.e., independent of dose).

c. Graphically, a semilogarithmic plot of plasma drug concentration versus time yields a straight line (Fig. 1-6B).

d. Elimination rate constant (K_{el})
  • Sum of all rate constants due to metabolism and excretion

$$K_{el} = K_m + K_{ex}$$

where K_m = metabolic rate constant; K_{ex} = excretion rate constant; K_{el} = elimination rate constant

e. Biologic or elimination half-life
  (1) Refers to the time required for drug concentration to drop by one half; independent of dose.
  (2) It is calculated using the following equation:

$$t_{1/2} = \frac{0.693}{K_{el}}$$

where K_{el} = elimination rate constant
  (3) Problem: What is the half-life ($t_{1/2}$) of a drug that has an elimination constant (K_{el}) of 0.05 hr^{-1}?
    • Solution:

$$t_{1/2} = 0.693/0.05 \text{hr}^{-1}$$

or

$$t_{1/2} = 13.9 \text{hr}$$

Constant half-life ($t_{1/2}$) with first order kinetics.

First-order: dose-independent pharmacokinetics

Know formula $t_{1/2} = 0.693/K_{el}$

3. Repetitive dosing kinetics; IV bolus or oral
   a. Refers to the attainment of a steady state of plasma concentration of a drug following first-order kinetics when a fixed drug dose is given at a constant time interval
   b. Concentration at steady state (C_{ss}) occurs when input equals output, as indicated by the following equation:

$$C_{ss} = \frac{\text{Input}}{\text{Output}} = \frac{F \times D/\tau}{Cl}$$

C_{ss} occurs when input equals output.

where F = bioavailability; D = dose; τ = dosing interval; Cl = clearance
   c. Problem: 100 mg of a drug with a bioavailability of 50% is given every half-life ($t_{1/2}$). The drug has a $t_{1/2}$ of 12 hours and a volume of distribution (V_d) of 100 L. What is the steady state concentration (C_{ss}) of this drug?
      (1) Solution: First substitute in clearance (Cl = $V_d \times K_{el}$) into the equation to get the new equation below:

$$C_{ss} = (F \times D/\tau)/(V_d \times K_{el})$$

Then substitute in the equation ($K_{el} = 0.693/t_{1/2}$) and rearrange to get:

$$C_{ss} = (1.44 \times F \times D/\tau \times t_{1/2})/V_d$$

or

$$C_{ss} = [1.44 \times 0.5 \times (100 \text{ mg}/12 \text{ hr}) \times 12 \text{ hr}]/100 \text{ L}$$

or

$$C_{ss} = 0.72 \text{ mg/L}$$

It takes 4 to 5 half-lives to reach steady state

Maintenance dose depends on clearance

      (2) The time required to reach the steady-state condition is 4 to 5 × $t_{1/2}$ (Table 1-5).
   d. The loading dose necessary to reach the steady-state condition immediately can be calculated using the following equation for intermittent doses (oral or IV bolus injection):

$$LD = 1.44 C_{ss} \times \frac{V_d}{F}$$

where LD = loading dose; C_{ss} = concentration at steady; V_d = volume of distribution; F = bioavailability
      (1) Problem: What loading dose (LD) can be given to achieve steady state concentration immediately for the problem above?
      (2) Solution:

$$LD = 1.44 \times C_{ss} \times (V_d/F)$$

or

$$LD = 1.44 \times 0.72 \text{ mg/L} \times (100 \text{ L}/0.5)$$

or

$$LD = \text{about } 200 \text{ mg}$$

Loading dose depends on volume of distribution
Loading dose is twice maintenance dose when given at drug's half-life

TABLE 1-5. **Number of Half-Lives ($t_{1/2}$) Required to Reach Steady-State Concentration (C_{ss})**

% C_{ss}	NUMBER OF $t_{1/2}$
50.0	1
75.0	2
87.5	3
93.8	4
98.0	5

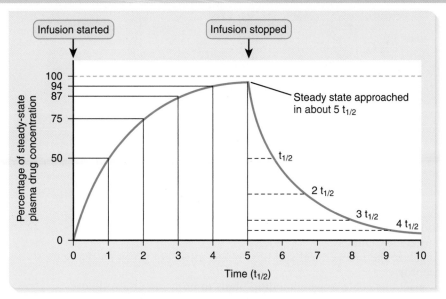

1-7: Drug accumulation to steady state as infusion is started and decline when infusion is stopped. *(From Brenner G and Stevens C. Pharmacology, 3rd ed. Philadelphia, Saunders, 2010, Figure 2-12.)*

4. Repetitive dosing kinetics; intravenous infusion

$$R_0 = C_{ss} \times K_{el} \times V_d$$

$$LD = C_{ss} \times V_d$$

where R_0 = rate of intravenous infusion; K_{el} = elimination constant; LD = loading dose; C_{ss} = concentration at steady; V_d = volume of distribution
   • Fig. 1-7 illustrates the accumulation of drug concentration during intravenous infusion and it its decline when infusion is stopped with respect to the half-life ($t_{1/2}$) of the drug.
5. Amount of drug in body at any time:

$$X_b = V_d \times C_p$$

where X_b = amount of drug in the body; V_d = volume of distribution; C_p = concentration in plasma

Know formula $X_b = V_d \times C_p$

   a. Problem: How much drug is in the body when the volume of distribution is 100 L and the plasma concentration 0.5 mg/L?
   b. Solution:

$$X_b = 100 \text{ L} \times 0.5 \text{ mg/L}$$

or

$$X_b = 50 \text{ mg}$$

CHAPTER 2

PHARMACODYNAMICS

I. Definitions

A. Pharmacodynamics
- Involves the biochemical and physiologic effects of drugs on the body.

B. Receptor
- A macromolecule to which a drug binds to bring about a response.

C. Agonist
- A drug that activates a receptor upon binding.

D. Pharmacological antagonist
- A drug that binds without activating its receptor and, thus, prevents activation by an agonist.

E. Competitive antagonist
- A pharmacological antagonist that binds reversibly to a receptor so it can be overcome by increasing agonist concentration.

F. Irreversible antagonist
- A pharmacological antagonist that cannot be overcome by increasing agonist concentration.

G. Partial agonist
- A drug that binds to a receptor but produces a smaller effect at full dosage than a full agonist.

H. Graded dose-response curve
- A graph of increasing response to increasing doses of a drug.

I. Quantal dose-response curve
- A graph of the fraction of a population that gives a specified response at progressively increasing drug doses.

II. Dose-Response Relationships

A. Overview
- These relationships are usually expressed as a log dose-response (LDR) curve.

B. Properties of LDR curves
1. LDR curves are typically S-shaped.
2. A steep slope in the midportion of the "S" indicates that a small increase in dosage will produce a large increase in response.
3. Types of log dose-response curves
   a. Graded response (Fig. 2-1)
      (1) Response in one subject or test system
      (2) Median effective concentration (EC_{50})
         - Concentration that corresponds to 50% of the maximal response
   b. All-or-none (quantal) response (Fig. 2-2)
      (1) Number of individuals within a group responding to a given dose
      (2) The end point is set, and an individual is either a *responder* or a *nonresponder*
      (3) This response is expressed as a *normal histogram* or *cumulative distribution* profile
      (4) The normal histogram is usually bell-shaped
      (5) Median effective dose (ED_{50})
         - Dose to which 50% of subjects respond
      (6) The therapeutic index (TI) and the margin of safety (MS) are based on quantal responses.
         (a) TI (therapeutic index): ratio of the lethal dose in 50% of the population (LD_{50}) divided by the effective dose for 50% of the population (ED_{50}), or

$$TI = \frac{LD_{50}}{ED_{50}}$$

Receptor is site that drug binds to, producing its actions.

Be able to distinguish reversible from irreversible binding drugs by how they affect log dose-response curves of an agonist (shown later in chapter).

Be able to distinguish a full agonist from a partial agonists from log dose-response curves (shown later in chapter).

Understand the difference between a graded and quantal log dose-response curve (shown later in chapter).

Graded response is in an individual subject.

Quantal (all-or-none) response is in a population of subjects.

Graded response measures degree of change; quantal measures frequency of response.

$TI = LD_{50} \div ED_{50}$

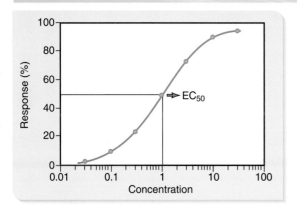

2-1: Log dose-response curve for an agonist-induced response. The median effective concentration (EC$_{50}$) is the concentration that results in a 50% maximal response.

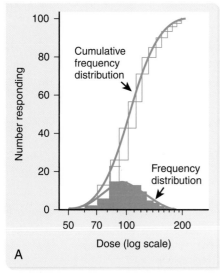

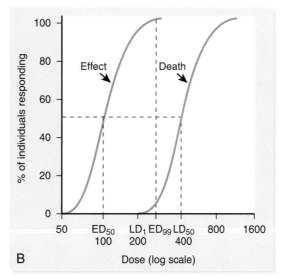

2-2: A, Cumulative frequency distribution and frequency distribution curves for a drug using a logarithmic dose scale. **B,** Cumulative frequency distribution curves for the therapeutic and lethal effects of a drug using a logarithmic dose scale.

    (b) MS (margin of safety): ratio of the lethal dose for 1% of the population (LD$_1$) divided by the effective dose for 99% of the population (LD$_{99}$), or

$$MS = \frac{LD_1}{ED_{99}}$$

MS = LD$_1$ ÷ ED$_{99}$

III. Drug Receptors
- Drug receptors are biologic components on the surface of or within cells that bind with drugs, resulting in molecular changes that produce a certain response.
A. Types of receptors and their signaling mechanisms (Table 2-1)
    1. Membrane receptors are coupled with a G protein, an ion channel, or an enzyme.
      a. G protein-coupled receptors (GPCRs) (Table 2-2)
        (1) These receptors are a superfamily of diverse guanosine triphosphate (GTP)-binding proteins that couple to "serpentine" (seven) transmembrane receptors.
        (2) G$_s$-coupled receptors (Fig. 2-3)
          (a) The G$_{s\alpha}$ subunits are coupled to adenylyl cyclase
          (b) Activation *stimulates* the formation of intracellular cyclic adenosine monophosphate (cAMP)
          (c) cAMP is responsible for numerous cellular responses (Table 2-3).
          (d) cAMP activates protein kinase A
        (3) G$_i$-coupled receptors
          (a) The G$_{i\alpha}$ subunits are coupled to adenylyl cyclase
          (b) Activation *inhibits* the formation of intracellular cyclic AMP (cAMP)
          (c) Whereas the G$_{i\beta\gamma}$ subunits open K$^+$ channels
        (4) G$_q$-coupled receptors (Fig. 2-4)
          (a) The G$_{q\alpha}$ subunits stimulate phospholipase C

GPCRs; Gs stimulates cAMP; Gi inhibits cAMP; Gq stimulates phospholipase C.

cAMP activates protein kinase A.

TABLE 2-1. **Drug Receptors and Mechanisms of Signal Transduction**

RECEPTOR	LIGAND	MECHANISM	TIME
G Protein–Coupled Receptors (GPCRs)			
α_1-Adrenergic receptors	Phenylephrine (agonist) Prazosin (antagonist)	Activation of phospholipase C	Sec
α_2-Adrenergic receptors	Clonidine (agonist) Yohimbine (antagonist)	Inhibition of adenylyl cyclase; open ion channels	Sec
β-Adrenergic receptors	Isoproterenol (agonist) Propranolol (antagonist)	Stimulation of adenylyl cyclase	Sec
Muscarinic receptors	Pilocarpine (agonist) Atropine (antagonist)	Activation of phospholipase C	Sec
Ligand-Gated Ion Channels			
GABA$_A$ receptors	Benzodiazepines (agonists) Flumazenil (antagonist)	Chloride flux	Msec
Nicotinic ACh receptors	Nicotine (agonist) Tubocurarine (antagonist)	Sodium flux	Msec
Membrane-Bound Enzymes			
Insulin receptors	Insulin	Activation of tyrosine kinase	Min
Cytokine receptors	Interleukin-2	Activation of tyrosine kinase	Min
Cytoplasmic Receptors			
Cytoplasmic guanylyl cyclase	Nitroglycerin (NO)	Activation of guanylyl cyclase	Min
Nuclear receptors			
Steroid receptors	Adrenal and gonadal steroids	Activation of gene transcription	Hr
Thyroid hormone receptors	Thyroxine	Activation of gene transcription	Hr

ACh, acetylcholine; GABA, γ-aminobutyric acid.

TABLE 2-2. **Major G Protein Signaling Pathways**

G_α TYPE	FUNCTION*	COUPLED RECEPTORS
G_s	Stimulates adenylyl cyclase ($\uparrow$ cAMP)	Dopamine (D$_1$), epinephrine (β_1, β_2), glucagon, histamine (H$_2$), vasopressin (V$_2$)
G_i	Inhibits adenylyl cyclase ($\downarrow$ cAMP)	Dopamine (D$_2$), epinephrine (α_2)
G_q	Stimulates phospholipase C ($\uparrow$ IP$_3$, DAG)	Angiotensin II, epinephrine (α_1), oxytocin, vasopressin (V$_1$), Histamine (H$_1$)

*In some signaling pathways, G_s and G_i are associated with ion channels, which open or close in response to hormone binding.
cAMP, cyclic adenosine monophosphate; DAG, diacylglycerol; IP$_3$, inositol triphosphate.
(Adapted from Pelley JW and Goljan EF: Rapid Review Biochemistry, 2nd ed. Philadelphia, Mosby, 2007, Table 3-3.)

IP$_3$ releases calcium from endoplasmic reticulum.

Calcium activates Ca^{2+}/Calmodulin kinase.

DAG activates protein kinase C.

Growth factors signal via ligand-regulated tyrosine kinases.

Cytokines signal via ligand-regulated tyrosine kinases.

cGMP activates protein kinase G.

(b) It cleaves PIP$_2$ (phosphatidyl inositol 4,5-bisphosphate) to yield two second messengers
- IP$_3$ (inositol 1,4,5-triphosphate), which can diffuse in the cytosol and release calcium from the endoplasmic reticulum
- DAG (diacylglycerol), which remains associated with the plasma membrane and activates protein kinase C

b. Ligand-gated channels (see Table 2-1)
  (1) Agonists change ion conductance and alter the electrical potential of cells.
  (2) The speed of the response is rapid (msec).

c. Receptor-linked enzymes (see Table 2-1)
  - These receptors contain a single transmembrane α-helix, an extracellular hormone-binding domain, and a cytosolic domain with tyrosine kinase catalytic activity.
  (1) Growth factors, such as the insulin receptor, signal via this pathway (Fig. 2-5)
  (2) Cytokines, such as interleukin-2, also signal via a pathway that is initiated by receptor tyrosine kinase driven pathway

2. Intracellular receptors; inside cells (see Table 2-1)
  a. Cytoplasmic guanylyl cyclase is activated by nitric oxide to produce cGMP
    - Nitroglycerin and sodium nitroprusside use this pathway
  b. Nuclear and cytosolic receptors (Fig. 2-6; also see Table 2-1)
    (1) Alter gene expression and protein synthesis
    (2) This mechanism is responsible for the biological actions of:
      (a) Steroid hormones

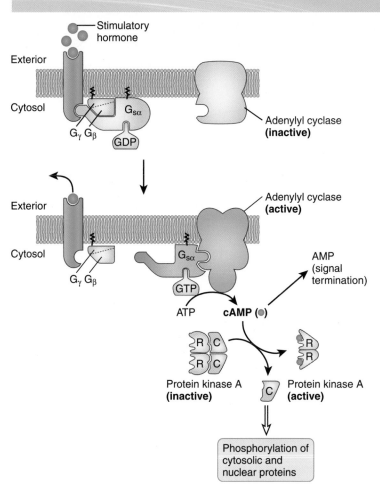

2-3: Cyclic adenosine monophosphate (cAMP) pathway. Following hormone binding, coupled G protein exchanges bound guanosine diphosphate (GDP) for guanosine triphosphate (GTP). Active $G_{s\alpha}$-GTP diffuses in the membrane and binds to membrane-bound adenylyl cyclase, stimulating it to produce cAMP. Binding of cAMP to the regulatory subunits (R) of protein kinase A releases the active catalytic (C) subunits, which mediate various cellular responses. *(From Pelley JW and Goljan EF: Rapid Review Biochemistry, 2nd ed. Philadelphia, Mosby, 2007, Figure 3-6.)*

TABLE 2-3. **Effects of Elevated cyclic adenoside monphosphate (cAMP) in Various Tissues**

TISSUE/CELL TYPE	HORMONE INCREASING cAMP	MAJOR CELLULAR RESPONSE
Adipose tissue	Epinephrine	↑ Hydrolysis of triglycerides
Adrenal cortex	Adrenocorticotropic hormone (ACTH)	Hormone secretion
Cardiac muscle	Epinephrine, norepinephrine	↑ Contraction rate
Intestinal mucosa	Vasoactive intestinal peptide, epinephrine	Secretion of water and electrolytes
Kidney tubules	Vasopressin (V_2 receptor)	Resorption of water
Liver	Glucagon, epinephrine	↑ Glycogen degradation ↑ Glucose synthesis
Platelets	Prostacyclin (PGI_2)	Inhibition of aggregation
Skeletal muscle	Epinephrine	↑ Glycogen degradation
Smooth muscle (bronchial and vascular)	Epinephrine	Relaxation (bronchial) Vasodilation (arterioles)
Thyroid gland	Thyroid-stimulating hormone	Synthesis and secretion of thyroxine

(Adapted from Pelley JW and Goljan EF: Rapid Review Biochemistry, 2nd ed. Philadelphia, Mosby, 2007, Table 3-4.)

    (b) Thyroid hormones
    (c) Retinoic acid
    (d) Vitamin D
  c. Other intracellular sites can serve as targets for drug molecules crossing cell membranes (e.g., structural proteins, DNA, RNA); drugs using these mechanisms include:
    (1) Antimicrobials
    (2) Anticancer drugs
    (3) Antiviral drugs

Steroid hormones, thyroid hormone, vitamin D and retinoic acid affect gene transcription via nuclear receptors.

Most antimicrobials, antivirals, and anticancer drugs act on intracellular sites: ribosomes; DNA pathways; RNA pathways; mitochondria; folate pathways.

2-4: Phosphoinositide pathway linked to G_q-coupled receptor. Top, The two fatty acyl chains of PIP_2 (phosphatidylinositol 4,5-bisphosphate) are embedded in the plasma membrane with the polar phosphorylated inositol group extending into the cytosol. Hydrolysis of PIP_2 (dashed line) produces DAG, which remains associated with the membrane, and IP_3, which is released into the cytosol. Bottom, Contraction of smooth muscle induced by hormones such as epinephrine (a_1 receptor), oxytocin, and vasopressin (V_1 receptor) results from the IP_3-stimulated increase in cytosolic Ca^{2+}, which forms a Ca^{2+}-calmodulin complex that activates myosin light-chain (MLC) kinase. MLC kinase phosphorylates myosin light chains, leading to muscle contractions. ER, endoplasmic reticulum. *(From Pelley JW and Goljan EF: Rapid Review Biochemistry, 2nd ed. Philadelphia, Mosby, 2007, Figure 3-7.)*

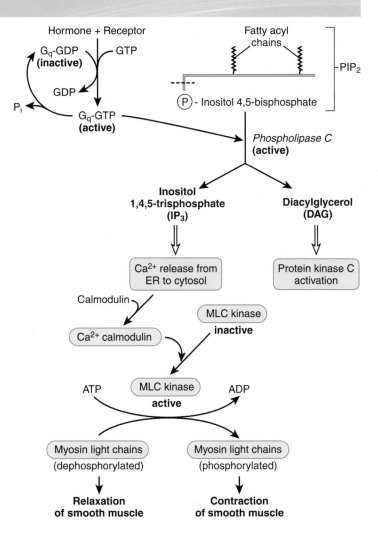

B. Degree of receptor binding

    1. Drug molecules bind to receptors at a rate that is dependent on drug concentration.

    2. The dissociation constant ($K_D = k_{-1}/k_1$) of the drug-receptor complex is inversely related to the affinity of the drug for the receptor.

       a. A drug with a K_D of 10^{-7} M has a higher affinity than a drug with a K_D of 10^{-6} M.

       b. k_1 is the rate of onset, and k_{-1} is the rate of offset for receptor occupancy.

    3. The intensity of response is proportional to the number of receptors occupied.

C. Terms used to describe drug-receptor interactions

    1. Affinity

       • Propensity of a drug to bind with a given receptor

    2. Potency

       • Comparative expression that relates the dose required to produce a particular effect of a given intensity relative to a standard reference (Fig. 2-7)

    3. Efficacy (intrinsic activity)

       • Maximal response resulting from binding of drug to its receptor (see Fig. 2-7)

    4. Full agonist

       • Drug that stimulates a receptor, provoking a maximal biologic response

    5. Partial agonist

       a. Drug that provokes a submaximal response

       b. In Figure 2-7, drug C is a partial agonist.

    6. Inverse agonist

       • Drug that stimulates a receptor, provoking a negative biologic response (e.g., a decrease in basal activity)

    7. Antagonist

       a. Drug that interacts with a receptor but does *not* result in a biologic response (*no* intrinsic activity)

Drug affinity for a receptor is inversely proportional to the dissociation constant ($K_D = k_{-1}/k_1$).

Be able to compare affinities, potencies, and intrinsic activities of drugs from LDR curves.

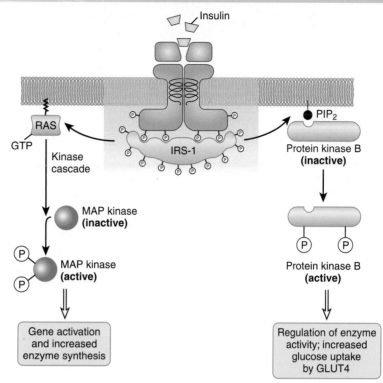

2-5: Signal transduction from an insulin receptor. Insulin binding induces autophosphorylation of the cytosolic domain. IRS-1 (insulin receptor substrate) then binds and is phosphorylated by the receptor's tyrosine kinase activity. Long-term effects of insulin, such as increased synthesis of glucokinase in the liver, are mediated via the RAS pathway, which is activated by MAP (mitogen-activated protein) kinase (left). Two adapter proteins transmit the signal from IRS-1 to RAS, converting it to the active form. Short-term effects of insulin, such as increased activity of glycogen synthase in the liver, are mediated by the protein kinase B (PKB) pathway (right). A kinase that binds to IRS-1 converts phosphatidylinositol in the membrane to PIP_2 (phosphatidylinositol 4,5-bisphosphate), which binds cytosolic PKB and localizes it to the membrane. Membrane-bound kinases then phosphorylate and activate PKB. *(From Pelley JW and Goljan EF: Rapid Review Biochemistry, 2nd ed. Philadelphia, Mosby, 2007, Figure 3-8.)*

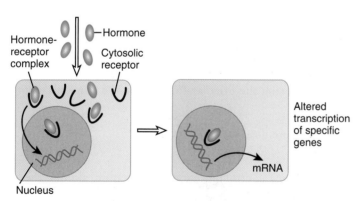

2-6: Signaling by hormones with intracellular receptors. Steroid hormones (e.g., cortisol) bind to their receptors in the cytosol, and the hormone-receptor complex moves to the nucleus. In contrast, the receptors for thyroid hormone and retinoic acid are located only in the nucleus. Binding of the hormone-receptor complex to regulatory sites in DNA activates gene transcription. *(From Pelley JW and Goljan EF: Rapid Review Biochemistry, 2nd ed. Philadelphia, Mosby, 2007, Figure 3-9.)*

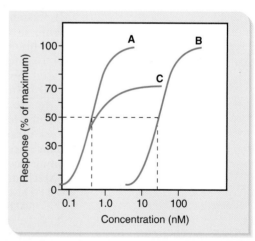

2-7: Dose-response curves of three agonists with differing potency and efficacy. Agonists A and B have the same efficacy but different potency; A is more potent than B. Agonists A and C have the same potency but different efficacy; A is more efficacious than C.

    b. Competitive antagonist (Fig. 2-8)
       (1) Binds reversibly to the same receptor site as an agonist
       (2) Effect can be overcome by increasing the dose of the agonist (reversible effect).
       (3) A fixed dose of a competitive antagonist causes the log dose-response curve of an agonist to make a parallel shift to the right.
       (4) A partial agonist may act as a competitive inhibitor to a full agonist.
    c. Noncompetitive antagonist (Fig. 2-9)

Propranolol is a competitive antagonist of epinephrine at β-adrenergic receptors.

Phentolamine is a competitive antagonist of epinephrine at α-adrenergic receptors.

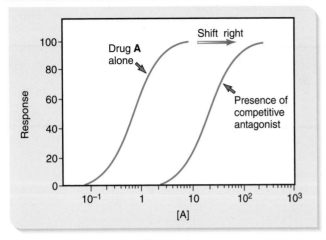

2-8: Competitive antagonism. The log dose-response curve for drug A shifts to the right in the presence of a fixed dose of a competitive antagonist.

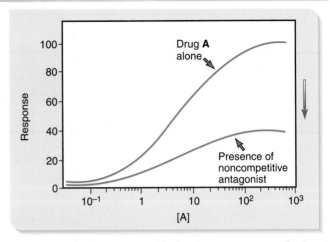

2-9: Noncompetitive antagonism. The log dose-response curve for drug A shifts to the right and downward in the presence of a fixed dose of a noncompetitive antagonist.

(1) Binds irreversibly to the receptor site for the agonist
(2) Its effects *cannot* be overcome completely by increasing the concentration of the agonist.
(3) A fixed dose of a noncompetitive antagonist causes a nonparallel, downward shift of the log dose-response curve of the agonist to the right.

IV. Pharmacodynamically Altered Responses

    A. Decreased drug activity

        1. Antagonism resulting from drug interactions

          a. Physiologic (functional) antagonism

            (1) This response occurs when two agonists with opposing physiologic effects are administered together.

            (2) Examples: histamine (vasodilation), norepinephrine (vasoconstriction)

          b. Competitive antagonism

            (1) This response occurs when a receptor antagonist is administered with an agonist.

            (2) Examples

               (a) Naloxone, when blocking the effects of morphine

               (b) Atropine, when blocking the effects of acetylcholine (ACh) at a muscarinic receptor

               (c) Flumazenil, when blocking the effects of diazepam at a benzodiazepine receptor

        2. Tolerance definition

          • Diminished response to the same dose of a drug over time

          a. Mechanisms of tolerance

            (1) Desensitization

               (a) Rapid process involving continuous exposure to a drug, altering the receptor so that it *cannot* produce a response

               (b) Example

                 • Continuous exposure to β-adrenergic agonist (e.g., use of albuterol in asthma) results in decreased responsiveness.

            (2) Down-regulation

               • Decrease in number of receptors caused by high doses of agonists over prolonged periods

            (3) Tachyphylaxis

               (a) Rapid development of tolerance

               (b) Indirect-acting amines (e.g., tyramine, amphetamine) exert their effects by releasing monoamines.

               (c) Several doses given over a short time deplete the monoamine pool, reducing the response to successive doses.

    B. Increased drug activity

        1. Supersensitivity or hyperactivity

Phenoxybenzamine is a noncompetitive antagonist of epinephrine at α-adrenergic receptors.

Anaphylactic reaction is produced by release of histamine; epinephrine is the drug of choice (DOC) for treatment.

Atropine is a competitive antagonist of ACh at muscarinic receptors.

Hexamethonium is a competitive antagonist of ACh at ganglionic nicotinic receptors.

Tubocurarine is a competitive antagonist of ACh at neuromuscular junction nicotinic receptors.

Continuous use of a β-adrenergic agonist involves both desensitization and down-regulation of receptors.

Multiple injections of tyramine in short time intervals produce tachyphylaxis.

a. Enhanced response to a drug may be due to an increase in the number of receptors (up-regulation).

b. Antagonists or denervation cause up-regulation of receptors.

2. Potentiation

a. Enhancement of the effect of one drug by another which has no effect by itself, when combined with a second drug (e.g., $5 + 0 = 20$, *not* 5)

b. Produces a parallel shift of the log dose-response curve to the left

c. Examples

(1) Physostigmine, an acetylcholinesterase inhibitor (AChEI), potentiates the response to acetylcholine (ACh).

(2) Cocaine (an uptake I blocker) potentiates the response to norepinephrine (NE).

(3) Clavulanic acid (a penicillinase inhibitor) potentiates the response to amoxicillin in penicillinase producing bacteria.

3. Synergism

- Production of a greater response than of two drugs that act individually (e.g., $2 + 5 = 15$, *not* 7)

C. Dependence

1. Physical dependence

- Repeated use produces an altered or adaptive physiologic state if the drug is *not* present.

2. Psychological dependence

a. Compulsive drug-seeking behavior

b. Individuals use a drug repeatedly for personal satisfaction.

3. Substance dependence (addiction)

- Individuals continue substance use despite significant substance-related problems.

V. Adverse Effects

A. Toxicity

1. Refers to dose related adverse effects of drugs

2. Benefit-to-risk ratio

- This expression of adverse effects is more useful clinically than therapeutic index

3. Overextension of the pharmacological response

- Responsible for mild, annoying adverse effects as well as severe adverse effects:

a. Atropine-induced dry mouth

b. Propranolol-induced heart block

c. Diazepam-induced drowsiness

4. Organ-directed toxicities

- Toxicity associated with particular organ or organ system

a. Aspirin-induced gastrointestinal toxicity

b. Aminoglycoside-induced renal toxicity

c. Acetaminophen-induced hepatotoxicity

d. Doxorubicin-induced cardiac toxicity

5. Fetal toxicity

- Some drugs are directly toxic whereas others are teratogenic

a. Directly toxic effects include:

(1) Sulfonamide-induced kernicterus

(2) Chloramphenicol-induced gray baby syndrome

(3) Tetracycline-induced teeth discoloration and retardation of bone growth

b. Teratogenic effects

- Causes physical defects in developing fetus; effect most pronounced during organogenesis (day 20 of gestation to end of first trimester in human) and include:

(1) Thalidomide

(2) Antifolates (methotrexate)

(3) Phenytoin

(4) Warfarin

(5) Isotretinoin

(6) Lithium

(7) Valproic acid

(8) Alcohol (fetal alcohol syndrome)

(9) Anticancer drugs

B. Drug allergies (hypersensitivity)

1. Abnormal response resulting from previous sensitizing exposure activating immunologic mechanism when given offending or structurally related drug

---

Continuous use of a β-adrenergic antagonist causes up-regulation of receptors.

Be able to depict drug potentiation, competitive antagonism, and noncompetitive antagonism from LDR curves.

Physostigmine potentiates the effects of ACh.

Cocaine potentiates the effects of NE.

Clavulanic acid potentiates the effects of amoxicillin.

Trimethoprim plus sulfamethoxazole are synergistic.

Drugs that may lead frequently to addiction: alcohol, barbiturates, benzodiazepines, opioid analgesics.

It is important to understand the benefit-to-risk ratio of every drug prescribed; all drugs can be harmful → some drugs can be beneficial if administered appropriately for the right situation

Aspirin can induce ulcers.

Aminoglycosides can produce kidney damage.

Acetaminophen can produce fatal hepatotoxicity.

Doxorubicin can produce heart failure.

Drug use should be minimized during pregnancy; some drugs are absolutely contraindicated.

Human teratogens: thalidomide; antifolates; phenytoin; warfarin; isotretinoin; lithium; valproic acid; fetal alcohol syndrome, anticancer drugs.

2. Examples
   a. Penicillins
   b. Sulfonamides
   c. Ester type local anesthetics

C. Drug idiosyncrasies
1. Refers to abnormal response *not* immunologically mediated; often caused by genetic abnormalities in enzymes or receptors; referred to as pharmacogenetic disorders
2. Classical idiosyncrasies include:
   a. Patients with abnormal serum cholinesterase develop apnea when given normal doses of succinylcholine.
   b. "Fast" and "slow" acetylation of isoniazid due to different expression of hepatic N-acetyltransferase (NAT)
   c. Hemolytic anemia elicited by primaquine in patients whose red cells are deficient in glucose-6-phosphate dehydrogenase
   d. Barbiturate-induced porphyria occurs in individuals with abnormal heme biosynthesis

VI. Federal Regulations
  • Safety and efficacy of drugs are regulated by the U.S. Food and Drug Administration (FDA)

A. Notice of Claimed Investigational Exemption for a New Drug (IND)
  • Filed with FDA once a potential drug is judged ready to administer to humans

B. Clinical trial phases
1. Phase 1
   • First time the agent is administered to humans
   a. First dose is placebo
   b. Goal is to find maximum tolerated dose
      • Usually involves 20 to 30 healthy volunteers
2. Phase 2
   a. First attempt to determine clinical efficacy of drug
   b. Tests may be single-blind or double-blind and involve hundreds of patients
3. Phase 3
   a. Large scale testing of a drug's efficacy and toxicity (few thousand patients)
   b. After completion, company files New Drug Application (NDA) with FDA
   c. Fewer than 10,000 subjects are usually tested
4. Phase 4 (post-marketing surveillance)
   a. Rare adverse effects and toxicity may become evident
   b. Example: incidence of aplastic anemia with chloramphenicol therapy is 1/40,000

Drug allergies are prominent with β-lactam antibiotics; drugs containing sulfonamide structure; ester-type local anesthetics.

Classical drug idiosyncrasies; primaquine-induced hemolytic anemia; isoniazid-induced peripheral neuropathy; succinylcholine-induced apnea; barbiturate-induced porphyria.

Phase 4 picks up rare adverse effects of a drug.

Drugs That Affect the Autonomic Nervous System and the Neuromuscular Junction

CHAPTER **3**

INTRODUCTION TO AUTONOMIC AND NEUROMUSCULAR PHARMACOLOGY

I. **Divisions of the Efferent Autonomic Nervous System (ANS)** (Fig. 3-1)
   A. **Parasympathetic nervous system (PSNS):** craniosacral division of the ANS
      1. Origin from spinal cord
         a. Cranial (midbrain, medulla oblongata)
         b. Sacral
      2. Nerve fibers
         a. Long preganglionic fibers
         b. Short postganglionic fibers
      3. Neurotransmitters
         a. Acetylcholine (ACh)
            (1) Ganglia (nicotinic receptors)
            (2) Somatic neuromuscular junction (nicotinic receptors)
            (3) Neuroeffector junction (muscarinic receptors)
         b. Actions terminated by acetylcholinesterase
         c. All ganglia and adrenal medulla have nicotinic receptors.
      4. Associated processes
         a. Digestion
         b. Conservation of energy
         c. Maintenance of organ function
   B. **Sympathetic nervous system (SNS):** thoracolumbar division of the ANS
      1. Origin from spinal cord
         a. Thoracic
         b. Upper lumbar regions
      2. Nerve fibers
         a. Short preganglionic nerve fibers, which synapse in the paravertebral ganglionic chain or in the prevertebral ganglia
         b. Long postganglionic nerve fibers
      3. Neurotransmitters
         a. ACh is the neurotransmitter at the ganglia (stimulates nicotinic receptors).
         b. Norepinephrine (NE) is usually the neurotransmitter at the neuroeffector junction (stimulates α- or β-adrenergic receptors).
            • Exception: ACh is the neurotransmitter found in sympathetic nerve endings at thermoregulatory sweat glands.

PSNS = craniosacral origin

ACh stimulates both nicotinic and muscarinic receptors.

PSNS conservation of energy at rest.

SNS = thoracolumbar origin

ACh is neurotransmitter at sympathetic thermoregulatory sweat glands

NE is neurotransmitter at sympathetic apocrine (stress) sweat glands

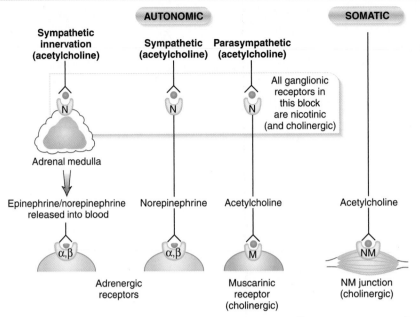

3-1: Schematic representation of sympathetic, parasympathetic, and somatic efferent neurons. α, α-adrenoreceptor; β, β-adrenoreceptor; M, muscarinic receptor; N, nicotinic receptor; NM, neuromuscular.

4. Associated processes
   • Mobilizing the body's resources to respond to fear and anxiety ("fight-or-flight" response)

II. Neurochemistry of the Autonomic Nervous System

A. Cholinergic pathways
   1. Cholinergic fibers
      a. Synthesis, storage, and release (Fig. 3-2A)
      b. Receptor activation and signal transduction
         (1) ACh activates nicotinic or muscarinic receptors (Table 3-1)
         (2) All ganglia, adrenal medulla, and neuromuscular junction have nicotinic receptor

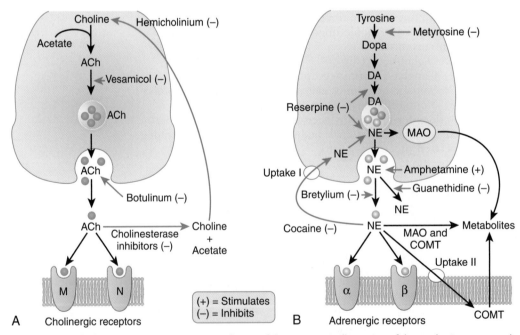

3-2: Cholinergic and adrenergic neurotransmission and sites of drug action. **A,** Illustration of the synthesis, storage, release, inactivation, and postsynaptic receptor activation of cholinergic neurotransmission. **B,** Illustration of the synthesis, storage, release, termination of action, and postsynaptic action of adrenergic neurotransmission. Uptake I is a transporter that transports NE into the presynaptic neuron. Uptake II is a transporter that transports NE into the postsynaptic neuron. α, α-adrenoreceptor; β, β-adrenoreceptor; ACh, acetylcholine; COMT, catechol-O-methyltransferase; DA, dopamine; M, muscarinic receptor; MAO, monoamine oxidase; N, nicotinic receptor; NE, norepinephrine.

TABLE 3-1. **Properties of Cholinergic Receptors**

TYPE OF RECEPTOR	PRINCIPAL LOCATIONS	MECHANISM OF SIGNAL TRANSDUCTION	EFFECTS
Muscarinic			
M_1	Autonomic ganglia Presynaptic nerve terminal CNS neurons	Increased IP_3 and DAG Increased intracellular calcium	Modulation of neurotransmission
M_2	Cardiac tissue (sinoatrial and atrioventricular nodes) Nerves	Increased potassium efflux Inhibition of cAMP	Slowing of heart rate and conduction
M_3	Smooth muscles and glands	Increased IP_3 and DAG Increased intracellular calcium	Contraction of smooth muscles Stimulation of glandular secretions
	Endothelium	Increased nitric oxide formation	Nitric oxide vasodilation
	Vascular smooth Muscle	Increased cGMP (from nitric oxide)	
Nicotinic			
N_M (muscle type)	Skeletal neuromuscular junctions	Increased sodium influx	Muscle contraction
N_N (neuron type)	Postganglionic cell body Dendrites	Increased sodium influx	Excitation of postganglionic neurons

cAMP, cyclic adenosine monophosphate; cGMP, cyclic guanosine monophosphate; CNS, central nervous system; DAG, diacylglycerol; IP_3, inositol triphosphate.

TABLE 3-2. **Drugs that Affect Autonomic Neurotransmission**

MECHANISM	DRUGS THAT AFFECT CHOLINERGIC NEUROTRANSMISSION	DRUGS THAT AFFECT ADRENERGIC NEUROTRANSMISSION
Inhibit synthesis of neurotransmitter	Hemicholinium*	Metyrosine
Prevent vesicular storage of neurotransmitter	Vesamicol*	Reserpine
Inhibit release of neurotransmitter	Botulinum toxin	Bretylium Guanethidine
Stimulate release of neurotransmitter	Black widow spider venom*	Amphetamine Tyramine
Inhibit reuptake of neurotransmitter	—	Tricyclic antidepressants Cocaine
Inhibit metabolism of neurotransmitter	Cholinesterase inhibitors (physostigmine, neostigmine)	Monoamine oxidase inhibitors (tranylcypromine)
Activate postsynaptic receptors	Acetylcholine (M, N) Bethanechol (M) Pilocarpine (M)	Albuterol (β_2) Dobutamine (β_1) Epinephrine (α, β)
Block postsynaptic receptors	Atropine (muscarinic receptors); hexamethonium (ganglia) and tubocurarine (NMJ) (nicotinic receptors)	Phentolamine (α-adrenergic receptors) and propranolol (β-adrenergic receptors)

*Used experimentally but not therapeutically.
M, muscarinic receptor; N, nicotinic receptor.

   c. Inactivation
      (1) ACh is metabolized to acetate and choline
      (2) Occurs by acetylcholinesterase (AChE) in the synapse
      (3) Occurs by pseudocholinesterase in the blood and liver
   2. Drugs that affect cholinergic pathways (Table 3-2)
      a. Botulinum toxin
         (1) Mechanism of action
            • Blocks release of ACh by degrading the SNAP-25 protein, inhibiting neurotransmitter transmission
         (2) Uses
            (a) Localized spasms of ocular and facial muscles
            (b) Lower esophageal sphincter spasm in achalasia
            (c) Spasticity resulting from central nervous system (CNS) disorders
      b. Cholinesterase inhibitors
         (1) Mechanism of action
            • Prevent breakdown of ACh
         (2) Examples of indirect-acting cholinergic receptor agonists:
            (a) Neostigmine
            (b) Physostigmine
            (c) Pyridostigmine
            (d) Donepezil

ACh action terminated by cholinesterases.

Botulinum toxin inhibits ACh release.

Physostigmine reverses the CNS effects of atropine poisoning.

Physostigmine crosses blood-brain barrier (BBB); neostigmine does *not*

c. Cholinergic receptor antagonists
  (1) Muscarinic receptor antagonists
      (a) Atropine
      (b) Scopolamine
  (2) Nicotinic receptor antagonists
      (a) Ganglionic blocker
        • Hexamethonium
      (b) Neuromuscular blocker
        • Tubocurarine

B. Adrenergic pathways
  1. Adrenergic fibers
    a. Synthesis, storage, and release (see Fig. 3-2B)
    b. Receptor activation and signal transduction
      • Norepinephrine or epinephrine binds to α or β receptors on postsynaptic effector cells (Table 3-3).
    c. Termination of action:
      (1) Reuptake by active transport (uptake I) is the primary mechanism for removal of norepinephrine from the synaptic cleft.
      (2) Monoamine oxidase (MAO) is an enzyme located in the mitochondria of presynaptic adrenergic neurons and liver.
      (3) Catechol-*O*-methyltransferase (COMT) is an enzyme located in the cytoplasm of autonomic effector cells and liver.
  2. Drugs that affect adrenergic pathways (see Fig. 3-2 and Table 3-2)
    a. Guanethidine
      (1) Effect involves active transport into the peripheral adrenergic neuron by the norepinephrine reuptake system (uptake I).
      (2) Mechanism of action
        (a) Guanethidine eventually depletes the nerve endings of norepinephrine by replacing norepinephrine in the storage granules.
        (b) Its uptake is blocked by reuptake inhibitors (e.g., cocaine, tricyclic antidepressants such as imipramine).
      (3) Use
        • Hypertension (discontinued in United States)
    b. Reserpine
      (1) Mechanism of action
        (a) Depletes storage granules of catecholamines by binding to granules and preventing uptake and storage of dopamine and norepinephrine
        (b) Acts centrally also to produce sedation, depression, and parkinsonian symptoms (due to depletion of norepinephrine, serotonin, and dopamine)
      (2) Uses
        (a) Mild hypertension (rarely used today)
        (b) Huntington's disease (unlabeled use)
        (c) Management of tardive dyskinesia (unlabeled use)
      (3) Adverse effects
        (a) Pseudoparkinsonism
        (b) Sedation
        (c) Depression

Atropine blocks muscarinic receptors.

Hexamethonium blocks ganglionic nicotinic receptors.

Tubocurarine-like drugs block nicotinic receptors in NMJ.

Epinephrine and norepinephrine both stimulate α- and β-adrenergic receptors.

Uptake 1 most important for termination of action.

Uptake 1 also referred to as NET (NorEpinephrine Transporter)

Guanethidine requires uptake I to enter presynaptic neuron to deplete NE.

Cocaine and tricyclic antidepressants (TCAs) block uptake I.

Reserpine used to treat Huntington's disease.

Guanethidine and reserpine are adrenergic nerve blocking agent

TABLE 3-3. **Properties of Adrenergic Receptors**

Type of Receptor	Mechanism of Signal Transduction	Effects
α_1	Increased IP$_3$ and DAG	Contraction of smooth muscles
α_2	Decreased cAMP	Inhibits norepinephrine release Decrease in aqueous humor secretion Decrease in insulin secretion Mediation of platelet aggregation and mediation of CNS effects
β_1	Increased cAMP	Increase in secretion of renin Increase in heart rate, contractility, and conduction
β_2	Increased cAMP	Glycogenolysis Relaxation of smooth muscles Uptake of potassium in smooth muscles
β_3	Increased cAMP	Lipolysis

cAMP, cyclic adenosine monophosphate; CNS, central nervous system; DAG, diacylglycerol; IP$_3$, inositol triphosphate.

    c. Adrenergic receptor antagonists
      (1) May be nonselective or selective for either α or β receptors
      (2) May be selective for a particular subtype of α or β receptor (see Chapter 5)

III. Physiologic Considerations
  A. Dual innervation
    1. Most visceral organs are innervated by both the sympathetic and parasympathetic nervous systems.
    2. Blood vessels are innervated *only* by the sympathetic system

> Most organs are dually innervated.

  B. Physiologic effects of autonomic nerve activity (Table 3-4)
    1. α responses
      • Usually excitatory (contraction of smooth muscle)

> Alpha responses are excitatory

    2. β_1 responses
      a. Located in the heart and are excitatory
      b. Cause renin secretion in the kidney
    3. β_2 responses
      • Usually inhibitory (relaxation of smooth muscle)

> β_2 responses are inhibitory.
>
> β_2 responses: bronchodilation and vasodilation

      a. Cause vasodilation in vasculature
      b. Cause bronchodilation in bronchi
      c. Responsible for metabolic effects in liver and adipocytes
    4. Adrenal medulla
      a. This modified sympathetic ganglion releases epinephrine and norepinephrine.
      b. These circulating hormones can affect α and β responses throughout the body.

> Epinephrine is main adrenergic hormone secreted from adrenal medulla.

    5. Heart
      a. Sympathetic effects increase cardiac output
        (1) Positive chronotropic effect (increased heart rate)
        (2) Positive inotropic effect (increased force of contraction)
        (3) Positive dromotropic effect (increased speed of conduction of excitation)
      b. Parasympathetic effects (M_2) decrease heart rate and cardiac output.
        (1) Negative chronotropic effect (decreased heart rate)
        (2) Negative inotropic effect (decreased force of contraction)
          • Exogenous ACh only (*no vagal innervation of the ventricular muscle*)
        (3) Negative dromotropic effect (decreased velocity of conduction of excitation)

> At rest, the predominant tone to the heart is parasympathetic.

    6. Blood pressure: the overall effects of autonomic drugs on blood pressure are complex and are determined by at least four parameters:
      a. Direct effects on the heart
        (1) β_1 stimulation leads to an increased heart rate and increased force: produces increased blood pressure and increased pulse pressure.
        (2) Muscarinic stimulation leads to a decreased heart rate and decreased force: produces decreased blood pressure.
      b. Vascular effects
        (1) Muscarinic stimulation results in dilation, which decreases blood pressure.
          • Exogenous muscarinic drugs *only* (*no PSNS innervation of the vascular system*)
        (2) Alpha (α) stimulation results in vascular constriction, which increases blood pressure; both venules and arterioles.
        (3) Beta (β_2) stimulation results in dilation, which decreases blood pressure; both venules and arterioles.

> α_1 stimulation vasoconstriction; β_2 stimulation vasodilation.

      c. Redistribution of blood
        (1) With increased sympathetic activity, the blood is shunted away from organs and tissues such as the skin, gastrointestinal tract, kidney, and glands and toward the heart and voluntary (e.g., skeletal) muscles.
        (2) This process occurs as a result of a predominance of β_2 vasodilation rather than α_1 constriction at these sites.

> The only tone to the vasculature is sympathetic.

      d. Reflex phenomena
        (1) A decrease in blood pressure, sensed by baroreceptors in the carotid sinus and aortic arch, causes reflex tachycardia.
        (2) An increase in blood pressure causes reflex bradycardia.

> Fall in blood pressure produces reflex tachycardia.
>
> Elevation in blood pressure produces reflex bradycardia.

    7. Eye
      a. Pupil (iris)
        (1) Sympathetic effects (α_1-adrenergic receptor) contract radial muscle (mydriasis).
        (2) Parasympathomimetic effects (M_3-muscarinic receptors) contract circular muscle (miosis).

TABLE 3-4. **Direct Effects of Autonomic Nerve Activity on Body Systems**

ORGAN/TISSUE	SYMPATHETIC RESPONSE			PARASYMPATHETIC RESPONSE	
	ACTION	RECEPTOR		ACTION	RECEPTOR
Eye: Iris					
Radial muscle	Contracts (mydriasis)	α_1		—	—
Circular muscle	—	—		Contracts	M_3
Ciliary muscle	Relaxes for far vision	β_2		Contracts for near vision	M_3
Heart					
Sinoatrial node	Accelerates	$\beta_1 > \beta_2$		Decelerates	M_2
Ectopic pacemakers	Accelerates	$\beta_1 > \beta_2$		—	—
Contractility	Increases	$\beta_1 > \beta_2$		Decreases (atria)	M_2
Arterioles					
Coronary	Dilation	β_2		Dilation	M_3*
	Constriction	$\alpha_1 > \alpha_2$		—	
Skin and mucosa	Constriction	$\alpha_1 > \alpha_2$		Dilation	M_3*
Skeletal muscle	Constriction	$\alpha_1 > \alpha_2$		Dilation	M_3*
	Dilation	β_2, M†		—	—
Splanchnic	Constriction	$\alpha_1 > \alpha_2$		Dilation	M_3*
Renal and mesenteric	Dilation	Dopamine, β_2		—	—
	Constriction	$\alpha_1 > \alpha_2$		—	—
Veins					
Systemic	Dilation	β_2		—	—
	Constriction	$\alpha_1 > \alpha_2$		—	—
Bronchiolar Muscle	Relaxes	β_2		Contracts	M_3
GI Tract					
Smooth muscle					
Walls	Relaxes	α_2, β_2		Contracts	M_3
Sphincters	Contracts	α_1		Relaxes	M_3
Secretion	Inhibits	α_2		Increases	M_3
Genitourinary Smooth Muscle					
Bladder wall	Relaxes	β_2		Contracts	M_3
Sphincter	Contracts	α_1		Relaxes	M_3
Uterus, pregnant	Relaxes	β_2		—	—
	Contracts	α_1		—	—
Penis, seminal vesicles	Ejaculation	α		Erection	M
Skin					
Pilomotor smooth muscle	Contracts	α_1		—	—
Sweat glands					
Thermoregulatory	Increases	M		—	—
Apocrine (stress)	Increases	α_1		—	—
Other Functions					
Muscle	Promotes K^+ uptake	β_2		—	—
Liver	Gluconeogenesis	α, β_2		—	—
	Glycogenolysis	α, β_2		—	—
Fat cells	Lipolysis	β_3		—	—
Kidney	Renin release Sodium reabsorption	β_1, α_1‡		—	—

*The endothelium of most blood vessels releases endothelium-derived releasing factor (EDRF), which causes vasodilation in response to muscarinic stimuli. However, these muscarinic receptors are not innervated and respond only to *circulating muscarinic agonists.*
†Vascular smooth muscle has sympathetic cholinergic dilator fibers.
‡α_1 inhibits; β_1 stimulates.
GI, gastrointestinal; M, muscarinic.

    b. Ciliary muscle
       (1) Sympathetic (β-adrenergic receptors) causes relaxation and facilitates the secretion of aqueous humor.
       (2) Parasympathetic (M_3-muscarinic receptors) causes contraction (accommodation for near vision) and opens pores facilitating outflow of aqueous humor into canal of Schlemm.
       (3) The predominant tone in the eye is PSNS

CHAPTER 4
CHOLINERGIC DRUGS

I. Cholinoreceptor Agonists
A. Muscarinic receptor agonists (Box 4-1)
- Physiologic muscarinic effects (Table 4-1)
1. Pharmacokinetics and classes
   a. Choline esters
      - Quaternary ammonium compounds
         (1) Do *not* readily cross the blood-brain barrier
         (2) Inactivation
            (a) Acetylcholinesterase (AChE)
            (b) Pseudocholinesterase
         (3) Carbachol should *not* be used systemically because it also has unpredictable nicotinic activity
   b. Plant alkaloids
      (1) Muscarine is used experimentally to investigate muscarinic receptors.
      (2) Pilocarpine
         (a) A tertiary amine
         (b) Can enter the central nervous system (CNS)
         (c) Used to treat glaucoma and increase secretions
   c. Synthetic drugs
      (1) Cevimeline, a tertiary amine
      (2) Binds to muscarinic receptors
      (3) Causes an increase in secretion of exocrine glands (including salivary glands)
2. Mechanism of action
   - Directly stimulate muscarinic receptors
3. Uses
   a. Bethanechol (selectively acts on smooth muscle of the gastrointestinal tract and the urinary bladder)
      (1) Urinary retention in the absence of obstruction
      (2) Postoperative ileus
      (3) Gastric atony and retention after bilateral vagotomy
   b. Pilocarpine
      (1) Glaucoma (ophthalmic preparation)
      (2) Xerostomia (dry mouth)
         - Given orally to stimulate salivary gland secretion
   c. Cevimeline used to treat dry mouth in Sjögren's syndrome
4. Adverse effects
   a. Due to overstimulation of parasympathetic effector organs
      (1) Nausea
      (2) Vomiting
      (3) Diarrhea
      (4) Salivation
      (5) Sweating
   b. Treatment of overdose
      (1) Atropine to counteract muscarinic effects
      (2) Epinephrine to overcome severe cardiovascular reactions or bronchoconstriction

Choline esters *do not* cross BBB.

Pilocarpine and nicotine cross BBB.

Pilocarpine used to treat glaucoma and increase secretions.

Bethanechol used to get GI and GU going.

Pilocarpine and cevimeline used to increase secretions.

Overdoses of muscarinic agonists can be treated with atropine and/or epinephrine.

BOX 4-1   MUSCARINIC AND NICOTINIC RECEPTOR AGONISTS

Choline Esters
Acetylcholine (M, N)
Bethanechol (M)
Carbachol (M)
Succinylcholine (N)

Plant Alkaloids
Muscarine (M)
Nicotine (N)
Pilocarpine (M)

Synthetic
Cevimeline (M)

M, muscarinic; N, nicotinic.

TABLE 4-1. **Effects of Muscarinic Receptor Agonists**

ORGAN/ORGAN SYSTEM	EFFECTS
Cardiovascular	Hypotension from direct vasodilation Bradycardia at high doses Slowed conduction and prolonged refractory period of atrioventricular node
Gastrointestinal	Increased tone and increased contractile activity of gut Increased acid secretion Nausea, vomiting, cramps, and diarrhea
Genitourinary	Involuntary urination from increased bladder motility and relaxation of sphincter Penile erection
Eye	Miosis: contraction of sphincter muscle, resulting in reduced intraocular pressure Contraction of ciliary muscle; accommodated for near vision
Respiratory system	Bronchoconstriction
Glands	Increased secretory activity, resulting in increased salivation, lacrimation, and sweating

B. **Cholinesterase inhibitors** (Box 4-2; Fig. 4-1; see also Fig. 3-2A)
   1. Pharmacokinetics
      a. Edrophonium is rapid and short-acting (i.e., effects last only about 10 minutes after injection).
      b. Physostigmine crosses the BBB.
      c. Drugs used in Alzheimer's disease cross the BBB.
   2. Mechanism of action
      a. Bind to and inhibit AChE, increasing the concentration of acetylcholine (ACh) in the synaptic cleft
      b. Stimulate responses at the muscarinic receptors as well as nicotinic receptors
      c. Stimulate responses at nicotinic receptors at the neuromuscular junction (NMJ), in the ganglia at higher doses and, those that cross the BBB, in the brain

AChE inhibitors used as drugs, insecticides and warfare agents.

BOX 4-2 CHOLINESTERASE INHIBITORS	
Reversible Inhibitors	**Irreversible Inhibitors**
Donepezil (A)	Echothiophate
Edrophonium (MG)	Isoflurophate
Galantamine (A)	Malathion
Neostigmine (C, MG)	Parathion
Physostigmine (C)	Sarin
Pyridostigmine (C, MG)	Soman
Rivastigmine (A,C)	
Tacrine (A)	

C, carbamate structure; A, used in Alzheimer's disease; MG, used in myasthenia gravis.

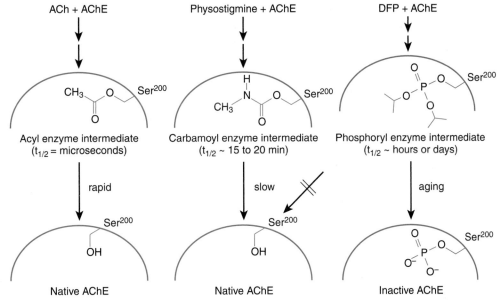

4-1: Interaction of acetylcholine (ACh), physostigmine, or isoflurophate (DFP) with the serine (Ser) hydroxyl at amino acid position 200 of the catalytic site of acetylcholine esterase (AChE).

3. Subsets of AChE inhibitors
   a. Reversible inhibitors
      (1) Truly reversible, compete with ACh at the enzyme active site
         (a) Edrophonium
         (b) Tacrine
         (c) Donepezil
         (d) Galantamine
      (2) Carbamates; carbamylate the serine hydroxyl at active site of enzyme which is slowly hydrolyzed (pseudoreversible)
         (a) Physostigmine
         (b) Rivastigmine
         (c) Neostigmine
         (d) Pyridostigmine
   b. Irreversible inhibitors (organophosphates)
      (1) Phosphorylate the serine hydroxyl at active site of enzyme
      (2) The phosphoryl group is *not* readily cleaved from the active site of cholinesterase
      (3) The enzyme can be reactivated by the early use of pralidoxime
      (4) Examples
         (a) Echothiophate (glaucoma)
         (b) Isoflurophate (DFP; experimental)
         (c) Malathion (insecticide)
         (d) Parathion (insecticide)
         (e) Sarin (war nerve agent)
         (f) Soman (war nerve agent)
4. Uses
   a. Alzheimer's disease
      (1) Donepezil
      (2) Tacrine
      (3) Rivastigmine
      (4) Galantamine
         • Galantamine may also increase glutamate and serotonin levels in the brain.
   b. Paralytic ileus and urine retention
      • Neostigmine
   c. Glaucoma
      (1) Physostigmine
      (2) Echothiophate

Edrophonium competes with ACh at AChE.

Carbamates form a covalent bond at AchE but are slowly hydrolyzed.

Physostigmine and rivastigmine cross BBB.

Neostigmine and pyridostigmine do *not* cross BBB.

Organophosphates form a covalent bond at AChE that does *not* readily hydrolyze, but AChE can be reactivated by pralidoxime prior to aging.

Tacrine may cause hepatotoxicity.

AChE inhibitors are beneficial in treating Alzheimer's and other dementias.

d. Myasthenia gravis
   (1) Edrophonium (short-acting; diagnosis only)
   (2) Pyridostigmine (treatment)
   (3) Neostigmine (treatment)
e. Insecticides and chemical warfare
   (1) Organophosphates used as insecticides
     (a) Malathion
     (b) Parathion
   (2) Organophosphates used as components in nerve gases
     (a) Sarin
     (b) Soman
5. Adverse effects
a. Due to overstimulation of parasympathetic effector organs
   (1) Nausea
   (2) Vomiting
   (3) Diarrhea
   (4) Urination
   (5) Salivation
   (6) Lacrimation
   (7) Constricted pupils (miosis)
   (8) Bronchoconstriction

b. Treatment
   (1) Atropine to counteract muscarinic effects
   (2) Pralidoxime to reactivate enzyme if toxicity due to an organophosphate
     (a) Prior to enzyme aging (Fig. 4-1)
     (b) Contraindicated for reversible inhibitors
   (3) Supportive therapy (check and support vital signs)

C. Ganglionic stimulants
1. Effects depend on the predominant autonomic tone at the organ system being assessed.
2. ACh
a. Much higher levels of ACh are required to stimulate nicotinic receptors in ganglia than muscarinic receptors at the neuroeffector junction.
b. Must pretreat with atropine to reveal ganglionic effects
3. Nicotine

a. Stimulates the ganglia at low doses
b. Blocks the ganglia at higher doses by persistent depolarization of nicotinic receptors and secondary desensitization of receptors (i.e., "depolarizing blocker")
c. Uses
   (1) Experimentally to investigate the autonomic nervous system (ANS)
   (2) Clinically as a drug to help smokers quit smoking
   (3) As an adjunct to haloperidol in the treatment of Tourette's syndrome
   (4) As an insecticide
4. Cholinesterase inhibitors
a. Increase the concentration of ACh at the ganglia
b. Tertiary amines also increase ACh in the brain

D. Neuromuscular junction (see Chapter 6)
1. ACh, nicotine and succinylcholine all are nicotinic agonists at the NMJ
  • Overstimulation produces a desensitizing or "depolarizing" blockade.
2. Succinylcholine is used as depolarizing neuromuscular blocker for:
a. Adjunct to general anesthesia
b. Endotracheal intubation
c. Reduction of intensity of muscle contractions of pharmacologically- or electrically-induced convulsions.

II. Cholinoreceptor Antagonists
A. Muscarinic receptor antagonists (Box 4-3)
1. Classes
a. Belladonna alkaloids
b. Synthetic muscarinic antagonists
c. Other classes of drugs with atropine-like effects, such as:
   (1) First generation antihistamines
   (2) Antipsychotics
   (3) Tricyclic antidepressants

BOX 4-3 MUSCARINIC RECEPTOR ANTAGONISTS

Belladonna Alkaloids
Atropine (Prototype)
Hyoscyamine (GI, B)
Scopolamine (A, O, MS)

Synthetic Muscarinic Antagonists
Benztropine (P)
Cyclopentolate (O)
Darifenacin (B)

Homatropine (O)
Ipratropium (L)
Oxybutynin (B; transdermal)
Solifenacin (B)
Tiotropium (L)
Trihexyphenidyl (P)
Tolterodine (B)
Tropicamide (O)

GI, Gastrointestinal tract; B, bladder; A, anesthesia; O, ophthalmic; MS, motion sickness; P, Parkinson's; L, lung.

---

       (4) Antiparkinsonian drugs
       (5) Quinidine
  2. Mechanism of action
    • Competitive inhibition of ACh at the muscarinic receptor
  3. Uses
    a. Chronic obstructive pulmonary disease (COPD)
       (1) Ipratropium
       (2) Tiotropium
    b. Asthma prophylaxis
      • Ipratropium
    c. Bradycardia
      • Atropine
    d. Motion sickness
      • Scopolamine
    e. Parkinson's disease
       (1) Benztropine
       (2) Trihexyphenidyl
    f. Bladder or bowel spasms and incontinence
       (1) Darifenacin
       (2) Oxybutynin
       (3) Solifenacin
       (4) Tolterodine
    g. Ophthalmic uses
       (1) Facilitation of ophthalmoscopic examinations when prolonged dilation is needed
       (2) Iridocyclitis
       (3) Examples
          (a) Atropine
          (b) Cyclopentolate
          (c) Homatropine
          (d) Scopolamine
          (e) Tropicamide
    h. "Colds" (over-the-counter remedies)
       (1) Some symptomatic relief as the result of a drying effect
       (2) Useful as sleep aids (diphenhydramine; see Chapter 7)
    i. Treatment of parasympathomimetic toxicity
      • Atropine
       (1) Overdose of AChE inhibitors
       (2) Mushroom *(Amanita muscaria)* poisoning
  4. Adverse effects
    a. Overdose
       (1) Common signs
          (a) Dry mouth
          (b) Dilated pupils
          (c) Blurring of vision
          (d) Hot, dry, flushed skin
          (e) Tachycardia

First generation antihistamine, many antipsychotics, tricyclic antidepressants, some antiparkinson drugs, and quinidine all have significant antimuscarinic effects.

Ipratropium and tiotropium are used for bronchodilation.

Atropine is an important drug for treating severe bradycardia.

Scopolamine is used as a patch behind the ear to treat motion sickness.

Benztropine and trihexyphenidyl are used to treat some Parkinson's symptoms.

Oxybutynin is available as a transdermal formulation; it has 1/5 the anticholinergic activity of atropine but has 4 to 10 times the antispasmodic activity; increases bladder capacity, decreases uninhibited contractions, and delays desire to void, therefore, decreases urgency and frequency.

Anticholinergics are useful in treating overactive bladder, Parkinson's disease, airway diseases, bradycardia, excess secretions, motion sickness

Anticholinergics are used to dilate pupil for eye examinations.

(f) Fever

(g) CNS changes

    (2) Death follows coma and respiratory depression.

  b. Treatment of overdose

    (1) Gastric lavage

    (2) Supportive therapy

    (3) Diazepam to control excitement and seizures

    (4) Effects of muscarinic receptor antagonists may be overcome by increasing levels of ACh in the synaptic cleft

      (a) Usually by administration of AChE inhibitors such as physostigmine

      (b) Physostigmine used only for pure anticholinergics and *not* for poisoning with:

        • Antihistamines

        • Antipsychotics

        • Tricyclic antidepressant drugs

B. Nicotinic receptor antagonists

  1. Ganglionic blockers

    a. Block nicotinic receptor at ganglion

    b. Primarily used in mechanistic studies

    c. Examples

      (1) Hexamethonium

        (a) Prototypic ganglionic blocking agent

        (b) Used experimentally

      (2) Trimethaphan

        (a) Used to control blood pressure during surgery

        (b) Discontinued in United States

  2. Neuromuscular blockers (see Chapter 6)

    a. Mechanism of action

      (1) Block nicotinic receptors at the neuromuscular junction

      (2) Examples

        (a) Cisatracurium

        (b) Tubocurarine

    b. Use

      (1) Relaxation of striated muscle

      (2) Relaxation may be reversed by cholinesterase inhibitors

        (a) Neostigmine

        (b) Pyridostigmine

III. Therapeutic summary of selected cholinergic drugs: (Table 4-2)

TABLE 4-2. **Therapeutic Summary of Selected Cholinergic Drugs**

DRUGS	CLINICAL APPLICATIONS	ADVERSE EFFECTS	CONTRAINDICATIONS
Mechanism: *Inhibits ACh release*			
Botulinum toxin	Strabismus Blepharospasm Cervical dystonia Wrinkles Hyperhydrosis	Arrhythmias Syncope Hepatotoxicity Anaphylaxis	Hypersensitivity
Mechanism: *Muscarinic receptor agonists*			
Bethanechol Carbachol Cevimeline	Urinary tract motility (bethanechol) Glaucoma (carbachol) Xerostomia (cevimeline and pilocarpine)	Rhinitis, nausea, dizziness ↑ frequency of urination (oral formulations)	Hypersensitivity Asthma Epilepsy Peptic ulcer disease
Mechanism: *AChE Inhibitors*			

Edrophonium
Neostigmine
Pyridostigmine
Physostigmine
	Diagnosis of myasthenia gravis (edrophonium)
	Treatment of myasthenia gravis (neostigmine, and
	  pyridostigmine)
	Reversal of anticholinergic effects (physostigmine)
		DUMBELS plus
		Seizures
		Bronchospasm
		Cardiac arrest
		Respiratory depression
			Intestinal or urinary
			  obstruction
			Cardiovascular disease

Mechanism: *AChE Inhibitors plus other mechanisms for treatment of Alzheimer's disease*			
Donepezil Galantamine Rivastigmine Tacrine	Alzheimer's disease Dementia	Anorexia, nausea and vomiting Cramps Vivid dreams Hepatotoxic (tacrine)	Tacrine in liver disease
Mechanism: *Nicotinic receptor agonist that produces a depolarizing blockade*			

Succinylcholine	Intubation
	Induction of neuromuscular blockade during
	  surgery
	Electroconvulsive therapy
		Cardiac slowing and arrest
		Malignant hyperthermia
		Respiratory depression
		↑ intraocular pressure,
		  Rhabdomyolysis
			History of malignant
			  hyperthermia

Mechanism: *Muscarinic receptor antagonists*			
Atropine (prototype)	AChEI overdose Acute bradycardia Anesthesia premedication Antidote for mushroom poisoning	Dry mouth Blurred vision Urinary retention Constipation Tachycardia ↑ intraocular pressure Hyperthermia	Narrow angle glaucoma
Mechanism: *Muscarinic receptor antagonists*			
Scopolamine	Motion sickness Nausea and vomiting	Like atropine, more sedation	Like atropine
Ipratropium Tiotropium	Asthma COPD	Like atropine	Like atropine
Mechanism: *Muscarinic receptor antagonists*			
Oxybutynin Tolterodine Darifenacin Solifenacin	Treat overactive bladder Urge incontinence	Like atropine	Like atropine
Mechanism: *Nicotinic receptor antagonists*			

Tubocurarine
Cisatracurium
Pancuronium
Rocuronium
Vecuronium
	Lethal injections (tubocurarine)
	All others are used for NMJ blockade during
	  surgery and intubation
		Apnea
		Bronchospasms
		Hypertension
		Arrhythmias
		Respiratory failure Histamine release
		  (tubocurarine)
			Hypersensitivity

ACh, acetylcholine; AChE, acetylcholine esterase; AChEI, acetylcholine esterase inhibitor; COPD, chronic obstructive pulmonary disease; DUMBELS: **D**efecation, **U**rination, **M**iosis, **B**ronchoconstriction, **E**mesis, **L**acrimation, **S**alivation; NMJ, neuromuscular junction.

CHAPTER 5
ADRENERGIC DRUGS

I. Adrenoreceptor Agonists
   A. General
   1. Endogenous catecholamines (norepinephrine, epinephrine, and dopamine) are found in peripheral sympathetic nerve endings, the adrenal medulla, and the brain.
   2. Catecholamines affect blood pressure and heart rate.
      a. Intravenous bolus injection (Fig. 5-1)
      b. Intravenous infusion for 20 min (Fig. 5-2)
   3. Some indirect agonists
      a. Potentiate the effects of catecholamines by decreasing their disappearance from the synaptic cleft
      b. Examples
         (1) Monoamine oxidase (MAO) inhibitors
         (2) Catechol-*O*-methyltransferase (COMT) inhibitors
         (3) Tricyclic antidepressants (TCAs)
         (4) Cocaine

   B. Physiological effects of selected agents (Table 5-1)
   C. Selected catecholamines (Box 5-1)
   1. Norepinephrine (NE)
      a. Stimulates β_1- and α_1-adrenergic receptors causing increased contractility and heart rate as well as vasoconstriction
      b. Clinically
         (1) Alpha effects (vasoconstriction) are greater than beta effects (inotropic and chronotropic effects)
         (2) Often resulting in reflex bradycardia (see Figs. 5-1, 5-2)
      c. Use
         • Occasionally to treat shock which persists after adequate fluid volume replacement
   2. Epinephrine (EPI)
      a. Pharmacokinetics
         (1) Usually injected subcutaneously
         (2) Given by intracardiac or intravenous route to treat cardiac arrest
      b. Uses
         (1) Treatment of asthma
         (2) Treatment of anaphylactic shock or angioedema
         (3) Prolongation of action of local anesthetics, due to the vasoconstrictive properties of EPI
         (4) Treatment of cardiac arrest, bradycardia, and complete heart block in emergencies
   3. Dopamine (DA)
      a. Mechanism of action
         • Stimulates D_1 specific dopamine receptors on renal vasculature, and at higher doses it also stimulates β_1- and α_1-adrenergic receptors
            (1) Low doses stimulate primarily renal dopamine receptors (0.5–2 µg/kg/min) causing vasodilation in the kidney.
            (2) Moderate doses also stimulate β_1-adrenergic receptors (2–10 µg/kg/min) increasing cardiac contractility.
            (3) High doses also stimulate α_1-adrenergic receptors (>10 µg/kg/min) causing vasoconstriction.

MAOI and COMT
inhibitors block the
metabolism of
catecholamines.

TCAs and cocaine block
the reuptake of some
catecholamines.

α-Effect: vasoconstriction

β-Effect: inotropic,
chronotropic

EPI used to treat
anaphylactic shock or
angioedema

EPI used to prolong
action of local
anesthetics.

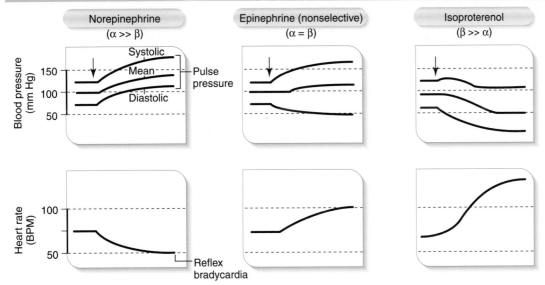

5-1: Graphic representations of the effects of three catecholamines given by intravenous bolus injection on blood pressure and heart rate. Note that the pulse pressure is greatly increased with epinephrine and isoproterenol. Norepinephrine causes reflex bradycardia.

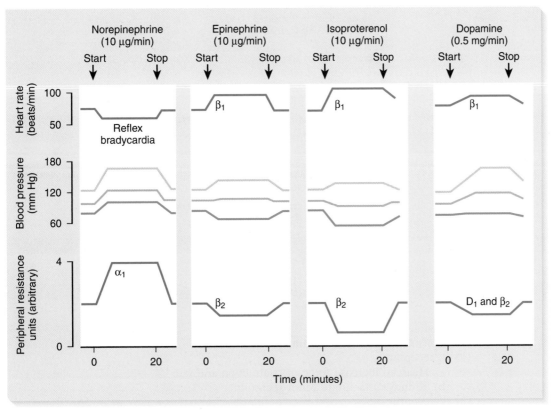

5-2: Comparison of the cardiovascular effects of four catecholamines when a low dose is given by intravenous infusion. *(From Brenner G and Stevens C: Pharmacology, 3rd ed. Philadelphia, Saunders, 2010, Figure 8-4.)*

   b. Uses
      (1) Cardiogenic and noncardiogenic shock
      (2) Dopamine increases blood flow through the kidneys
   c. Adverse effects
      (1) Premature ventricular tachycardia, sinus tachycardia
      (2) Angina pectoris

Dopamine increases renal blood flow; important in preventing ischemic kidney.

TABLE 5-1. **Pharmacologic Effects and Clinical Uses of Adrenoreceptor Agonists**

DRUG DIRECT-ACTING ADRENORECEPTOR AGONISTS	EFFECT AND RECEPTOR SELECTIVITY	CLINICAL APPLICATION
Catecholamines		
Dobutamine	Cardiac stimulation (β_1) $\beta_1 > \beta_2$	Shock, heart failure
Dopamine	Renal vasodilation (D_1) Cardiac stimulation (β_1) Increased blood pressure (α_1) $D_1 = D_2 > \beta_1 > \alpha_1$	Shock, heart failure
Epinephrine	Increased blood pressure (α_1) Cardiac stimulation (β_1) Bronchodilation (β_2) Vasodialtion (β_2) General agonist ($\alpha_1, \alpha_2, \beta_1, \beta_2$)	Anaphylaxis, open-angle glaucoma, asthma, hypotension, cardiac arrest, ventricular fibrillation, reduction in bleeding in surgery, prolongation of local anesthetic action
Isoproterenol	Cardiac stimulation (β_1) $\beta_1 = \beta_2$	Atrioventricular block, bradycardia
Norepinephrine	Increased blood pressure (α_1) $\alpha_1, \alpha_2, \beta_1$	Hypotension, shock
NONCATECHOLAMINES		
Albuterol	Bronchodilation (β_2) $\beta_2 > \beta_1$	Asthma
Clonidine	Decreased sympathetic outflow (α_2)	Chronic hypertension
Oxymetazoline	Vasoconstriction (α_1)	Decongestant
Phenylephrine	Vasoconstriction, increased blood pressure, and mydriasis (α_1) $\alpha_1 > \alpha_2$	Pupil dilation, decongestion, mydriasis, neurogenic shock, blood pressure maintenance during surgery
Ritodrine	Bronchodilation and uterine relaxation (β_2)	Premature labor
Terbutaline	Bronchodilation and uterine relaxation (β_2) $\beta_2 > \beta_1$	Asthma, premature labor
Fenoldopam	Dilates renal and mesenteric vascular beds D_1-agonist	Hypertensive emergency
INDIRECT-ACTING ADRENORECEPTOR AGONISTS		
Amphetamine	Increased norepinephrine release General agonist ($\alpha_1, \alpha_2, \beta_1, \beta_2$)	Narcolepsy, obesity, attention deficit disorder
Cocaine	Inhibited norepinephrine reuptake General agonist ($\alpha_1, \alpha_2, \beta_1, \beta_2$)	Local anesthesia
MIXED-ACTING ADRENORECEPTOR AGONISTS		
Ephedrine	Vasoconstriction (α_1) General agonist ($\alpha_1, \alpha_2, \beta_1, \beta_2$)	Decongestant
Pseudoephedrine	Vasoconstriction (α_1)	Decongestant

Potency of α_1-adrenoreceptor agonists: EPI > NE >> DA >>>> ISO

Potency of β_1-adrenoreceptor agonists: ISO >> EPI > NE = DA

Potency of β_2-adrenoreceptor agonists: ISO > EPI >>> NE > DA

4. Isoproterenol (ISO)
   a. Mechanism of action is to stimulate
     (1) β_1 receptors
       (a) Heart to increase force of contraction and rate
       (b) Kidney to facilitate renin secretion
     (2) β_2 receptors
       (a) Vasculature (vasodilation)
       (b) Bronchioles (bronchodilation)
     (3) β_3 receptors
       Adipocytes to increase lipolysis
 D. α-Adrenergic receptor agonists (see Box 5-1)
   1 α_1-Adrenergic receptor agonists
    a. Examples
     (1) Phenylephrine
     (2) Naphazoline
     (3) Oxymetazoline

BOX 5-1   ADRENORECEPTOR AGONISTS

Direct-Acting Agonists and Receptor Selectivity
Catecholamines
Dobutamine β_1 (α_1)
Dopamine (DA) D_1 (α_1 and β_1 at high doses)
Epinephrine (EPI) α_1, α_2, β_1, β_2
Isoproterenol (ISO) β_1, β_2
Norepinephrine (NE) α_1, α_2, β_1
Noncatecholamines
Albuterol β_2
Clonidine α_2
Methyldopa (prodrug) α_2
Oxymetazoline α_1
Naphazoline α_1
Phenylephrine α_1
Ritodrine β_2
Salmeterol β_2
Terbutaline β_2

Indirect-Acting Agonists
Releasers
   Amphetamine
   Tyramine
Monoamine Oxidase Inhibitors
   Phenelzine (MAO-A, -B)
   Selegiline (MAO-B)
   Tranylcypromine (MAO-A, -B)
Catechol-O-methyltransferase Inhibitors
   Entacapone
   Tolcapone
Reuptake Inhibitors
   Cocaine
   Imipramine
Mixed-Acting Agonists
   Ephedrine
   Pseudoephedrine

   b. Mechanism of action
      (1) Directly stimulate α_1-receptors
      (2) Phenylephrine when injected intravenously produces effects similar to NE
   c. Uses
      (1) Blood pressure elevation (phenylephrine only)
      (2) Nasal decongestant
      (3) Mydriasis induction
      (4) Relief of redness of eye due to minor eye irritations
  2. α_2-Adrenergic receptor agonists
   a. Examples
      (1) Methyldopa (prodrug)
      (2) Clonidine
      (3) Guanabenz
      (4) Guanfacine
      (5) Tizanidine
   b. Used to treat hypertension (see Chapter 13)
   c. Clonidine is used unlabeled for several central effects:
      (1) Heroin or nicotine withdrawal
      (2) Severe pain
      (3) Dysmenorrhea
      (4) Vasomotor symptoms associated with menopause
      (5) Ethanol dependence
      (6) Prophylaxis of migraines
      (7) Glaucoma
      (8) Diabetes-associated diarrhea
      (9) Impulse control disorder

Phenylephrine is sometimes injected IV to rapidly elevate blood pressure.

Naphazoline and oxymetazoline get the red out of the eyes.

α_2-Adrenergic receptor agonists are centrally acting sympatholytic agents that decrease sympathetic outflow from the brain.

(10) Attention-deficit/hyperactivity disorder (ADHD)
(11) Clozapine-induced sialorrhea
d. Tizanidine is a centrally acting skeletal muscle relaxant used for the treatment of muscle spasms

Clonidine has many central actions

Tizanidine used to treat muscle spasms.

E. **β-Adrenergic receptor agonists** (see Box 5-1)
   1. β$_1$-Adrenergic receptor agonists
      a. Example
         • Dobutamine
      b. Use
         • Selective inotropic agent in the management of advanced cardiovascular failure associated with low cardiac output

Dobutamine increases cardiac output.

   2. β$_2$-Adrenergic receptor agonists (See Chapter 20)
      a. Examples
         (1) Terbutaline
         (2) Albuterol
         (3) Salmeterol
      b. Uses
         (1) Asthma and chronic obstructive pulmonary disease (COPD)
            (a) Albuterol
            (b) Salmeterol
            (c) Terbutaline
         (2) Treatment of hyperkalemia
            (a) Terbutaline subcutaneously
            (b) Redistributes potassium into the intracellular compartment
         (3) Reduce uterine tetany
            (a) Terbutaline
            (b) Ritodrine
      c. Adverse effects
         (1) Fine skeletal muscle tremor (most common)
         (2) Minimal cardiac adverse effects (palpitations)
         (3) Nervousness

Many β$_2$-adrenergic receptor agonists used in treatment of asthma and COPD.

Tremor common complaint of those who use β$_2$-adrenergic receptor agonists for asthma.

Fenoldopam used for the acute treatment of severe hypertension.

F. **Dopamine D$_1$ agonist**
   • Fenoldopam; an intravenous dopamine D$_1$ agonist used for the acute treatment of severe hypertension

G. **Indirect stimulants** (see Box 5-1)
   1. Tyramine
      a. Releases norepinephrine from storage granules, thus producing both α and β stimulation
      b. Leads to tachyphylaxis, because of depletion of norepinephrine stores after repeated use
      c. Results in hypertensive crisis in patients who are taking MAO inhibitors when tyramine is ingested (foods, wine)
      d. Often used experimentally to understand mechanisms

Rapid repetitive injections of tyramine results in tachyphylaxis

Hypertensive crisis: MAO inhibitors and tyramine-rich foods ("cheese effect")

   2. Amphetamine
      a. Mechanism of action
         (1) Indirect-acting amine
         (2) Releases norepinephrine, epinephrine, and dopamine (brain)
      b. Uses
         (1) Central nervous system (CNS) stimulant
            • Stimulates mood and alertness
         (2) Appetite suppression
         (3) ADHD disorder in children
            • Methylphenidate is preferable
      c. Adverse effects (due to sympathomimetic effects)
         (1) Nervousness, insomnia, anorexia
         (2) Growth inhibition (children)

Methylphenidate for ADHD.

MAO-A metabolizes norepinephrine and serotonin; thus, inhibition is useful in depression.

MAO-B metabolizes dopamine; thus, inhibition is useful in Parkinson's disease.

   3. MAO inhibitors
      a. Examples
         (1) Phenelzine (MAO-A & B)
         (2) Tranylcypromine (MAO-A & B)
         (3) Selegiline (MAO-B)

b. Uses (see Chapters 10 and 11)
   (1) Occasional treatment of depression (MAO-A & B)
   (2) Parkinson's disease (MAO-B)
c. Adverse effects
   • Due to sympathomimetic effects
4. Catechol-*O*-methyltransferase (COMT) inhibitors
  a. Examples
   (1) Tolcapone
   (2) Entacapone
  b. Use
   • Parkinson's disease (see Chapter 11)
5. Norepinephrine reuptake (uptake I) inhibitors
  a. Examples
   (1) Cocaine
   (2) Imipramine (a TCA)
  b. Potentiate effects of norepinephrine, epinephrine, and dopamine, but *not* isoproterenol (*not* taken up by uptake I) (see Fig. 3-2B)

H. Direct and indirect stimulants (see Box 5-1)
1. Examples
  a. Ephedrine
  b. Pseudoephedrine
2. Mechanism of action
  a. Releases norepinephrine (like tyramine)
  b. Also has a direct effect on α- and β-adrenergic receptors
3. Uses
  a. Mild asthma
  b. Nasal decongestion
4. Restrictions
  a. Herbal products with ephedrine have been banned in the United States
  b. Pseudoephedrine over-the-counter products are restricted because it is used to make methamphetamine in home laboratories

II. Adrenoreceptor Antagonists (Box 5-2)
  A. α-Adrenergic receptor antagonists
   1. Mechanism of action
    a. Blocks α-mediated effects of sympathetic nerve stimulation
    b. Blocks α-mediated effects of sympathomimetic drugs
   2. Nonselective α-adrenergic receptor antagonists (see Box 5-2)
    a. Phentolamine
     (1) Pharmacokinetics
      • Reversible, short-acting
     (2) Uses
      (a) Diagnosis and treatment of pheochromocytoma
      (b) Reversal of effects resulting from accidental subcutaneous injection of epinephrine
    b. Phenoxybenzamine
     (1) Pharmacokinetics
      • Irreversible, long-acting
     (2) Use
      • Preoperative management of pheochromocytoma
   3. Selective α$_1$-adrenergic receptor antagonists (see Box 5-2)
    a. Examples
     (1) Doxazosin
     (2) Prazosin
     (3) Terazosin
     (4) Tamsulosin
     (5) Alfuzosin
    b. Mechanism of action
     (1) Block α$_1$ receptors selectively on arterioles and venules
     (2) Produce less reflex tachycardia than nonselective α-receptor antagonists
    c. Uses
     (1) Hypertension
      (a) Doxazosin

COMT inhibition useful in Parkinson's disease.

Cocaine and TCAs potentiate catecholamine actions by blocking uptake I.

Herbal ephedra containing products banned in the United States.

Pseudoephedrine is starting material for making illicit methamphetamine.

Phentolamine is a reversible alpha blocker; thus, competitive kinetics.

Phenoxybenzamine is the only irreversible alpha blocker; thus, noncompetitive kinetics.

Note: -sin ending

BOX 5-2 ADRENORECEPTOR ANTAGONISTS

Nonselective α-Receptor Antagonists
Phenoxybenzamine (irreversible)
Phentolamine (reversible)

α₁-Receptor Antagonists
Alfuzosin (prostate specific)
Doxazosin
Prazosin
Tamsulosin (prostate specific)
Terazosin

α₂-Receptor Antagonists
Yohimbine

Nonselective β-Receptor Antagonists
Propranolol
Nadolol
Timolol

β₁-Receptor Antagonists
Atenolol
Esmolol
Metoprolol

Nonselective α- and β-Receptor Antagonists
Carvedilol
Labetalol

β-Receptor Antagonists with Intrinsic Sympathomimetic Activity (ISA)
Acebutolol (β₁-selective)
Penbutolol (nonselective)
Pindolol (nonselective)

β-Receptor Antagonists with Nitric Oxide Production
Nebivolol

Large "first-dose" effect

Tamsulosin and alfuzosin, which relaxes the bladder neck and the prostate, is used to treat BPH.

      (b) Prazosin
      (c) Terazosin
    (2) Benign prostatic hyperplasia (BPH)
      (a) Doxazosin
      (b) Tamsulosin
      (c) Alfuzosin
  d. Adverse effects
    (1) Orthostatic hypotension
    (2) Impaired ejaculation
  4. Selective α₂-adrenergic receptor antagonist
    • Yohimbine
      a. *No* clinical use
        (1) Ingredient in herbal preparations
        (2) Marketed for treatment of impotence
      b. May inhibit the hypotensive effect of clonidine or methyldopa
B. β-Adrenergic receptor antagonists (beta blockers)
  1. Pharmacologic properties
    a. Mechanism of action
      (1) Block β-receptor sympathomimetic effects
      (2) Cardiovascular effects
        (a) Decreased cardiac output and renin secretion
        (b) Decreased vasodilation

    (c) Decreased salt and water retention
    (d) Decreased heart and vascular remodeling
    (e) Decreased sympathetic outflow from the brain
  b. Uses
   (1) Cardiac problems
    (a) Arrhythmias
    (b) "Classic" angina (angina of effort)
    (c) Hypertension
    (d) Moderate heart failure
   (2) Thyrotoxicosis
   (3) Performance anxiety
   (4) Essential tremor (propranolol, metoprolol)
   (5) Migraine (prevention; propranolol, timolol)
  c. Adverse effects
   (1) Bradycardia, heart block
   (2) Bronchiolar constriction
   (3) Increased triglycerides, decreased high-density lipoprotein (HDL) levels
   (4) Mask symptoms of hypoglycemia (in diabetics)
   (5) Sedation; "tired or exhausted feeling"
   (6) Depression
   (7) Hyperkalemia
  d. Precautions
   (1) Abrupt withdrawal of β-adrenoreceptor antagonists can produce nervousness, increased heart rate, and increased blood pressure.
   (2) These drugs should be used with caution in patients with:
    (a) Asthma
    (b) Heart block
    (c) COPD
    (d) Diabetes
 2. Nonselective β-adrenergic receptor antagonists (see Box 5-2)
  a. Propranolol
   • β_1- and β_2-receptor antagonist
   (1) Mechanism of action
    (a) Decreases heart rate and contractility
     • Reduces myocardial oxygen consumption
    (b) Decreases cardiac output, thus reducing blood pressure
    (c) Decreases renin release
   (2) Uses
    (a) Arrhythmias
    (b) Hypertension
    (c) Angina
    (d) Heart failure
    (e) Tremor
    (f) Migraine prophylaxis
    (g) Pheochromocytoma
    (h) Thyrotoxicosis
  b. Timolol
   (1) Mechanism of action
    (a) Lowers intraocular pressure
    (b) Presumably by reducing production of aqueous humor
   (2) Uses
    (a) Wide-angle glaucoma (topical preparation)
    (b) Migraine prophylaxis
    (c) Hypertension
  c. Nadolol
   (1) Pharmacokinetics
    • Long half-life (17 to 24 hrs)
   (2) Uses
    (a) Hypertension
    (b) Angina
    (c) Migraine headache prophylaxis

Metoprolol, carvedilol and bisoprolol reduce mortality in patients with chronic heart failure.

Use beta blockers with caution in the following conditions: heart block, asthma, COPD, diabetes.

Note: -olol ending.

Timolol is in many ophthalmic preparations for treatment of wide-angle glaucoma

Timolol has no local anesthetic effect

3. Selective β_1-adrenergic receptor antagonists (see Box 5-2)
   a. Metoprolol and atenolol
      • Cardioselective β_1-adrenergic blockers
      (1) Uses
         (a) Hypertension
         (b) Angina
         (c) Acute myocardial infarction (MI)
            • Prevention and treatment
         (d) Heart failure
         (e) Tachycardia
      (2) These β_1-adrenergic blockers may be safer than propranolol for patients who experience bronchoconstriction because they produce less β_2-receptor blockade.
   b. Esmolol
      (1) Pharmacokinetics
         (a) Short half-life (9 min)
         (b) Given by intravenous infusion
      (2) Uses
         (a) Hypertensive crisis
         (b) Acute supraventricular tachycardia
4. Nonselective β- and α_1-adrenergic receptor antagonists (see Box 5-2)
   a. Labetalol
      (1) Mechanism of action
         (a) α and β blockade (β blockade is predominant)
         (b) Reduces blood pressure without a substantial decrease in resting heart rate, cardiac output, or stroke volume
      (2) Uses
         (a) Hypertension and hypertensive emergencies
         (b) Pheochromocytoma
   b. Carvedilol
      (1) Mechanism of action
         • α and β blockade
      (2) Use
         • Heart failure
5. β-Adrenoreceptor antagonists with intrinsic sympathomimetic activity (ISA) (see Box 5-2)
   a. Examples
      (1) Acebutolol (selective β_1)
      (2) Penbutolol (nonselective)
      (3) Pindolol (nonselective)
   b. These agents have partial agonist activity
   c. Uses
      (1) Preferred in patients with moderate heart block
      (2) May have an advantage in the treatment of patients with asthma, diabetes, and hyperlipidemias
6. β-Adrenoreceptor antagonist with nitric oxide release
   a. Example
      • Nebivolol
   b. Mechanism of action
      (1) Selective β_1-adrenergic blockade
      (2) Release of nitric oxide from endothelial cells resulting in reduction of systemic vascular resistance
   c. Use
      • Treatment of hypertension, alone or in combination with other drugs
III. Therapeutic summary of selected adrenergic drugs: (Table 5-2)

Use selective β_1-adrenergic receptor antagonists with caution in the following conditions: asthma, COPD

Atenolol has minimal CNS effects

Esmolol short-acting intravenous beta blocker used to slow the heart.

Note labetalol and carvedilol **don't end in -olol;** block both α and β receptors

TABLE 5-2. **Therapeutic Summary of Selected Adrenergic Drugs**

DRUGS	CLINICAL APPLICATIONS	ADVERSE EFFECTS	CONTRAINDICATIONS
Mechanism: *α₁-Adrenergic receptor agonists*			
Phenylephrine Naphazoline Oxymetazoline	Hypotension (phenylephrine) Nasal congestion Eye hyperemia	Arrhythmias Hypertension Nervousness Rebound nasal congestion	Severe hypertension Narrow-angle glaucoma
Mechanism: *α₂-Adrenergic receptor agonists*			

Clonidine
Guanabenz
Methyldopa
  (prodrug)
Tizanidine
	Hypotension (not
	  tizanidine)
	CNS effects
	  (clonidine)
	Muscle spasms
	  (tizanidine)
		Bradycardia
		Dry mouth
		Constipation
		Sedation
		Autoimmune hemolytic anemia
		  (methyldopa)
			Abrupt withdrawal

Mechanism: *β₁-Adrenergic agonists*			

Dobutamine	Cardiac
	  decompensation
		Tachycardia
		Hypertension
		Dyspnea
			Idiopathic hypertrophic subaortic
			  stenosis
			Hypersensitivity to dobutamine or
			  sulfites

Mechanism: *β₂-Adrenergic agonists*			
Albuterol Salmeterol Terbutaline Ritodrine	Asthma COPD Tocolytic (terbutaline and ritodrine)	Tremors Nervousness Xerostomia Tachycardia Hypertension	Hypersensitivity
Mechanism: *D₁-agonist*			
Fenoldopam	Emergency hypertension	Arrhythmias Angina Facial flushing Hypokalemia	Hypersensitivity
Mechanism: *Non-selective alpha blockers*			
Phentolamine Phenoxybenzamine (irreversible)	Pheochromocytoma Extravasation of alpha agonists Sweating	Postural hypotension Tachycardia Inhibition of ejaculation Nasal congestion	Shock Coronary artery disease
Mechanism: *α₁-antagonists*			

Prazosin
Terazosin
Doxazosin
	Hypertension	First-dose postural hypotension
		↑ urinary frequency
		Nasal congestion
		Hepatotoxicity
		Pancreatitis
			Concurrent use with
			  phosphodiesterase-5 (PDE-5)
			  inhibitors such as sildenafil

Mechanism: *α₁-antagonists*			

Doxazosin
Tamsulosin
  (prostate
  specific)
Alfuzosin (prostate
  specific)
	Benign prostatic
	  hyperplasia (BPH)
		Same as doxazosin but tamsulosin
		  and alfuzosin produce less
		  hypotension
			Hypersensitivity

Mechanism: *Non-selective beta blockers*			

Propranolol
Nadolol
Timolol
	Hypertension
	Angina
	Supraventricular
	  arrhythmias
	Migraine headache
	  (propranolol)
	Essential tremor
	  (propranolol)
	Glaucoma (timolol)
		AV block
		Bronchospasm
		Sedation
		Wheezing
		Mask hypoglycemia
			Lung disease
			Cardiogenic shock
			Heart block

Mechanism: *Selective β₁-blockers*			

Metoprolol
Atenolol
Esmolol
  (short acting)
	Angina
	Hypertension
	Essential tremor
	Arrhythmias
	Migraine prophylaxis
		Same as propranolol but less
		  bronchospasm
			Same as propranolol

Mechanism: *Beta blockers with intrinsic sympathomimetic activity (ISA)*			

Acebutolol
  (β₁-blocker)
Penbutolol
Pindolol
	Hypertension
	Arrhythmias
		Less likely to cause heart block
		  than other beta blockers	

(Continued)

TABLE 5-2. **Therapeutic Summary of Selected Adrenergic Drugs—Cont'd**

DRUGS	CLINICAL APPLICATIONS	ADVERSE EFFECTS	CONTRAINDICATIONS
Mechanism: *Beta blockers that also block alpha receptors*			
Labetalol	Hypertension	Hepatotoxicity (labetalol)	Same as propranolol
Carvedilol	Angina	Same as propranolol	
Mechanism: *Beta blockers that also release nitric oxide*			
Nebivolol	Hypertension	Similar to propranolol	Similar to propranolol
			Liver disease
Mechanism: *Beta blockers for patients with chronic heart failure*			
Metoprolol	Reduces mortality in	Similar to propranolol	Similar to propranolol
Carvedilol	patients with heart		
Bisoprolol	failure		

AV, atrioventricular node; CNS, central nervous system, COPD, chronic obstructive pulmonary disease.

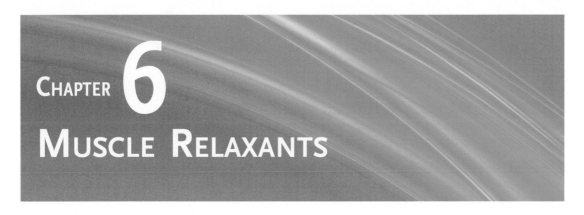

CHAPTER 6
MUSCLE RELAXANTS

I. **Spasmolytics** (Box 6-1)
  • Certain chronic diseases (e.g., cerebral palsy, multiple sclerosis) and spinal cord injuries are associated with abnormally high reflex activity in neuronal pathways controlling skeletal muscles, resulting in painful spasms or spasticity.
  A. **Goals of spasmolytic therapy**
    1. Reduction of excessive muscle tone without reduction in strength
    2. Reduction in spasm, which reduces pain and improves mobility
  B. **γ-Aminobutyric acid (GABA)-mimetics** (see Box 6-1)
    1. Baclofen (GABA$_B$ agonist)
      a. Mechanism of action
        • Interferes with release of excitatory transmitters in the brain and spinal cord
      b. Uses
        • Spasticity in patients with central nervous system (CNS) disorders, such as:
          (1) Multiple sclerosis
          (2) Spinal cord injuries
          (3) Stroke
      c. Adverse effects
        (1) Sedation
        (2) Hypotension
        (3) Muscle weakness
    2. Diazepam
      a. Benzodiazepine, which acts on the GABA$_A$ receptor
      b. Facilitates GABA-mediated presynaptic inhibition in the brain and spinal cord (see Chapter 7)
  C. **Other relaxants** (see Box 6-1)
    1. Botulinum toxin (Botox)
      a. Mechanism of action
        (1) Type A toxin blocks release of acetylcholine (ACh) by degrading the SNAP-25 protein
        (2) Inhibiting neurotransmitter release
      b. Uses
        (1) Spasticity associated with cerebral palsy (pediatrics) or stroke (adults)
        (2) Sialorrhea (excessive drooling)
        (3) Facial wrinkles
        (4) Cervical dystonia
        (5) Strabismus
        (6) Hyperhydrosis
        (7) Migraine prophylaxis
    2. Cyclobenzaprine
      a. Relieves local skeletal muscle spasms, associated with acute, painful musculoskeletal conditions, through central action, probably at the brain-stem level
      b. Ineffective in spasticity caused by CNS disorders, such as:
        (1) Multiple sclerosis
        (2) Spinal cord injuries
        (3) Stroke
      c. Sedating

Maintenance intrathecal infusion can be administered via an implanted pump delivering the drug to a selective site of the spinal cord.

Diazepam acts on GABA$_A$; baclofen acts on GABA$_B$ receptors.

Botox popular wrinkle remover

Cyclobenzaprine is sedating.

BOX 6-1 SPASMOLYTICS	
GABA-Mimetics	**Other Relaxants**
Baclofen	Botulinum toxin
Diazepam	Cyclobenzaprine
	Dantrolene
	Tizanidine

3. Dantrolene
    a. Mechanism of action
      (1) Decreases the release of intracellular calcium from the sarcoplasmic reticulum
      (2) "Uncoupling" the excitation-contraction process
    b. Uses
      (1) Spasticity from CNS disorders
        (a) Cerebral palsy
        (b) Spinal cord injury
      (2) Malignant hyperthermia after halothane/succinylcholine exposure
      (3) Neuroleptic malignant syndrome caused by antipsychotics
    c. Adverse effects
      (1) Hepatotoxicity
      (2) Significant muscle weakness
4. Tizanidine
    a. Mechanism of action
      (1) Stimulates presynaptic α_2 adrenoreceptors
      (2) Inhibits spinal interneuron firing
    b. Use
      • Spasticity associated with conditions such as cerebral palsy and spinal cord injury
    c. Adverse effects
      (1) Sedation
      (2) Hypotension
      (3) Muscle weakness (less than with baclofen)

II. Pharmacology of Motor End Plate
    A. General:
      1. ACh acts on nicotinic receptors at the motor end plate or neuromuscular junction (NMJ); see Chapter 4 for further discussion on cholinergic drugs.
      2. Several drugs and toxins alter the release of ACh (Fig. 6-1).
      3. Neuromuscular blockers may be classified as either depolarizing or nondepolarizing drugs (Box 6-2, Table 6-1).

Dantrolene for malignant hyperthermia.

Dantrolene is not effective in serotonin syndrome.

Tizanidine good for spasticity associated with spinal cord injuries.

Tizanidine is similar to clonidine with fewer peripheral effects.

ACh acts on nicotinic receptors at motor end plate or NMJ.

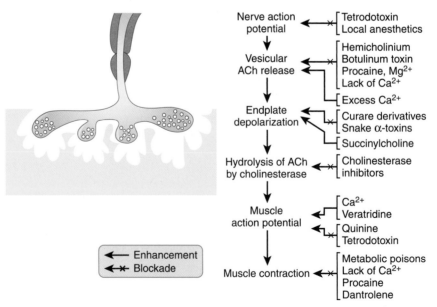

6-1: Pharmacology of motor end plate. ACh, acetylcholine. *(From Hardman JG, Limbird LE: Goodman and Gilman's The Pharmacologic Basis of Therapeutics, 10th ed. New York, McGraw-Hill, 2001. Reproduced with permission of The McGraw-Hill Companies.)*

BOX 6-2   NEUROMUSCULAR BLOCKERS

Nondepolarizing Drugs
Cisatracurium
Mivacurium
Pancuronium
Rocuronium
Tubocurarine
Vecuronium

Depolarizing Drugs
Succinylcholine

TABLE 6-1. Comparison of Nondepolarizing and Depolarizing Neuromuscular Blockers

EFFECT	COMPETITIVE	DEPOLARIZING
Action at receptor	Antagonist	Agonist
Effect on motor end plate depolarization	None	Partial persistent depolarization
Initial effect on striated muscle	None	Fasciculation
Muscles affected first	Small muscles	Skeletal muscle
Muscles affected last	Respiratory	Respiratory
Effect of AChE inhibitors	Reversal	No effect or increased duration
Effect of ACh agonists	Reversal	No effect
Effect on previously administered D-tubocurarine	Additive	Antagonism
Effect on previously administered succinylcholine	No effect of antagonism	Tachyphylaxis or no effect
Effect of inhalational anesthetics	Increase potency	Decrease potency
Effect of antibiotics	Increase potency	Decrease potency
Effect of calcium channel blockers	Increase potency	Increase potency

ACh, acetylcholine; AChE, acetylcholinesterase.

B. Nondepolarizing neuromuscular blockers
- Also known as curariform drugs, of which tubocurarine is the prototype
  1. Mechanism of action
     - These drugs compete with ACh at nicotinic receptors at the neuromuscular junction, producing muscle relaxation and paralysis.
  2. Uses
     a. Induction of muscle relaxation during surgery
     b. Facilitation of intubation
     c. Adjunct to electroconvulsive therapy for prevention of injury
     d. Tubocurarine is only used in the United States today for executions by lethal injections
  3. Drug interactions
     a. Muscle relaxation is reversed by acetylcholinesterase (AChE) inhibitors such as neostigmine.
     b. Use with inhaled anesthetics, such as isoflurane, or aminoglycoside antibiotics, such as gentamicin, may potentiate or prolong blockade.
  4. Adverse effects
     a. Respiratory paralysis
        - Can be reversed with neostigmine
     b. Blockade of autonomic ganglia
        - Produce hypotension
     c. Histamine release (most profound with tubocurarine)
        (1) Flushing
        (2) Hypotension
        (3) Urticaria
        (4) Pruritus
        (5) Erythema
        (6) Bronchospasms

C. Depolarizing neuromuscular blockers
- Succinylcholine
  1. Mechanism of action
     a. Binds to nicotinic receptors in skeletal muscle, causing persistent depolarization of the neuromuscular junction.

MOA: compete with ACh at nicotinic receptors at NMJ

Nondepolarizing neuromuscular blockers are reversed by AChE inhibitors.

Tubocurarine is noted for histamine release.

b. This action initially produces an agonist-like stimulation of skeletal muscles (fasciculations) followed by sustained muscle paralysis.

c. The response changes over time.

(1) Phase I

(a) Continuous depolarization at end plate

(b) Cholinesterase inhibitors prolong paralysis at this phase

(2) Phase II

(a) Resistance to depolarization

(b) Cholinesterase inhibitors may reverse paralysis at this phase

Depolarizing neuromuscular blockers may be potentiated by AChE inhibitors.

2. Uses

a. Muscle relaxation during surgery or electroconvulsive therapy

b. Routine endotracheal intubation

3. Adverse effects

a. Hyperkalemia

b. Muscle pain

Succinylcholine may cause malignant hyperthermia.

c. Malignant hyperthermia

4. Precaution

• Blockade may be prolonged if the patient has a genetic variant of plasma cholinesterase (pseudocholinesterase) that metabolizes the drug very slowly

III. Therapeutic summary of selected muscle relaxants: (Table 6-2)

TABLE 6-2. Therapeutic Summary of Selected Muscle Relaxants

DRUGS	CLINICAL APPLICATIONS	ADVERSE EFFECTS	CONTRAINDICATIONS
Mechanism: *Inhibits acetylcholine (Ach) release*			
Botulinum toxin	Strabismus Blepharospasm Cervical dystonia Wrinkles Hyperhydrosis	Arrhythmias Syncope Hepatotoxicity Anaphylaxis	Hypersensitivity
Mechanism: *γ-Aminobutryic acid $_B$ (GABA$_B$) agonist*			
Baclofen	Spasticity associated with multiple sclerosis or spinal cord lesions	Sedation Slurred speech Hypotension Polyuria	Hypersensitivity
Mechanism: *GABA$_A$ agonist*			
Diazepam	Skeletal muscle relaxant (see Chapter 7 for other uses)	Amnesia Sedation Slurred speech Paradoxical excitement	Hypersensitivity Narrow-angle glaucoma Pregnancy
Mechanism: *Centrally-acting skeletal muscle relaxant*			
Cyclobenzaprine	Muscle spasm associated with acute painful musculoskeletal conditions	Drowsiness Xerostomia Dyspepsia Blurred vision	Hypersensitivity Hyperthyroidism Don't use with MAO inhibitors Heart disease
Mechanism: *Prevents release of calcium from the sarcoplasmic reticulum*			
Dantrolene	Spasticity associated with: spinal cord injury, stroke, cerebral palsy, or multiple sclerosis Malignant hyperthermia	Drowsiness Headache Blurred vision Diarrhea (severe) Respiratory depression	Hepatic disease
Mechanism: *α$_2$-Adrenergic agonist that acts as a centrally acting muscle relaxant*			
Tizanidine	Skeletal muscle relaxant for muscle spasticity	Hypotension Somnolence Xerostomia	Hypersensitivity Concomitant therapy with ciprofloxacin or fluvoxamine (potent *CYP1A2* inhibitors)

(Continued)

TABLE 6-2. **Therapeutic Summary of Selected Muscle Relaxants—Cont'd**

DRUGS	CLINICAL APPLICATIONS	ADVERSE EFFECTS	CONTRAINDICATIONS
Mechanism: *Nicotinic receptor antagonists*			
Tubocurarine Cisatracurium Pancuronium Rocuronium Vecuronium	Lethal injections (tubocurarine), All others are used for NMJ blockade during surgery and intubation	Apnea Bronchospasms Hypertension Arrhythmias Respiratory failure Histamine release (tubocurarine)	Hypersensitivity
Mechanism: *Nicotinic receptor agonist that produces a depolarizing blockade*			
Succinylcholine	Intubation Induction of neuromuscular blockade during surgery Electroconvulsive therapy	Hyperkalemia Muscle pain Malignant hyperthermia	History of malignant hyperthermia

NMJ, neuromuscular junction.

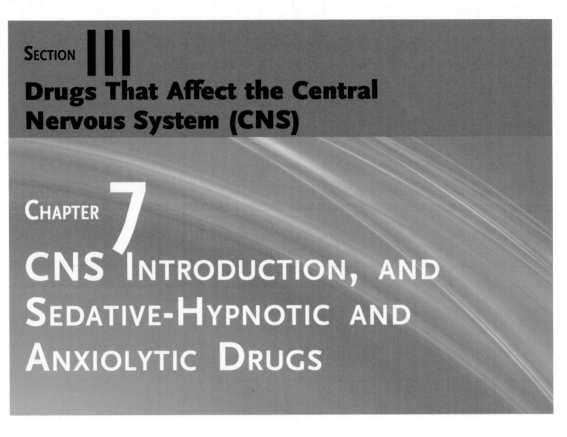

CHAPTER **7**

CNS INTRODUCTION, AND SEDATIVE-HYPNOTIC AND ANXIOLYTIC DRUGS

I. CNS Introduction: See Rapid Review Neuroscience, Chapters 4 to 6, for a review of principles needed to understand how drugs affect neurobiological processes.

    A. Synaptic Transmission

        1. Electrical synapses (Fig. 7-1)

            a. Important mechanism for rapid cell communication

            b. Minimal impact of drugs on this process

        2. Chemical synapses (Fig. 7-2)

            a. Slower and more complex signaling process than via electrical synapses; important for actions of most CNS drugs

                (1) Release of neurotransmitter from the presynaptic terminal requires calcium; enters through voltage-dependent calcium channels.

                (2) Voltage-dependent calcium channels open when action potentials depolarize the terminal.

                (3) Synaptic cleft

                    • Space between presynaptic axon terminal and postsynaptic membrane through which transmitter diffuses

                (4) Postsynaptic responses depend on receptor subtype.

            b. Direct gating

                • Ligand-gated receptors

                (1) Binding of neurotransmitter opens or closes an ion channel within the receptor.

                (2) Activation results in a rapid change in postsynaptic membrane potential.

                (3) Neurotransmitters that activate gated channels:

                    (a) Glutamate

                    (b) Acetylcholine (ACh)

                    (c) γ-Aminobutyric acid (GABA)

                    (d) Glycine

                    (e) Serotonin

            c. Indirect gating

                • Non-channel-linked receptors

                (1) Binding of neurotransmitter activates second-messenger pathways by way of guanosine triphosphate-binding (G proteins).

Mechanisms of signal transduction processes at synapses is high yield for Board Exams.

Glutamate the most important excitatory amino acid in brain.

GABA the most important inhibitory amino acid in brain.

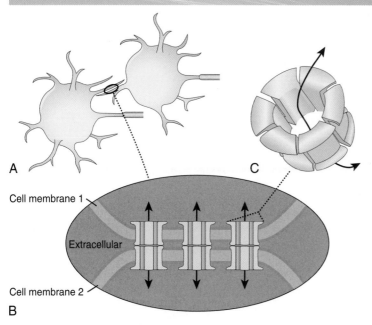

7-1: Electrical synapse. Ions diffuse through central pore of connexon (arrows). **A**, Gap junction forms between dendrites of two neurons. **B**, Gap junction. **C**, Connexon. *(From Nolte J: The Human Brain, 5th ed. Philadelphia, Mosby, 2002.)*

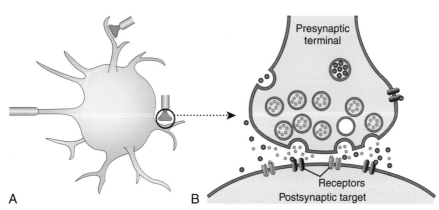

7-2: Chemical synapse. **A**, Axon terminal forms chemical synapse on dendrite of another neuron. **B**, Two neurotransmitters (gray and orange dots) are released by presynaptic terminal. One (orange) has postsynaptic effect. The other (gray), by binding both to postsynaptic receptors and presynaptic autoreceptors, can affect both postsynaptic target and activities of the presynaptic terminal. *(From Nolte J: The Human Brain, 5th ed. Philadelphia, Mosby, 2002.)*

(2) Signal transduction pathways activated by second messengers have multiple and lasting effects.

(3) Important signaling pathways

    (a) Cyclic adenosine monophosphate (cAMP)

    (b) Polyphosphoinositide products
        Diacylglycerol (DAG)
        Inositol-trisphosphate (IP_3)

    (c) Ca^{2+} conductance

    (d) K^+ conductance (hyperpolarization)

    (e) Cation conductance, mainly Na^+ (depolarization)

    (f) Cl^- conductance (hyperpolarization)

B. Important small-molecule neurotransmitters

  1. Acetylcholine (ACh); review Fig. 3-2A for synthesis, storage, release and inactivation.

    a. Activation of M_1 muscarinic receptors is excitatory.

      (1) Decreases K^+ conductance

      (2) Increases IP_3 and DAG

    b. Activation of M_2 muscarinic receptors is inhibitory.

      (1) Increases K^+ conductance

      (2) Decreases cAMP

Increased intracellular Ca^{2+} important for smooth muscle contraction, secretions, and transmitter release.

Learn how CNS drugs affect the chemical synapse as you study these drugs.

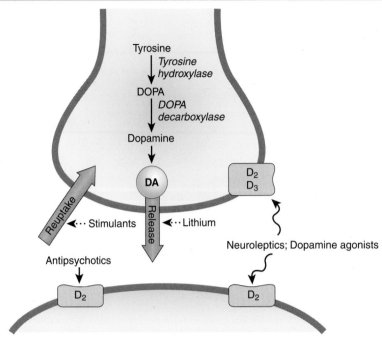

7-3: Chemistry and pharmacology of the dopamine (DA) synapse. Almost all antipsychotics bind to the D_2 receptor, and some bind to the D_1 receptor. *(From Hardman JG, Limbird LE: Goodman and Gilman's The Pharmacologic Basis of Therapeutics, 10th ed. New York, McGraw-Hill, 2001. Reproduced with permission of The McGraw-Hill Companies.)*

Reduction in the activity of the cholinergic neurons occurs in Alzheimer's disease; drugs are used to increase CNS cholinergic activity.

Dopamine is responsible for reward, drive, and in various feelings such as euphoria, orgasm, anger, addiction, love, pleasure.

Activations of adrenergic receptors elevate mood and increase wakefulness and attention.

Serotonin modulates anger, aggression, body temperature, mood, sleep, human sexuality, appetite, and metabolism, as well as stimulates vomiting.

    c. Activation of nicotinic receptors is excitatory.
- Increases cation conductance

2. Dopamine (DA); Fig. 7-3
    a. Activation of D_1 receptors is stimulatory.
- Increases cAMP

    b. Activation of D_2 receptors is inhibitory.
      (1) Presynaptic
- Decreases Ca^{2+} conductance

      (2) Postsynaptic
        (a) Increases K^+ conductance
        (b) Decreases cAMP

3. Norepinephrine (NE); Fig. 7-4; also review Fig. 3-2B for syntheses, storage release and inactivation
    a. Activation of α_1 receptors is excitatory.
      (1) Decreases K^+ conductance
      (2) Increases IP_3 and DAG

    b. Activation of α_2 receptors is inhibitory
      (1) Presynaptic
- Decreases Ca^{2+} conductance

      (2) Postsynaptic
        (a) Increases K^+ conductance
        (b) Decreases cAMP

4. Serotonin (5-HT); Fig. 7-5
    a. Activation of 5-HT_{1A} receptors is inhibitory.
      (1) Increases K^+ conductance
      (2) Decreases cAMP

    b. Activation of 5-HT_{2A} receptors is excitatory.
      (1) Decreases K^+ conductance
      (2) Increases IP_3 and DAG

    c. Activation of 5-HT_3 receptors is excitatory.
- Increases cation conductance

    d. Activation of 5-HT_4 receptors is excitatory.
- Decreases K^+ conductance

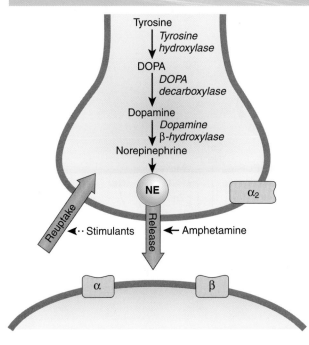

7-4: Chemistry and pharmacology of the norepinephrine (NE) synapse. Note that the conversion of dopamine to NE takes place inside the NE granules. DET, dopamine transporter. *(From Weyhenmeyer JA and Gallman EA: Rapid Review Neuroscience. Philadelphia, Mosby, 2007, Figure 6-3.)*

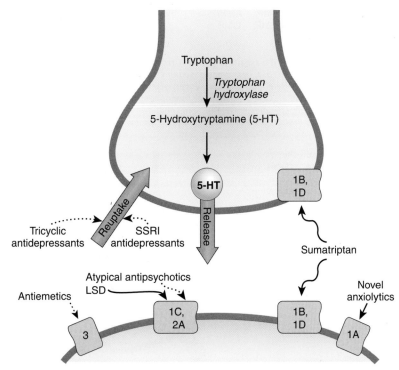

7-5: Chemistry and pharmacology of the serotonin (5-HT) synapse. 5-HT, 5-hydroxytryptamine; LSD, lysergic acid diethylamide; SSRI, selective serotonin reuptake inhibitor; 1A, 1B, 1C, 1D, 2, and 3, are receptor subtypes. Reuptake transporter is currently referred to as SERT (serotonin reuptake transporter). *(From Weyhenmeyer JA and Gallman EA: Rapid Review Neuroscience. Philadelphia, Mosby, 2007, Figure 6-4.)*

5. Glutamate (GLU); Fig. 7-6
    a. Activation of N-methyl-D-aspartate (NMDA) receptors is excitatory.
        • Increases Ca^{2+} conductance
    b. Activation of α-amino-3-hydroxyl-5-methyl-4-isoxazole-propionate (AMPA) or kainite receptors is excitatory.
        • Increases cation conductance
    c. Activation of metabotropic presynaptic receptor is inhibitory.
        (1) Decreases Ca^{2+} conductance
        (2) Decreases cAMP

Glutamate is the major excitatory neurotransmitter in brain.

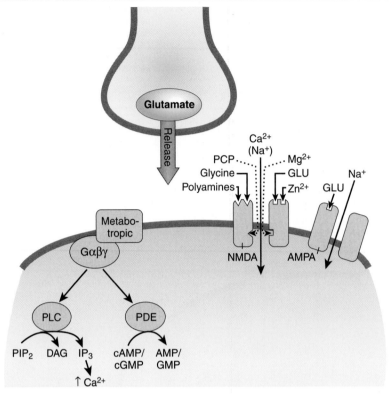

7-6: Classes of glutamate receptors. N-methyl-D-aspartate (NMDA) receptor is primarily a calcium channel. Aminohydroxy-methylisoxazole propionate (AMPA) receptor is a ligand-gated sodium channel. Metabotropic receptors are coupled to G protein (Gαβγ), and each is coupled to a different second messenger system. AMP, adenosine monophosphate; cAMP, cyclic AMP; DAG, diacylglycerol; Glu, glutamate; GMP, guanosine monophosphate; cGMP, cyclic GMP; IP$_3$, inositol 1,4,5-triphosphate; PCP, phencyclidine; PDE, phosphodiesterase; PIP$_2$, phosphatidylinositol phosphate; PLC, phospholipase C. *(From Weyhenmeyer JA and Gallman EA: Rapid Review Neuroscience. Philadelphia, Mosby, 2007, Figure 6-5.)*

7-7: Chemistry and pharmacology of the γ-aminobutyric acid (GABA) synapse. *(From Weyhenmeyer JA and Gallman EA: Rapid Review Neuroscience. Philadelphia, Mosby, 2007, Figure 6-6.)*

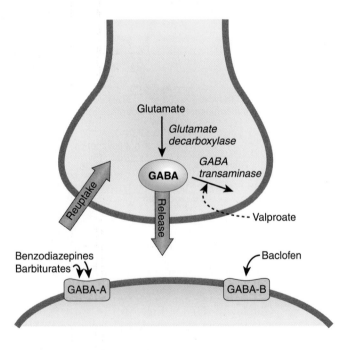

d. Activation of metabotropic postsynaptic receptor is excitatory.
  (1) Decreases K$^+$ conductance
  (2) Increases IP$_3$, DAG
6. GABA; Fig. 7-7
  a. Activation of GABA$_A$ receptors is inhibitory.
    • Increases Cl$^-$ conductance

Glutamate-induced excitatory effect is involved in both acute and chronic brain injury.

      b. Activation of GABA$_B$ presynaptic receptors is inhibitory.
         • Decreases Ca^{2+} conductance
      c. Activation of GABA$_B$ postsynaptic receptors is inhibitory.
         • Increases K$^+$ conductance
   7. Histamine (H)
      a. Activation of H$_1$ receptors is excitatory.
         (1) Decreases K$^+$ conductance
         (2) Increases IP$_3$ and DAG
      b. Activation of H$_2$ receptors is excitatory.
         (1) Decreases K$^+$ conductance
         (2) Increases cAMP
   8. Opioid peptides
      a. Activation of mu presynaptic receptors is inhibitory.
         (1) Decreases Ca^{2+} conductance
         (2) Decreases cAMP
      b. Activation of delta postsynaptic receptors is inhibitory.
         (1) Increases K$^+$ conductance
         (2) Decreases cAMP
      c. Activation of kappa postsynaptic receptors is inhibitory.
         (1) Increases K$^+$ conductance
         (2) Decreases cAMP
   9. Endocannabinoids (CB)
      • Activation of CB$_1$ presynaptic receptors is inhibitory.
        a Decreases Ca^{2+} conductance
        b. Decreases cAMP

II. **Basic Properties of CNS Depressant Drugs**
   A. **General**
      1. Sedative-hypnotics and anxiolytics are used to reduce anxiety or to induce sleep (Box 7-1).
      2. These agents, especially the barbiturates, produce CNS depression at the level of the brain, spinal cord, and brain stem.
      3. These agents cause tolerance and physical dependence (withdrawal symptoms) if used for long periods.
      4. Barbiturates and other older sedative-hypnotics cause complete CNS depression, whereas benzodiazepines do not (Fig. 7-8).
   B. **Pharmacokinetics**
      1. Metabolism primarily occurs by the microsomal system in the liver.
      2. Duration of action is variable.
         a. The half-life ($t_{1/2}$) of these drugs ranges from minutes to days.
         b. Many benzodiazepine metabolites are active, thus increasing the duration of action of the parent drug.

GABA is the major inhibitory neurotransmitter in brain.

Decreased GABA activity or increased glutamate activity lead to seizures.

Inhibition of the H$_1$ receptor in the brain is responsible for sedative adverse effects of many drugs.

Drugs that target the opioid receptors are used to treat pain.

Rimonabant, an inverse agonist of the CB$_1$ receptor, is being evaluated for treatment of weight loss, drug addictions and the metabolic syndrome; not approved in the United States.

Sedative-hypnotic drugs should not be used in combination with alcohol.

Barbiturates induce cytochrome P-450 drug metabolizing enzymes but benzodiazepines do not; so minimal drug-drug interactions with bezodiazepines compared with barbiturates.

BOX 7-1 SEDATIVE-HYPNOTICS AND ANXIOLYTICS

Benzodiazepines
Alprazolam
Chlordiazepoxide
Clorazepate
Diazepam
Estazolam
Flurazepam
Lorazepam
Midazolam
Oxazepam
Prazepam
Quazepam
Temazepam
Triazolam

Barbiturates
Pentobarbital
Phenobarbital
Secobarbital
Thiopental
Methohexital

Other Sedative-Hypnotics
Chloral hydrate
Diphenhydramine
Eszopiclone
Meprobamate
Paraldehyde
Propranolol
Ramelteon
Zaleplon
Zolpidem

Nonsedating Anxiolytic
Buspirone

Benzodiazepine Antagonist
Flumazenil

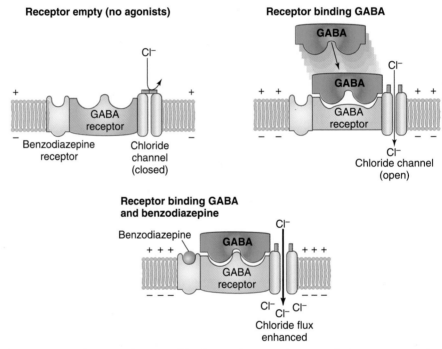

7-8: Dose-response curves for barbiturates and for benzodiazepines. Barbiturates produce complete central nervous system depression leading to anesthesia, coma, and death, even when given orally. Benzodiazepines may cause anesthesia and respiratory depression with intravenous, but not oral, administration.

7-9: Benzodiazepine-γ-aminobutyric acid (GABA)-chloride ionophore complex. Benzodiazepines increase the frequency of channel opening. Barbiturates increase the length of time that the channels remain open.

C. **Mechanism of action**
1. Sedative-hypnotics facilitate Cl⁻ flux through the GABA receptor chloride channel complex (Fig. 7-9).
2. This hyperpolarizes the neuron

D. **Uses**
- Sedation, hypnosis, or anesthesia, depending on dose
1. Sleep induction (hypnosis)
2. Anxiety relief (anxiolytic)
3. Sedation
4. Preanesthesia (see Chapter 8)
5. Anticonvulsant properties (see Chapter 9)
- Phenobarbital, clonazepam, and diazepam are used clinically.
6. Central-acting muscle relaxants (see Chapter 6)

E. **Adverse effects**
- Chronic use may lead to toxicity
1. General effects
a. Drowsiness
b. Impaired performance and judgment

      c. "Hangover"

      d. Risk of drug abuse and addiction

      e. Withdrawal syndrome (most frequently seen with short-acting sedative-hypnotics that are used for long periods)

   2. Overdose results in severe CNS depression, which may manifest as coma, hypotension, and respiratory cessation, especially when agents are given in combination.

   3. Treatment of overdose

      a. Observe continuously

      b. Prevent absorption of ingested drug (charcoal, lavage)

      c. Support respiration

      d. Prevent or treat hypotension or shock

      e. Maintain renal function

      f. Flumazenil in benzodiazepine overdose

      g. Increase rate of drug excretion

         (1) Alkaline diuresis

            • Useful for a few barbiturates, such as phenobarbital

         (2) Peritoneal dialysis

         (3) Hemodialysis

  F. Precautions

   1. Porphyria or a family history of porphyria may be a problem

      • Barbiturates may increase porphyrin synthesis

   2. Hepatic or renal insufficiency requires a reduced dose.

   3. Additive effect of CNS depressant drugs in combination may have serious consequences.

III. Benzodiazepines (see Box 7-1)

  A. General

   1. These CNS depressant drugs are associated with a reduced risk of respiratory depression and coma, which gives them a major advantage over the barbiturates (see Fig. 7-8).

   2. The incidence of dependence is probably lower with benzodiazepines than with barbiturates.

  B. Pharmacokinetics

   1. Many have active metabolites

   2. Enterohepatic circulation with many agents

   3. Variable duration of action

      • Most agents or their metabolites accumulate with multiple dosing as a result of long plasma half-lives.

      a. Short-acting agents

         (1) Triazolam

         (2) Midazolam

      b. Intermediate-acting agents

         (1) Alprazolam

         (2) Estazolam

         (3) Lorazepam

         (4) Oxazepam

         (5) Temazepam

      c. Long-acting agents

         (1) Chlordiazepoxide

         (2) Clorazepate

         (3) Diazepam

         (4) Flurazepam

         (5) Prazepam

         (6) Quazepam

  C. Mechanism of action (see Fig. 7-9)

   1. Benzodiazepines bind to specific receptors on the $GABA_A$ receptor-ionophore complex.

   2. Benzodiazepines potentiate the activity of GABA on chloride ion influx by increasing the frequency of the openings of the chloride channels.

   3. Alcohols, as well as barbiturates, also interact at these receptors leading to cross tolerance.

  D. Uses: All of the general uses listed in Section IID, plus the following indications

   1. Alcohol withdrawal

   2. Status epilepticus (intravenous diazepam or lorazepam)

Chronic use of a drug that decreases CNS activity often leads to weight gain.

Benzodiazepines are incomplete CNS depressants; so are much less likely to cause death from overdose compared with complete CNS depressants such as barbiturates and alcohol.

Don't use barbiturates in patients with porphyria.

Benzodiazepines increase the frequency of chloride channel opening.

E. **Adverse effects**
   1. Ataxia
   2. Retrograde amnesia
   3. Moderate addictive potential
      a. Physical dependence when used in high doses for several months
      b. Withdrawal symptoms
         (1) Anxiety
         (2) Agitation
         (3) Depression
         (4) "Rebound" insomnia
F. **Benzodiazepine antagonist**
   1. Flumazenil, a benzodiazepine antagonist, stops action or reverses toxicity.
   2. Flumazenil can produce seizures if administered for drug over-doses that are not benzodiazepine-related drugs.
G. **BZ_1 benzodiazepine agonists**
   1. These drugs act on the BZ_1 subset of benzodiazepine receptors.
   2. Unlike the benzodiazepines, these drugs produce muscle relaxation and anticonvulsant effects only at doses much higher than the hypnotic dose.
   3. Effects are reversed by flumazenil
   4. Drugs
      a. Zolpidem
         (1) Short-acting
         (2) Nonbenzodiazepine
         (3) Sedative-hypnotic for the short-term treatment of insomnia
      b. Zaleplon
         (1) Also, short-acting
         (2) Nonbenzodiazepine
         (3) Sedative-hypnotic for the short-term treatment of insomnia
            • Zaleplon has a faster onset of action and a shorter terminal elimination half-life than zolpidem.
      c. Eszopiclone
         (1) Longer acting
         (2) Nonbenzodiazepine
         (3) Sedative-hypnotic
            • First agent indicated for chronic treatment of insomnia
         (4) Properties similar to the BZ_1 agonists
            • *But* is a nonselective agonist at BZ_1 and BZ_2 receptors

IV. **Barbiturates**
   A. **Pharmacokinetics**
      1. Elimination occurs by metabolism in the liver and excretion of the parent compound or its metabolites in the urine.
         a. Phenobarbital is a weak organic acid, whose excretion is enhanced by alkalinization of urine.
         b. The effects of thiopental and methohexital are terminated by redistribution.
      2. Duration of action
         a. Ultrashort-acting
            (1) Thiopental
            (2) Methohexital
         b. Intermediate-acting
            (1) Pentobarbital
            (2) Secobarbital
         c. Long-acting
            • Phenobarbital
   B. **Mechanism of action**
      1. Barbiturates facilitate the actions of GABA; unlike benzodiazepines, these agents increase the length of time that the GABA-gated chloride channel remains open.
      2. The multiplicity of barbiturate binding sites is the basis of the ability to induce full surgical anesthesia (see Fig. 7-9).
   C. **Effects**
      1. Low doses
         a. Depression of sensory function

Triazolam is noted for causing traveler's amnesia.

It is possible to reduce rebound effects by slowly reducing the dose of longer-acting benzodiazepines.

Although nonbenzodiazepines are less amnestic than benzodiazepines, amnestic behaviors are reported with zolpidem and zaleplon.

Barbiturates increase the length of time that the chloride channel remains open.

Barbiturates are complete CNS depressants.

    b. Sedation without analgesia
      • May be hyperalgesic
    c. Drowsiness
  2. High doses
    a. Depression of motor function
    b. Depression of medullary centers of brain (circulatory and respiratory depression)
    c. Marked sedation
    d. Sleep
    e. Anesthesia
  3. Induce cytochrome P450 metabolizing enzymes
    • Many drug-drug interactions
V. **Other Sedative-Hypnotics**
  • Some of these agents are structurally related to the barbiturates and have similar
    properties.
  A. **Diphenhydramine**
    1. An antihistamine found in over-the-counter (OTC) "sleep aids"
    2. Other antihistamines are found in OTC night time cold treatments
  B. **Buspirone**
    1. Mechanism of action
      • Partial agonist at 5-hydroxytryptamine (5-HT$_{1A}$) serotonin receptors in the brain
    2. Uses
      a. Antianxiety (several days of use required for the drug to become effective)
      b. *No* hypnotic, anticonvulsant, or muscle relaxant properties
    3. Adverse effects
      a. Some sedation but less than most benzodiazepines
      b. *No* evidence of tolerance, rebound anxiety on withdrawal of drug, cross-tolerance to
        benzodiazepines, drug abuse, or additive effects
  C. **Chloral hydrate**
    1. General
      a. Structurally related to alcohol, with trichloroethanol as active metabolite
      b. Paraldehyde is a short-acting congener.
    2. Use
      a. Very rapid-acting hypnotic
        • Often used in children in the past
      b. Low incidence of abuse
    3. Adverse effect
      a. Bad taste and smell
      b. CNS depression
  D. **Meprobamate**
    1. Oral anxiolytic
    2. Use replaced by benzodiazepines
  E. **Propranolol**
    • Used to treat performance anxiety
  F. **Ramelteon**
    1. A potent, selective agonist of melatonin receptors (MT$_1$ and MT$_2$) that regulate
      circadian rhythms.
    2. Used to treat insomnia characterized by difficulty with sleep onset.
VI. **Alcohols**
  A. **Ethanol**
    1. Pharmacokinetics
      a. Rapid, complete absorption
      b. Metabolism: Conversion to acetate by two enzymes
        (1) Alcohol dehydrogenase
        (2) Acetaldehyde dehydrogenase
      c. Often used as an example to illustrate zero-order kinetics
    2. Mechanism of action
      a. Potentiates actions at the GABA receptor
      b. CNS depressant with synergistic effects with many other CNS depressants
      c. Cross-tolerant with other sedative-hypnotic drugs
    3. Adverse effects
      a. Liver

Adverse effects of barbiturates: ataxia, retrograde amnesia, impaired performance, dependence, withdrawal symptoms.

Barbiturates induce drug metabolism; benzodiazepines do not.

Buspirone is the only *non-sedating* anxiolytic drug available.

Alcoholic drinks spiked with chloral hydrate were referred to as *Mickey Finns*; used for amnestic properties as a "date-rape" drug.

Flunitrazepam and GHB (γ-hydroxy butyrate) are also misused in this manner.

Propranolol used to treat performance anxiety.

Ramelteon useful for treatment of disrupted sleep cycles due to shift work.

Ethanol eliminated by zero-order kinetics

               (1) Fatty liver

               (2) Alcoholic hepatitis

               (3) Cirrhosis

          b. Gastrointestinal

               (1) Nutritional deficiencies (malabsorption)

               (2) Bleeding

          c. Nervous system

Give thiamine to alcoholics who present for emergency treatment.

               (1) Peripheral neuropathy ("stocking glove" pattern)

               (2) Wernicke-Korsakoff syndrome due to thiamine deficiency

                   (a) Ataxia

                   (b) Confusion

                   (c) Ophthalmoplegia

                   (d) Retrograde and antegrade memory deficits

          d. Endocrine

               (1) Gynecomastia

               (2) Testicular atrophy related to hyperestrinism

          e. Cancer

              • Squamous cancers

               (1) Mouth

               (2) Esophagus

               (3) Larynx

         f. Fetal alcohol syndrome

               (1) Teratogenic effects when used during pregnancy

               (2) Symptoms include:

                   (a) Mental retardation

                   (b) Growth retardation

                   (c) Microcephaly

Avoid alcohol during pregnancy.

                   (d) Wide-spaced eyes

                   (e) Congenital heart defects

         g. Alcoholism

               (1) Withdrawal syndrome

                   (a) Insomnia

                   (b) Tremor, anxiety, seizures, hallucinations, delirium tremens

                   (c) Diarrhea, nausea

               (2) Management

                   (a) Benzodiazepines (only in abstinent patients)

                   (b) Antihypertensives

      4. Drug interactions

         a. Drugs that inhibit acetaldehyde dehydrogenase

               (1) Disulfiram, which is used in the treatment of alcoholism

               (2) Some drugs have a disulfiram-like effect:

Disulfiram use leads to nausea, hypotension, headache, and flushing when patients drink alcohol; thus, it is used to help patients stop drinking.

                   (a) Metronidazole

                   (b) Oral hypoglycemic agents (chlorpropamide)

                   (c) Some cephalosporins (cefamandole, cefotetan, cefoperazone)

         b. Acute alcohol suppresses cytochrome P-450 activities

         c. Chronic alcohol enhances cytochrome P-450 activities

               (1) Especially, *CYP2E1*

               (2) This potentiates acetaminophen hepatotoxicity

  B. Other alcohols

    1. Methanol

         a. Conversion to formic acid by alcohol dehydrogenase can lead to:

               (1) Blindness

               (2) Severe anion gap metabolic acidosis

Methanol produces CNS toxicity and blindness.

         b. Intoxicated patients are treated with ethanol or fomepizole

            • Ethanol competes with methanol for the dehydrogenase enzymes.

    2. Ethylene glycol

         a. Found in antifreeze

          b. Adverse effects

               (1) Severe anion gap metabolic acidosis due to alcohol dehydrogenase conversion into oxalic acid

               (2) Hypocalcemia

Ethylene glycol produces kidney toxicity.

               (3) Renal damage

         c. Intoxicated patients are treated with ethanol or fomepizole.

  VII. Therapeutic summary of selected sedative-hypnotic drugs: (Table 7-1)

TABLE 7-1. **Therapeutic Summary of Selected Sedative-Hypnotic drugs**

DRUGS	CLINICAL APPLICATIONS	ADVERSE EFFECTS	CONTRAINDICATIONS
Mechanism: *Allosteric agonist of GABA$_A$ receptors that increase the frequency of chloride channel opening*			
Short-acting benzodiazepines Triazolam Midazolam *Intermediate-acting benzodiazepines* Alprazolam Estazolam Lorazepam Oxazepam Temazepam *Long-acting benzodiazipines* Chlordiazepoxide Clorazepate Diazepam Flurazepam Prazepam Quazepam	Hypnotic (triazolam and many others) Amnesia induction and anesthesia (midazolam) Absence seizures (clorazepate) Insomnia (many) Anxiety (many but especially alprazolam) Alcohol withdrawal (diazepam, chlordiazepoxide) Status epilepticus (diazepam, lorazepam) Muscle relaxant (diazepam)	Respiratory depression Drowsiness Physical and psychological dependence Blurred vision	Hypersensitivity Children <6 months of age (oral) Pregnancy
Mechanism: *Enhance GABA$_A$ receptors by increasing duration of chloride channel open time*			
Ultrashort-acting barbiturates Thiopental Methohexital	Induction and maintenance of anesthesia Treatment of elevated intracranial pressure (thiopental)	Respiratory depression Cardiac depression CNS depression Hematologic depression	Porphyria Respiratory disease Liver disease
Intermediate-acting barbiturates Secobarbital Pentobarbital	Preanesthetic agent Short-term treatment of insomnia Treatment of elevated intracranial pressure (pentobarbital)	Same as above	Same as above
Long-acting barbiturates Phenobarbital	Management of generalized tonic-clonic (grand mal) and partial seizures Sedative	Same as above	Same as above
Mechanism: *BZ, benzodiazepine agonists*			
Zolpidem Zaleplon Eszopiclone	Insomnia	Drowsiness Drugged feeling	Hypersensitivity
Mechanism: *Central H$_1$ receptor blocker*			
Diphenhydramine Other antihistamines	OTC sleeping aid	See chapter 20	See chapter 20
Mechanism: *Selective agonist of melatonin receptors (MT$_1$ and MT$_2$)*			
Ramelteon	Insomnia	Drowsiness	Hypersensitivity Concurrent use with fluvoxamine
Mechanism: *Partial agonist at 5-HT$_{1A}$ serotonin receptors in the brain*			
Buspirone	Management of generalized anxiety disorder (GAD)	Dizziness	Hypersensitivity
Mechanism: *Benzodiazepine antagonist*			
Flumazenil	Reverse benzodiazepine effects in conscious sedation and general anesthesia Treatment of benzodiazepine overdose	GI distress CNS agitation Seizures	Serious tricyclic-antidepressant overdoses Seizure disorders

CNS, central nervous system; GABA, γ-aminobutyric acid; GI, gastrointestinal; OTC, over the counter

CHAPTER 8

ANESTHETICS

I. **General Anesthetics**
  A. **Goals of balanced anesthesia**
    1. Analgesia
       • Elimination of perception and reaction to pain
    2. Amnesia
       • Loss of memory, which is *not* essential but desirable during most surgical procedures
    3. Loss of consciousness
       • Essential for many surgical procedures (e.g., cardiac, orthopedic)
    4. Muscle relaxation
       a. Occurs in varying degrees
       b. Usually has to be further supplied by neuromuscular relaxants (See Chapter 6)
    5. Suppression of autonomic and sensory reflexes
       • Requires use of additional medications to suppress the enhanced autonomic and sensory reactions that occur during surgical procedures
  B. **Inhalation anesthetics** (Box 8-1 and Table 8-1)
    1. General considerations
       a. Depth of anesthesia directly relates to the partial pressure of the anesthetic in the brain.
       b. Anesthetic potency is expressed as the minimum alveolar concentration (MAC).
          (1) 1 MAC is the concentration in inspired air at which 50% of patients have *no* response to a skin incision.
          (2) The higher the lipid solubility
              (a) The greater the potency
              (b) The lower the MAC (See Table 8-1).
          (3) Inhalational anesthetics exert additive synergism
              • 0.5 MAC from two anesthetics together will produce 1 MAC anesthesia.
       c. Speed of induction is influenced by several factors.
          (1) Higher inspired concentration equals more rapid induction.
          (2) Lower solubility in blood equals more rapid induction.
          (3) Higher ventilation rate equals more rapid induction.
          (4) Lower pulmonary blood flow equals more rapid induction.
       d. The lower the blood-gas partition coefficient, the more rapid is the onset and recovery from anesthesia (See Table 8-1).
       e. Mechanism of action
          (1) Usually described as nonspecific interaction with lipid bilayer of neuronal membrane (Meyer-Overton principle)
          (2) Recent evidence suggest that Cl^- and K^+ fluxes are increased (hyperpolarization)
    2. Nitrous oxide (N_2O)
       • *Only* gaseous anesthetic used
         a. Characteristics
            (1) *Cannot* produce surgical anesthesia by itself
            (2) To produce unconsciousness, N_2O must be used with other anesthetics.
            (3) Significantly reduces the required concentration of halogenated anesthetics when used as an adjunct to anesthesia

---

Multiple drugs are required for balanced anesthesia.

Depth of anesthesia relates to partial pressure of the anesthetic in brain.

MAC is concentration in inspired air where 50% of patients have no response to skin incision; thus, surgery must be performed above 1 MAC.

MACs are additive.

Low partition coefficient for nitrous oxide (0.47) and desflurane (0.42) leads to rapid onset and recovery

N_2O only gaseous anesthetic used

A mixture of O_2 and N_2O often used as a carrier gas for halogenated anesthetics.

N_2O has excellent analgesic properties.

64

BOX 8-1   GENERAL ANESTHETICS

Inhalation Anesthetics
Desflurane
Enflurane
Halothane
Isoflurane
Nitrous oxide
Sevoflurane
Methohexital

Parenteral Anesthetics
Alfentanil
Etomidate
Fentanyl
Ketamine
Lorazepam
Midazolam
Propofol
Sufentanil
Thiopental

TABLE 8-1. Properties of Inhalation Anesthetics

AGENT	MAC (% VOL/VOL)	BLOOD:GAS PARTITION COEFFICIENT	RATE OF INDUCTION AND EMERGENCE	AMOUNT METABOLIZED	SKELETAL MUSCLE RELAXATION	EFFECT ON CARDIOVASCULAR SYSTEM	EFFECT ON LIVER AND KIDNEY
Nonhalogenated (Gaseous)							
Nitrous oxide	>100	0.47	Rapid	None	None	↓ Heart rate No arrhythmias	None
Halogenated (Volatile)							
Desflurane	6.0	0.42	Rapid	<2%	Medium	↑ Heart rate and blood pressure (transient)	None
Enflurane	1.7	1.9	Medium	5% (fluoride)	Medium	↓ Heart rate No arrhythmias; does *not* sensitize heart to catecholamines	Hepatotoxic
Halothane	0.75	2.3	Slow	20%	Low	Sensitizes heart to catecholamine	Hepatotoxic
Isoflurane	1.3	1.4	Medium	<2% (fluoride)	Medium	↑ Heart rate No arrhythmias; does *not* sensitize heart to catecholamines	None
Sevoflurane	1.9	0.65	Rapid	<2%	Medium	None	Nephrotoxic (rare)

MAC, minimum alveolar concentration.

  b. Pharmacokinetics
    (1) Extremely fast absorption and elimination
    (2) Resulting in rapid:
      (a) Induction
      (b) Recovery from anesthesia
  c. Uses
    (1) Has good analgesic properties
    (2) Therefore, used to decrease pain in:
      (a) Obstetrics
      (b) Procedure that does *not* require unconsciousness
        Dental procedures
  d. Contraindications
    (1) Head injury
    (2) Preexisting increased intracranial pressure
    (3) Brain tumors.
      • N_2O can raise intracranial pressure.

  3. Volatile halogenated hydrocarbons (see Box 8-1 and Table 8-1)
    a. These agents are of variable potency (MAC) and blood solubility.
    b. Use
      • Part of balanced anesthesia
    c. Adverse effects
      (1) They may sensitize the heart to the arrhythmogenic effects of catecholamines.
      (2) Varied affects on cardiovascular system (See Table 8-1)
      (3) Halothane noted for its idiosyncratic hepatotoxicity
      (4) Some nephrotoxicity with sevoflurane (rare)
      (5) May trigger malignant hyperthermia, especially in patients susceptible to malignant hyperthermia

N_2O contraindicated with head injuries.

The use of halothane may lead to hepatotoxicity and malignant hyperthermia.

C. **Parenteral anesthetics** (see Box 8-1)
   1. These anesthetics are useful for:
      a. Procedures of short duration
      b. Induction for inhalation anesthesia (wide use)
      c. Supplementation of weak inhalation agents such as N_2O
   2. Ultrashort-acting barbiturates
      a. Thiopental
      b. Methohexital
         • Both have *no* analgesic activity, may be hyperalgesic
      c. Pharmacokinetics
         (1) Extremely rapid onset and action due to high lipid solubility
         (2) Brief duration of action due to redistribution from brain to other tissues
      d. Primary uses
         (1) Induction of anesthesia
         (2) Procedures of short duration
   3. Propofol
      a. Preferred for 1-day surgical procedures because patients can ambulate sooner and recover from the effects of anesthesia more rapidly
      b. May cause hypotension
      c. Has antiemetic activity
   4. Dissociative anesthetics
      a. General
         (1) During induction, patients feel dissociated from the environment (i.e., in trance-like states).
         (2) Good analgesic properties
         (3) Examples
            (a) Ketamine
            (b) Phencyclidine, a veterinary anesthetic
               • Both are abused as a street drugs
      b. Mechanism of action
         • Blocks the *N*-methyl-D-aspartate (NMDA) receptor
      c. Uses
         (1) Allows patients, particularly children, to be awake and respond to commands yet endure painful stimuli
         (2) Example is changing painful burn dressings
      d. Adverse effects
         (1) Increases:
            (a) Heart rate
            (b) Cardiac output
            (c) Arterial blood pressure
         (2) Postoperative psychotic phenomena (hallucinations)
            • Rarely used in adults because of this effect
   5. High-potency opioid analgesics
      a. Examples
         (1) Fentanyl
         (2) Alfentanil
         (3) Sufentanil
      b. Uses
         (1) Cardiothoracic surgery
         (2) Especially bypass surgery
         (3) Avoids cardiac effects of many inhalation agents (see Chapter 19)
   6. Midazolam or lorazepam
      a. Used for procedures that require consciousness
      b. Excellent for producing amnesia
   7. Etomidate
      a. A short-acting, intravenous general anesthetic
      b. *Minimal* cardiovascular effects
      c. *No* histamine release
      d. Useful for patients with compromised cardiopulmonary function

---

Thiopental often used for induction; halogenated hydrocarbons for maintenance anesthesia.

Thiopental's action is terminated by redistribution.

Patients ambulate more rapidly after propofol than after thiopental.

Most anesthetics cause nausea and vomiting upon emergence: propofol has antiemetic actions.

Like phencyclidine (Angel dust), ketamine (Special K) is also used for recreational purposes.

Dissociative anesthetics are noncompetitive inhibitors of the NMDA receptor calcium ionophore; especially in hippocampus.

Dissociative anesthetics have excellent analgesic actions.

High-potency opioids are preferred anesthetics for bypass surgery.

Etomidate preferred for patients with impaired cardiopulmonary function

TABLE 8-2. **Preanesthetic Drugs**

DRUG CLASS	SPECIFIC AGENT	EFFECT(S)
Opioids	Morphine	Sedation to decrease tension and anxiety
	Meperidine	Analgesia
	Fentanyl	
Barbiturates	Pentobarbital	Decreased apprehension
	Secobarbital	Sedation
	Thiopental	Rapid induction
	Methohexital	
Benzodiazepines	Diazepam	Decreased apprehension
	Lorazepam	Sedation
		Amnesia
		Rapid induction
Phenothiazines	Prochlorperazine	Antiemetic
	Promethazine	Antihistaminic effect
		Antiemetic
		Decreased motor activity
Anticholinergic drugs	Atropine	Inhibition of secretions, vomiting, and laryngospasms
	Scopolamine	
	Glycopyrrolate	
Antiemetics	Droperidol	Prevention of postoperative vomiting
	Hydroxyzine	
	Benzquinamide	
	Ondansetron	

D. **Preanesthetic medications** (Table 8-2) used to:
1. Increase analgesia
2. Produce amnesia
3. Enhance muscle relaxation
4. Decrease vagal reflexes
5. Prevent postoperative nausea and vomiting

II. **Local Anesthetics** (Box 8-2)
A. General
- Local anesthetics reversibly abolish sensory perception, especially pain, in restricted areas of the body.
B. Pharmacokinetics
1. Epinephrine is often added to:
a. Localize the anesthetic to the injection site
b. Prolong the anesthetic effect
c. Slow absorption
d. Thus, minimizing systemic toxicity
2. Epinephrine combination is *not* used for anesthesia in acral regions (ear, nose, fingers, penis etc.).
3. Route of administration
a. Topical application
b. Local injection
4. Metabolism
a. Esters are metabolized by plasma pseudocholinesterases.
(1) Therefore, many have a shorter duration of action (minutes) than amides.
(2) All ester-type local anesthetics, *except* cocaine, are metabolized to *p*-aminobenzoic acid (PABA) derivatives.
- These metabolites are allergenic.

Midazolam is an excellent amnestic agent.

Epinephrine often localizes anesthetics to the injection site; prolongs the anesthetic effect, and slows systemic absorption.

Ester local anesthetics are more allergenic than amides.

BOX 8-2 LOCAL ANESTHETICS	
Esters	**Amides**
Benzocaine	Bupivacaine
Cocaine	Lidocaine
Procaine	Mepivacaine
Tetracaine	Prilocaine
	Ropivacaine

b. Amides are metabolized by cytochrome P450s or amidases in the liver.
  • Therefore, many have a longer duration of action (hours) than esters.

C. **Mechanism of action:** Local anesthetics cause reversible blockade of nerve conduction (Fig. 8-1).
  1. Decrease the nerve membrane permeability to sodium by binding to inactivated sodium channels ("use-dependent" binding)
     a. Diffuse across the nerve membrane in the nonionized form
     b. Then, block the channel in the ionized form
     c. From the inside of the nerve membrane
  2. Reduce the rate of membrane depolarization
  3. Raise the threshold of electrical excitability
  4. Affect pain fibers first because they are small and unmyelinated
  5. Some agents, such as lidocaine, have antiarrhythmic effects and are used to treat ventricular arrhythmias.

D. Adverse effects
  1. Central nervous system (CNS)
     a. Seizures
     b. Lightheadedness
     c. Sedation
  2. Cardiovascular system
     a. Myocardial depression
     b. Hypotension
     c. Cardiac arrest

E. **Specific local anesthetics** (see Box 8-2)
  1. Esters
     a. Examples
        (1) Procaine
        (2) Tetracaine
        (3) Benzocaine
        (4) Cocaine

Infections that increase the acidity on the outside of nerve membranes decrease the effectiveness of local anesthetics because more is in the ionized form on the outside of the nerve membrane.

Local anesthetics block the Na$^+$ channel from inside the neuronal membrane.

With local anesthetics, loss of sensation occurs in the following sequence: pain, temperature, touch, movement.

Use of cocaine on the mucosa of the nose and paranasal sinuses causes shrinkage and minimizes bleeding.

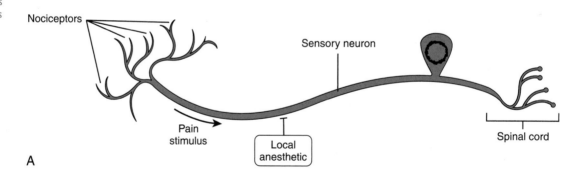

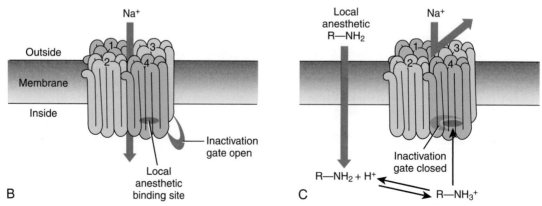

8-1: Mechanism of action of local anesthetics. **A,** Peripheral neuron, **B,** Schematic of sodium channel, and **C,** Illustration of how local anesthetics block the sodium channel from inside-to-out. *(From Brenner G and Stevens C: Pharmacology, 3rd ed. Philadelphia, Saunders, 2010, Figure 21-2.)*

   b. Uses
      (1) Topical anesthesia
      (2) Infiltration anesthesia
      (3) Nerve block
      (4) Spinal anesthesia
      (5) Cocaine is also a vasoconstrictor because it blocks norepinephrine uptake
   c. Adverse effects
      (1) CNS stimulation
      (2) Higher incidence of seizures; especially cocaine
2. Amides
   a. These agents are preferred for all types of infiltration, nerve blocks, and spinal anesthesia because of their slower metabolism and longer half-life ($t_{1/2}$).
   b. Examples
      (1) Lidocaine
      (2) Bupivacaine
      (3) Mepivacaine
      (4) Prilocaine
      (5) Ropivacaine

The names of all amides contain letter "i" twice (e.g., lidocaine).

CHAPTER 9
ANTICONVULSANT DRUGS

I. Anticonvulsant Therapy
- Seizures are episodes of abnormal electrical activity in the brain that may lead to involuntary movements and sensations, which are accompanied by characteristic changes on electroencephalography (EEG).
  - **A. Classification of seizures** (Table 9-1)
  - **B. Drugs used in the treatment of seizures** (Table 9-2)
    1. Mechanism of action (Fig. 9-1)
    2. Summary of therapeutic effects (see Table 9-3)
    3. Antiepileptics
       - Increased risk of suicidal behavior or ideation (U.S. Food and Drug Administration [FDA] Special Alert; February 2008)

II. Drugs Used in the Treatment of Partial Seizures and Generalized Tonic-Clonic Seizures
(Box 9-1; see also Table 9-2)
  - **A. Phenytoin and fosphenytoin**
    1. Pharmacokinetics
       a. High plasma protein-binding
          (1) Affects drug levels and activity
          (2) Site of drug-drug interactions
       b. First-order kinetics (low blood levels) can switch to zero-order kinetics (high blood levels), i.e., dose-dependent pharmacokinetics.
       c. Fosphenytoin, a prodrug to phenytoin, is preferred for parenteral administration.
       d. Metabolism in the liver
       e. Causes many drug-drug interactions because it induces cytochrome P-450 system
    2. Mechanism of action
       - Block voltage-sensitive sodium channels in the neuronal membrane (see Fig. 9-1)
    3. Uses (see Table 9-2)
       a. To treat partial and generalized tonic-clonic seizures
       b. Fosphenytoin is given to control generalized convulsive status epilepticus and prevent and treat seizures occurring during neurosurgery
    4. Adverse effects
       a. Central nervous system (CNS) effects
          (1) Sedation
          (2) Cerebellar ataxia
          (3) Nystagmus
          (4) Diplopia
       b. Induction of liver enzymes, which leads to vitamin D deficiency
          (1) Increases conversion of calcidiol to an inactive metabolite
          (2) Affects mineralization of the epiphyseal plate in children (rickets) and osteomalacia in adults
       c. Gingival hyperplasia
       d. Hirsutism
       e. Folate deficiency, leading to megaloblastic anemia
       f. Teratogenic ability (fetal hydantoin syndrome)
          (1) Nail and distal phalanx hypoplasia
          (2) Cleft lip and palate
          (3) Neuroblastoma in children
          (4) Vitamin K deficiency (bleeding diathesis)
       g. Atypical lymphocytosis

Many patients receive two anticonvulsant drugs, because decreased doses of each individual drug can be given, minimizing adverse effects.

Sulfonamides may displace phenytoin from plasma proteins increasing the free level as well as toxicity.

Many anticonvulsants (phenytoin, carbamazepine, phenobarbital, primidone) induce drug-metabolizing, enzymes decreasing the effects of concomitantly administered drugs including oral contraceptives.

Anticonvulsants that block sodium channels: phenytoin, carbamazepine, lamotrigine, felbamate, valproic acid, topiramate, zonisamide

Phenytoin powerful inducer of drug metabolism.

Phenytoin may produce gingival hyperplasia and hirsutism; unpleasant adverse effects for young girls.

Most anticonvulsants are relatively contraindicated during pregnancy.

TABLE 9-1. **International Classification of Partial and Generalized Seizures**

CLASSIFICATION	ORIGIN AND FEATURES
Partial (Focal) Seizures	**Arising in one cerebral hemisphere**
Simple partial seizure	No alteration of consciousness
Complex partial seizure	Altered consciousness, automatisms, and behavioral changes
Secondarily generalized seizure	Focal seizure becoming generalized and accompanied by loss of consciousness
Generalized seizures	Arising in both cerebral hemispheres and accompanied by loss of consciousness
Tonic-clonic (grand mal) seizure	**Increased muscle tone followed by spasms of muscle contraction and relaxation**
Tonic seizure	Increased muscle tone
Clonic seizure	Spasms of muscle contraction and relaxation
Myoclonic seizure	Rhythmic, jerking spasms
Atonic seizure	Sudden loss of all muscle tone
Absence (petit mal) seizure	Brief loss of consciousness, with minor muscle twitches and eye blinking

TABLE 9-2. **Choice of Antiepileptic Drugs for Seizure Disorders**

DRUG	PARTIAL SEIZURES	GENERALIZED SEIZURES				STATUS EPILEPTICUS
		TONIC-CLONIC	ABSENCE	MYOCLONIC	ATONIC	
Carbamazepine	1	1	W	—	—	—
Phenytoin	1	1	W	—	—	2
Phenobarbital	2	2	—	—	—	3
Primidone	2	2	—	—	—	—
Gabapentin	A	—	—	—	—	—
Lamotrigine	A	A	—	—	A	—
Topiramate	A	—	—	—	—	—
Levetiracetam	A	—	—	—	—	—
Vigabatin	A	—	—	—	—	—
Zonisamide	A	—	—	—	—	—
Ethosuximide	—	—	1*	—	—	—
Valproate	2	1	2*	1	1	—
Clonazepam	—	W	3	2	1	—
Diazepam	—	—	—	—	—	1
Lorazepam	—	—	—	—	—	1

*For absence seizures in children, ethosuximide is the drug of first choice and valproate is the drug of second choice. For absence seizures in adults, valproate is probably the drug of first choice.

1, Drugs of first choice; 2, drug of second choice; 3, drug of third choice; A, drug for adjunct use with other drugs; W, drug that may worsen seizure.

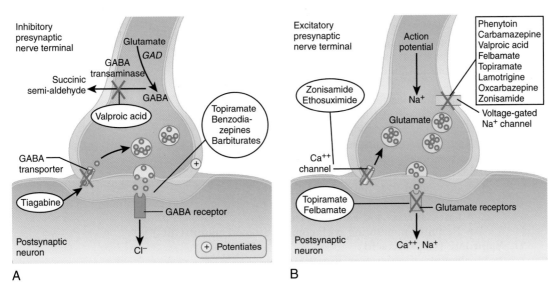

9-1: Mechanisms for anticonvulsant drugs. Note that many drugs have multiple mechanisms of action. GAD, glutamic acid decarboxylase; GABA, γ amino-butyric acid. *(From Kester M, et al.: Elsevier's Integrated Pharmacology. Philadelphia, Mosby, 2007, Figure 13-3.)*

BOX 9-1 ANTICONVULSANTS

Drugs Used to Treat Partial and Generalized Tonic-Clonic Seizures
Carbamazepine/oxcarbazepine
Phenobarbital
Phenytoin/fosphenytoin
Primidone
Valproate

Adjunct Drugs Used to Treat Partial Seizures
Clorazepate
Felbamate
Gabapentin
Pregabalin
Lamotrigine
Levetiracetam
Tiagabine
Topiramate
Vigabatrin
Zonisamide

Drugs Used to Treat Absence, Myoclonic, or Atonic Seizures
Clonazepam
Ethosuximide
Lamotrigine
Valproate

Drugs Used to Treat Status Epilepticus
Diazepam
Lorazepam
Fosphenytoin
Phenobarbital
Phenytoin

Phenobarbital induces cytochrome P-450 drug metabolizing enzymes.

Phenobarbital most sedating amongst the anticonvulsants.

Anticonvulsants that potentiate GABA mechanisms: barbiturates, primidone, benzodiazepines, vigabatrin, gabapentin, tiagabine, valproic acid

Oxcarbazepine is an active metabolite of carbamazepine.

Carbamazepine interacts with phenobarbital, phenytoin, primidone, and valproic acid, reducing their therapeutic effect.

Monitor blood counts when patients are taking carbamazepine.

B. **Phenobarbital** (see Chapter 7)
  1. Mechanism of action
     • Enhances the inhibitory action of the γ-aminobutyric acid (GABA) receptor by increasing the time that the chloride channel remains open (see Fig. 7-1)
  2. Use
     a. Management of generalized tonic-clonic and partial seizures
     b. Febrile seizures in children and neonatal seizures (unlabeled uses)
  3. Adverse effects
     a. Induction of liver cytochrome P-450 enzymes
     b. Sedation (high)
     c. Increase in irritability and hyperactivity in children (paradoxical effect)
     d. Agitation and confusion in the elderly
     e. Contraindicated in patients with porphyria
C. **Carbamazepine/oxcarbazepine**
  1. General
     a. Structurally related to imipramine and other tricyclic antidepressants
     b. Pharmacological activity results from its metabolite oxcarbazepine and its monohydroxy metabolite
     c. Oxcarbazepine is also available as a drug
  2. Mechanism of action (see Fig. 9-1)
     a. Blocks voltage-sensitive sodium channels
     b. Inhibits sustained, repetitive firing
  3. Uses
     a. Drug of choice for partial seizures
        • Often used first if the patient also has generalized tonic-clonic seizures.
     b. Trigeminal neuralgia and neuropathic pain
     c. Bipolar affective disorder (alternative to lithium)
  4. Adverse effects
     a. Diplopia and ataxia (most common)
     b. Induction of liver microsomal enzymes
        • Carbamazepine accelerates its own metabolism and the metabolism of other drugs.
     c. Aplastic anemia and agranulocytosis
        • Requires monitoring with complete blood count (CBC)
D. **Valproate (valproic acid)**
  1. Mechanism of action (see Fig. 9-1)
     a. Increases concentrations of GABA in the brain
     b. Suppresses repetitive neuronal firing through inhibition of voltage-sensitive sodium channels
     c. Blocks T-type calcium channels

2. Uses
   a. Absence seizures
      - Valproate is the preferred agent if the patient also has generalized tonic-clonic seizures.
   b. Complex partial seizures and myoclonic seizures
   c. Mania associated with bipolar disorder
   d. Migraine prophylaxis
3. Adverse effects
   a. Liver failure most serious adverse reaction
      - Highest incidence in young children
   b. High incidence of:
      (1) Mild CNS effects
      (2) Gastrointestinal (GI) effects
   c. Valproate inhibits its own metabolism as well as the metabolism of other drugs
   d. Folate antagonist
   e. Teratogenic
      (1) Open neural tube defects (folate antagonist)
      (2) Autism

E. Primidone
1. The action of primidone is due both to the parent compound and to its active metabolites
   a. Phenobarbital
   b. Phenylethylmalonamide (PEMA)
2. This drug is frequently added to the regimen when satisfactory seizure control is *not* achieved with phenytoin or carbamazepine.

F. Vigabatrin
1. Mechanism of action
   - Potentiates GABA by irreversibly inhibiting GABA-transaminase
2. Use
   - Most effective in the management of partial seizures

G. Gabapentin
1. Mechanism of action
   - May alter GABA metabolism or its nonsynaptic release
2. Uses
   a. Adjunctive management of partial seizures with or without secondary generalized tonic-clonic seizures
   b. Neuropathic pain
   c. Management of postherpetic neuralgia in adults

H. Pregabalin
1. Mechanism of action
   a. Binds to voltage-gated calcium channels, inhibiting excitatory neurotransmitter release
   b. Although structurally related to GABA, it does *not* bind to GABA or benzodiazepine receptors
   c. Exerts antinociceptive and anticonvulsant activity
2. Uses
   a. Adjunctive therapy for partial seizure disorder in adults
   b. Management of postherpetic neuralgia
   c. Management of pain associated with diabetic peripheral neuropathy
   d. Management of fibromyalgia

I. Lamotrigine
1. Mechanism of action
   - Acts at voltage-sensitive sodium channels to stabilize neuronal membranes (see Fig. 9-1)
2. Uses
   a. Primary generalized tonic-clonic seizures
   b. Adjunctive management for refractory partial seizures with or without secondary generalized tonic-clonic seizures
   c. Maintenance treatment of bipolar disorder
3. Adverse effects
   a. Watch for skin rashes
      - Boxed warning; may cause Stevens-Johnson syndrome
   b. CNS depression

J. Tiagabine
1. Mechanism of action
   - Inhibits neuronal and glial uptake of GABA (see Fig. 9-1)

Valproic acid treats both grand mal and petit mal seizures.

Valproic acid, a folate antagonist, may cause neural tube defects when used during pregnancy.

Valproate inhibits the metabolism of phenytoin, phenobarbital, and carbamazepine, increasing the toxicity of these drugs.

Primidone is converted to phenobarbital and PEMA; all 3 compounds have anticonvulsant properties.

Vigabatrin inhibits GABA-transaminase.

Gabapentin widely used to treat neuropathic pain.

Many anticonvulsants are used to treat neuropathic pain.

Patients taking lamotrigine need to be monitored for skin rashes; can be severe.

Tiagabine inhibits GABA reuptake.

2. Use
  • Adjunctive treatment of partial seizures

K. Felbamate
  1. Mechanism of action (see Fig. 9-1)
    a. Unknown but has weak inhibitory effects on:
      (1) GABA-receptor binding
      (2) Benzodiazepine receptor binding
    b. Devoid of activity at the MK-801 receptor binding site of the N-methyl-D-aspartate (NMDA) receptor-ionophore complex
  2. Uses
    a. Approved for the management of:
      (1) Partial seizures in adults
      (2) Lennox-Gastaut syndrome in children and adults
    b. Due to the occurrence of aplastic anemia and acute hepatic failure, use is limited to management of seizures refractory to other agents

L. Levetiracetam
  1. Mechanism of action
    • Unknown but does alter inhibitory and excitatory neurotransmission
  2. Uses
    a. Adjunctive therapy in the management of partial seizures with or without secondary generalization
    b. Bipolar disorder (unlabeled use)

M. Zonisamide
  1. Mechanism of action (see Fig. 9-1)
    a. Acts at sodium and calcium channels
    b. Stops the spread of seizures
    c. Suppresses the seizure focus
  2. Uses
    a. Approved for adjunctive management of partial seizures in adults 16 years and older with epilepsy
    b. Bipolar disorder (unlabeled use)

N. Topiramate
  1. Mechanism of action (see Fig. 9-1)
    a. Reduces sodium currents through voltage-gated sodium channels
    b. Activates a hyperpolarizing potassium current
    c. Enhances $GABA_A$ receptor activity
  2. Uses
    a. Refractory partial seizures
    b. Refractory generalized tonic-clonic seizures
    c. Migraine prophylaxis
    d. Adjunctive treatment of seizures associated with Lennox-Gastaut syndrome
    e. Unlabeled uses
      (1) Infantile spasms
      (2) Neuropathic pain
      (3) Cluster headache
  3. Adverse effects
    a. Drowsiness
    b. Dizziness
    c. Ataxia

III. **Absence (Petit Mal) Seizures and Drugs Used in their Treatment** (see Box 9-1 and Table 9-2)
  A. Absence seizures are primarily a childhood disorder
  B. Features
    1. Brief lapses of consciousness
    2. Characteristic spike-and-wave pattern on EEG (3/sec)
  C. Therapeutic drugs
    1. Ethosuximide
      • Effective in a high percentage of cases
        a. Mechanism of action (see Fig. 9-1)
          • Reduces current in T-type calcium channel found on primary afferent neurons

---

Use of felbamate limited because of it can cause aplastic anemia and liver failure.

Topiramate is used in migraine prophylaxis.

Anticonvulsants that reduce T-type calcium currents: ethosuximide, valproic acid, zonisamide are effective in absence seizures.

   b. Adverse effects
      (1) GI upset
      (2) Drowsiness
   2. Valproate (used for both tonic-clonic and absence seizures)
   3. Clonazepam
      a. Tolerance develops within a few months
      b. Makes the drug inappropriate for long-term therapy (see Chapter 7)
IV. **Status Epilepticus and Drugs Used in Its Treatment** (see Box 9-1 and Table 9-2)
   A. **Status epilepticus is a life-threatening emergency involving repeated seizures.**
   B. **Treatment of choice**
      1. Diazepam (intravenous)
      2. Lorazepam (intravenous)
   C. **Other therapeutic drugs**
      1. Fosphenytoin or phenytoin (intravenous) given by loading dose over 20 to 30 minutes
      2. Phenobarbital
      3. Midazolam (intravenous)
V. **Therapeutic Summary of Selected Anticonvulsant Drugs used in Treatment of Epilepsy**
   (Table 9-3)

Treatment of absence seizures with ethosuximide often unmasks tonic-clonic seizures.

Lorazepam and diazepam are preferred agents for treatment of status epilepticus.

TABLE 9-3. **Therapeutic Summary of Selected Anticonvulsant Drugs used in Treatment of Epilepsy**

DRUGS	CLINICAL APPLICATIONS IN EPILEPSY	ADVERSE EFFECTS	CONTRAINDICATIONS
Mechanism: *Inhibits voltage-gated Na⁺ channels*			
Phenytoin	Generalized tonic-clonic or partial seizures	Nystagmus, ataxia, dysarthria, sedation, confusion, gingival hyperplasia, hirsutism, megaloblastic anemia, blood dyscrasias, skin rashes, fever, systemic lupus erythematosus, lymphadenopathy, peripheral neuropathy, dyskinesias	Hypersensitivity Pregnancy
Fosphenytoin	Status epilepticus		
Carbamazepine	Generalized tonic-clonic or partial seizures	Nystagmus, dysarthria, diplopia, ataxia, drowsiness, nausea, blood dyscrasias, hepatotoxicity, hyponatremia.	Hypersensitivity Bone marrow depression
Oxcarbazepine		May exacerbate myoclonic seizures	With or within 14 days of MAO inhibitor use Concurrent use of nefazodone
Valproic acid; also has other mechanisms	Generalized tonic-clonic or partial seizures Absence seizures	Nausea, vomiting, diarrhea, drowsiness, alopecia, weight gain, hepatotoxicity, thrombocytopenia, tremor, pancreatitis	Hypersensitivity Hepatic disease Pregnancy
Lamotrigine; also has other mechanisms	Generalized tonic-clonic or partial seizures	Sedation, skin rash, visual disturbances, dyspepsia, ataxia, Stevens-Johnson syndrome	Hypersensitivity
Topiramate; also has other mechanisms	Generalized tonic-clonic or partial seizures	Somnolence, nausea, dyspepsia, irritability, dizziness, ataxia, nystagmus, diplopia, glaucoma, renal calculi, weight loss, hypohidrosis, hyperthermia	Hypersensitivity
Zonisamide; also has other mechanisms	Generalized tonic-clonic or partial seizures	Somnolence, ataxia, anorexia, nausea, vomiting, rash, confusion, renal calculi. Do not use in patients with sulfonamide allergy.	Sulfonamide hypersensitivity
Mechanism: *Potentiates GABA activity*			
Phenobarbital Primidone; also has other mechanisms	Generalized tonic-clonic or partial seizures	Drowsiness, nystagmus, ataxia, skin rashes, learning difficulties, hyperactivity.	Hypersensitivity Marked hepatic impairment Dyspnea or airway obstruction Porphyria Pregnancy

Continued

TABLE 9-3. **Therapeutic Summary of Selected Anticonvulsant Drugs used in Treatment of Epilepsy—Cont'd**

DRUGS	CLINICAL APPLICATIONS IN EPILEPSY	ADVERSE EFFECTS	CONTRAINDICATIONS
Mechanism: *Potentiates GABA activity*			
Clonazepam Diazepam Lorazepam	Short term therapy for absence seizures (clonazepam) Status epilepticus	Drowsiness, ataxia, irritability, behavioral changes, exacerbation of tonic-clonic seizures	Hypersensitivity Marked hepatic impairment Narrow-angle glaucoma Pregnancy
Mechanism: *Potentiates GABA activity by blocking GABA reuptake*			
Tiagabine	Partial seizures	Somnolence, anxiety, dizziness, poor concentration, tremor, diarrhea	Hypersensitivity
Mechanism: *Potentiates the release of GABA*			
Gabapentin Pregabalin	Partial seizures	Sedation, fatigue, ataxia, nystagmus	Hypersensitivity
Mechanism: *Inhibits T-type calcium channels*			
Ethosuximide	Absence seizures	Nausea, vomiting, anorexia, headache, lethargy, unsteadiness, blood dyscrasias, systemic lupus erythematosus, urticaria, pruritus	Hypersensitivity

GABA, γ-aminobutyric acid.

CHAPTER 10

PSYCHOTHERAPEUTIC DRUGS

I. **Antipsychotic Drugs, Sometimes Referred to as Neuroleptic Drugs** (Box 10-1)
  A. **General**
   1. Neuroleptics are useful in the treatment of schizophrenia.
   2. These drugs reduce positive symptoms (e.g., paranoia, hallucinations, delusions) more than negative symptoms (e.g., emotional blunting, poor socialization, cognitive deficit) in patients with schizophrenia.
   3. The newer "atypical" antipsychotics are more effective, especially against negative symptoms, and less toxic than the older but less expensive conventional antipsychotics.
   4. Late in 2003, the U.S. Food and Drug Administration (FDA) requested all manufacturers to include product label warnings about the potential for an increased risk of hyperglycemia and diabetes with the use of "atypical" antipsychotics.
   5. April 2005, FDA issued a boxed warning that "atypical" antipsychotics increased risk of death in patients treated with certain "atypical" antipsychotics for dementia-related behavioral disorders.
   6. June 2008, this boxed warning was extended to conventional antipsychotics (e.g., haloperidol, fluphenazine) as well.
  B. **Pharmacokinetics**
   1. Immediate onset after intramuscular or intravenous injection
   2. Slow and variable absorption after oral administration
   3. Most antipsychotics are metabolized to active and inactive metabolites.
   4. Haloperidol (every 4 weeks) and fluphenazine (every 2 weeks) decanoate salts are available as depot preparations for noncompliant patients.
   5. Risperidone is also available as an intramuscular preparation that can be given every 2 weeks.
  C. **Mechanism of action** (Table 10-1)
   1. All antipsychotics alter dopamine pathways; the antipsychotic activity correlates best with changes in mesolimbic and mesocortical pathways where adverse effects are often due to changes in nigrostriatal and tuberoinfundibular pathways (Table 10-2 and Fig. 10-1)
   2. Blockade of dopamine D_2 receptor correlates best with antipsychotic activity.
   3. Blockade of dopamine D_3 and D_4 receptors may also contribute to therapeutic effects.
   4. Blockade of serotonin receptors may contribute to benefits against negative symptoms.
   5. Blockade of other receptors also occurs (see Table 10-1).
  D. **Uses**
   1. Schizophrenic reactions, mania, psychosis
     • The actions of the neuroleptic agents in the mesolimbic and mesocortical pathways are most important for their antipsychotic effects.
   2. Nausea (antiemetic)
     a. Prochlorperazine
     b. Benzquinamide
     c. Droperidol
   3. Intractable hiccoughs
     • Chlorpromazine
   4. Antipruritic
     • Promethazine

Neuroleptics useful in treatment of schizophrenia

"Atypical" antipsychotics better for negative symptoms, especially clozapine.

"Atypical" antipsychotics may increase risk of metabolic syndrome including diabetes mellitus.

Antipsychotics may increase risk of death in patients with dementia-related behavioral disorders.

Intramuscular "depot" preparations good for noncompliant patients.

Antipsychotic effects of neuroleptic agents are related to blockade of dopamine receptors.

BOX 10-1	ANTIPSYCHOTIC DRUGS
Phenothiazines (Conventional) Chlorpromazine Fluphenazine Thioridazine Trifluoperazine	**Benzisoxazoles ("Atypical")** Risperidone Paliperidone
Thioxanthenes (Conventional) Thiothixene	**Azepines ("Atypical")** Clozapine Olanzapine Quetiapine
Butyrophenones (Conventional) Droperidol Haloperidol	**Other Drugs ("Atypical")** Aripiprazole (partial dopamine agonist) Ziprasidone

TABLE 10-1. Mechanisms and Effects of Neuroleptic Agents

MECHANISM	ACTION
Blockade of dopamine D_1 and D_2 receptors	Antipsychotic, extrapyramidal, and endocrine effects
Blockade of α-adrenergic receptors	Hypotension, failure to ejaculate
Blockade of histamine H_1 receptors	Sedation
Blockade of muscarinic receptors	Anticholinergic effects (e.g., dry mouth, urinary retention)
Blockade of serotonin receptors	Antipsychotic effects

TABLE 10-2. Central Dopamine Pathways

DOPAMINE TRACT	ORIGIN	INNERVATION	BEHAVIORAL RESPONSE	AFFECT OF DOPAMINE ANTAGONISTS
Mesolimbic	Ventral tegmental area	Limbic area Amygdala Olfactory tubercle	Memory Arousal Stimulus processing	Antipsychotic
Mesolimbic	Ventral tegmental area	Cingulated gyrus Septal nuclei	Motivational Behavior	Antipsychotic
Mesocortical	Ventral tegmental area	Prefrontal and frontal cortex	Stress response Communication Cognition Social function	Antipsychotic
Nigrostriatal	Substantia nigra	Basal ganglia	Abnormal movements Extrapyramidal symptoms	Acute dystonic Akathisia Parkinsonian syndrome Perioral tremor Tardive dyskinesia
Tuberoinfundibular	Arcuate nucleus of the hypothalamus	Anterior pituitary	Inhibition of prolactin release	Increased prolactin release (galactorrhea, menstrual disorders)

Many adverse effects of phenothiazines associated with blocking alpha, muscarinic or histaminergic receptors.

Antipsychotics with strongest D_2 blocking actions have highest incidence of extrapyramidal adverse effects.

E. **Adverse effects**
  • Neuroleptics cause unpleasant effects, thus have *no* abuse potential.
  1. Behavioral effects, such as *pseudodepression*
  2. Phenothiazines and related compounds produce many adverse effects by antagonizing:
     a. Alpha adrenergic receptors
     b. Muscarinic cholinergic receptors
     c. Histamine receptors
  3. Neurologic effects
     a. Extrapyramidal effects and iatrogenic Parkinsonism
     b. Dystonic reactions and akathisia
        • The best treatment is diphenhydramine or benztropine (antimuscarinic action).
        (1) Acute dystonic reactions (1–5 days)
           • Involvement of neck and head muscles

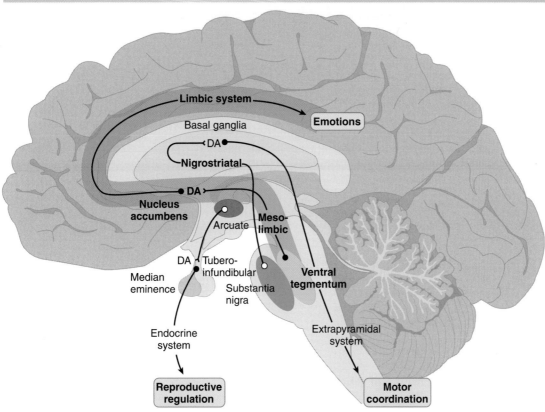

10-1: Dopaminergic (DA) pathways in the brain responsible for the beneficial and adverse effects of many antipsychotic drugs. *(From Kester M, et al.: Elsevier's Integrated Pharmacology. Philadelphia, Mosby, 2007, Figure 13-6.)*

(2) Akathisia (5–60 days)
   • Restlessness and agitation seen as continuous movement
(3) Parkinsonian syndrome (5–30 days)
   (a) Extrapyramidal effects
   (b) Tremors
   (c) Rigidity
   (d) Shuffling gait
   (e) Postural abnormalities
(4) Neuroleptic malignant syndrome (weeks)
   (a) Catatonia
   (b) Stupor
   (c) Fever
   (d) Unstable blood pressure (autonomic instability)
      • May be fatal
      • Treatment involves stopping the neuroleptic drug and using dantrolene and/or bromocriptine.
(5) Perioral tremor (months or years)
   (a) Rabbit syndrome (involuntary movement of the lips)
   (b) Treatment involves the use of anticholinergic agents.
(6) Tardive dyskinesia (months or years) producing stereotypical involuntary movements
   (a) Frequently irreversible
   (b) Results from effects on dopamine D_2 receptors
   (c) Treatment involves clozapine or diazepam
c. Decrease in seizure threshold
   (1) Use caution when giving neuroleptics to individuals with epilepsy.
   (2) Avoid giving these drugs to patients who are undergoing withdrawal from central nervous system (CNS) depressants.
d. Weight gain is high with many
   (1) Olanzapine
   (2) Quetiapine

Acute dystonia, akathisia, and Parkinsonian extrapyramidal adverse effects of antipsychotics can be treated with anticholinergics.

Neuroleptic malignant syndrome is treated with dantrolene and/or bromocriptine.

Tardive dyskinesia is associated with prolonged use of traditional neuroleptics; especially those with strong dopamine receptor antagonism

Extensive weight gain with olanzapine and quetiapine.

e. QT_c prolongation
  (1) Ziprasidone
  (2) Thioridazine
  (3) Haloperidol
 f. Elevated serum prolactin

F. Specific drugs (Table 10-3)
  1. Aliphatic phenothiazines (e.g., chlorpromazine)
    • Least potent phenothiazine
  2. Piperidine phenothiazines (e.g., thioridazine)
    a. Generally low incidence of acute extrapyramidal effects
    b. Requires regular eye examinations because of retinitis pigmentosa
  3. Piperazine phenothiazines (e.g., fluphenazine)
    • Generally high incidence of acute extrapyramidal effects
  4. Butyrophenones
    a. Examples
      (1) Haloperidol
      (2) Droperidol
    b. Additional uses for haloperidol
      (1) Tourette's syndrome
      (2) Acute psychosis
      (3) Alcoholic hallucinosis
      (4) Antiemetic
    c. Extremely high incidence of acute extrapyramidal effects
  5. Azepines ("atypical" agents)
    a. Clozapine
      (1) Mechanism of action
        (a) Blocks serotonin and dopamine (especially, D_1 and D_4) receptors, with a greater effect on the serotonin receptors (5-hydroxytryptamine [5-HT$_{2A}$])
        (b) Has less effect on dopamine D_2 receptors than conventional antipsychotics
        (c) Has a greater effect on negative symptoms of schizophrenia than the older conventional antipsychotics
      (2) Adverse effects
        (a) Low incidence of extrapyramidal effects
        (b) High incidence of agranulocytosis (1–2%), which necessitates regular (weekly) complete blood counts (CBCs)
        (c) Very sedating
    b. Olanzapine
      • Newer clozapine-like agent with *no* notable incidence of agranulocytosis

Use of neuroleptics leads to hyperprolactinemia, which results in amenorrhea-galactorrhea syndrome and infertility in women and loss of libido, impotence, and infertility in men.

Thioridazine noted for causing retinitis pigmentosa (irreversible).

Clozapine is associated with agranulocytosis.

Clozapine is very sedating.

Olanzapine is worst for producing weight gain.

TABLE 10-3. Effects of Antipsychotic Drugs

DRUG	RELATIVE POTENCY*	EXTRAPYRAMIDAL EFFECTS	SEDATIVE ACTION	HYPOTENSIVE ACTIONS	ANTICHOLINERGIC EFFECTS
Phenothiazines					
Chlorpromazine (aliphatic)	Low	Medium	High	High	Medium
Fluphenazine (piperazine)	High	High	Low	Very low	Low
Thioridazine (piperidine)	Low	Low	High	High	Very high
Trifluoperazine (piperazine)	High	High	Low	Low	Medium
Thioxanthenes					
Thiothixene	High	Medium-high	Low	Medium	Very low
Butyrophenones					
Haloperidol	High	Very high	Low	Very low	Very low
"Atypicals"					
Aripiprazole	High	Very low	Very low	Low	Very low
Clozapine	Medium	Very low	High	Medium	High
Olanzapine	High	Very low	Low	Low	Medium
Risperidone	High	Low	Low	Low	Very low
Ziprasidone	Medium	Very low	Low	Very low	Very low

*Potency: low = 50–2000 mg/d; medium = 20–250 mg/d; high = 1–100 mg/d.

    c. Quetiapine
- Newer "atypical" antipsychotic agent structurally similar to clozapine, a dibenzodiazepine structure

6. Benzisoxazoles ("atypical" agents)
    a. Examples
        (1) Risperidone
        (2) Paliperidone
    b. Monoaminergic antagonist with a high affinity for both serotonin 5-HT_{2A} and dopamine D_2 receptors
    c. Widely used for long-term therapy (risperidone)
    d. Associated with fewer extrapyramidal symptoms
    e. Paliperidone, the primary active metabolite of risperidone, is now available as a drug
        (1) Like risperidone, it has high affinity to α_1, D_2, H_1, and 5-HT_{2C} receptors, and low affinity for muscarinic and 5-HT_{1A} receptors.
        (2) In contrast to risperidone, it displays nearly 10-fold lower affinity for α_2 and 5-HT_{2A} receptors, and nearly 3- to 5-fold less affinity for 5-HT_{1A} and 5-HT_{1D}, respectively.

> Risperidone is one of the more widely used "atypical" antipsychotics.

7. Dihydroindolone ("atypical"; ziprasidone)
    a. An atypical antipsychotic, pharmacologically distinct from conventional agents such as the phenothiazines or haloperidol
    b. This drug offers advantages over others by causing less weight gain and greater effects against depressive symptoms in patients with schizophrenia or schizoaffective disorders.
    c. A serious adverse effect of ziprasidone is QTc interval prolongation.

> Ziprasidone, thioridazine, and haloperidol are associated with prolonged QTc intervals.

8. Dihydrocarbostyril ("atypical"; aripiprazole)
    a. A new class of atypical antipsychotic drugs known as dopamine system stabilizers (i.e., partial agonist)
    b. Approved for several treatments
        (1) Schizophrenia
        (2) Mania
        (3) Bipolar disorders
        (4) Depression (adjunctive)

> Aripiprazole is partial agonist at dopamine receptors.

G. Therapeutic summary of selected antipsychotic drugs: (Table 10-4)

II. Antidepressants and Mood Stabilizers (Box 10-2)
A. General
1. Depression can be classified as:
    a. Reactive (i.e., response to grief or illness)
    b. Endogenous (i.e., genetically determined biochemical condition)
    c. Bipolar affective (i.e., manic-depressive disorder)
2. Features of depressive disorders overlap with those of anxiety disorders
    a. Panic-agoraphobia syndrome
    b. Generalized anxiety disorder
    c. Social anxiety disorder
    d. Posttraumatic stress disorder
    e. Obsessive-compulsive disorder (OCD)
3. Antidepressant drugs are used to treat endogenous and bipolar affective forms of depression and anxiety disorders.
4. The FDA has issued a boxed warning that all antidepressants increase the risk of suicidal thinking and behavior in children, adolescents, and young adults (18–24 years of age) with major depressive disorder (MDD) and other psychiatric disorders.

> Anxiety and depression are co-morbid states.

> Selective serotonin reuptake inhibitors (SSRIs) are now used for long-term treatment of anxiety disorders.

> Antidepressants may increase suicide risk.

B. Tricyclic antidepressants (TCAs) (see Box 10-2)
1. Pharmacokinetics
    a. Tricyclics are well absorbed and are metabolized; many metabolites are active
    b. Most have a half-life of 24 hours or longer.
    c. Clinical improvement requires use for 2–3 weeks, thus reducing compliance.
2. Mechanism of action
    a. Most TCAs block the reuptake of serotonin and norepinephrine, causing accumulation of these monoamines in the synaptic cleft.
    b. Accumulation of monoamines in the synaptic cleft produces multiple adaptations in receptor and transport systems, such as:
        (1) Desensitization of adenylyl cyclase
        (2) Down regulation of β-adrenergic receptors

> TCAs block presynaptic reuptake of norepinephrine and serotonin.

TABLE 10-4. **Therapeutic Summary of Selected Antipsychotic Drugs:**

DRUGS	CLINICAL APPLICATIONS	ADVERSE EFFECTS	CONTRAINDICATIONS
Mechanism: *Therapeutic effect due to blocking D_2 and $5\text{-}HT_2$ receptors; many adverse effects associated with blocking α adrenergic, muscarinic and histaminic receptors*			

Phenothiazines
Chlorpromazine
Prochlorperazine
Thioridazine
Fluphenazine
Trifluoperazine
	Schizophrenia
	Acute psychosis
	Severe agitation
	Intractable hiccoughs
	   (Chlorpromazine)
	Nausea and vomiting
	   (Prochlorperazine)
		Anticholinergic effects
		Orthostatic hypotension
		Sedation
		Failure to ejaculate
		Extrapyramidal effects
		Endocrine effects
			Hypersensitivity
			Liver disease
			Coma
			Long QT syndrome
			   (thioridazine)

Mechanism: *Strong D_2 receptor blockers*			
Butyrophenones Droperidol Haloperidol	Schizophrenia Acute psychosis Severe agitation Tourette's syndrome (haloperidol)	Extrapyramidal effects Endocrine effects Sedation	Hypersensitivity Liver disease Coma Parkinson's disease
Mechanism: *More equal D_2 and $5\text{-}HT_2$ receptor blocking actions*			
Benzisoxazoles *(Atypical)* Risperidone Paliperidone	Schizophrenia Acute psychosis Severe agitation	Fewer extrapyramidal effects; fewer autonomic effects	Hypersensitivity
Mechanism: *Greater $5\text{-}HT_2$ than D_2 receptor blocking actions*			

Azepines
(Atypical)
Clozapine
Olanzapine
Quetiapine
	Schizophrenia
	Acute psychosis
	Severe agitation
	Clozapine's use is restricted to
	   those who failed other agents
	Bipolar disorder (olanzapine)
		Fewer extrapyramidal effects;
		   fewer autonomic effects
		Strong sedation
		Weight gain
		Agranulocytosis (clozapine)
			History of agranulocytosis
			   or granulocytopenia

Mechanism: *Greater $5\text{-}HT_2$ than D_2 receptor blocking actions*			

Ziprasidone
(Atypical)
	Schizophrenia
	Acute psychosis
	Severe agitation
		Less weight gain than other
		   "atypicals"
		QT prolongation
			Prolonged QT
			Use with other drugs that
			   prolong QT

Mechanism: *Partial dopamine agonists*			
Aripiprazole *(Atypical)*	Schizophrenia Acute psychosis Severe agitation	Hypotension Somnolence	Hypersensitivity Immediately after strong dopamine antagonists

D_1, D_2, dopamine receptors; 5-HT, 5-hydroxytryptamine.

BOX 10-2   ANTIDEPRESSANTS

Tricyclic Antidepressants
Amitriptyline
Clomipramine
Desipramine
Imipramine
Nortriptyline

Selective Serotonin Reuptake Inhibitors (SSRIs)
Citalopram
Escitalopram
Fluoxetine
Fluvoxamine
Paroxetine
Sertraline

Monoamine oxidase (MAO) Inhibitors
Phenelzine
Tranylcypromine

Other Antidepressants
Amoxapine
Bupropion
Desvenlafaxine
Duloxetine
Maprotiline
Mirtazapine
Nefazodone
Trazodone
Venlafaxine

Amitriptyline for chronic pain.

Trazodone to aid in sleep during hospitalization.

Imipramine used to treat bed-wetting in children.

Clomipramine and fluvoxamine are drugs for OCD.

(3) Down-regulation of serotonin receptors
(4) Upregulation of neurotrophic factors such as brain-derived neurotropic factor (BDNF)
3. Uses
   a. Depression
   b. Chronic pain (amitriptyline)
   c. Insomnia (trazodone)
   d. Enuresis (imipramine)
   e. OCD (clomipramine)

4. Adverse effects
   a. Sedation, which is due to blockade of histamine H_1 receptors
   b. Full range of anticholinergic effects, such as dry mouth, because agents are potent anticholinergics
   c. Full range of phenothiazine-like effects, especially orthostatic hypotension, resulting from α_1-adrenergic receptor blockade
   d. Rare acute extrapyramidal signs, because these agents are *not* potent dopamine blockers
   e. Overdose
      (1) Electrical cardiac conduction problems, increased QT_c interval and widened QRS (correct with sodium bicarbonate)
      (2) Convulsions (treat with diazepam)
   C. **Selective serotonin reuptake inhibitors (SSRIs)** (Table 10-5; see also Box 10-2)
   1. Mechanism of action
      a. Highly specific serotonin reuptake blockade at the neuronal membrane
      b. Dramatically decreased binding to histamine, acetylcholine, and norepinephrine receptors, which leads to less sedative, anticholinergic, and cardiovascular effects when compared with TCAs
   2. Uses
      a. Depression
      b. OCD
      c. Panic disorders
      d. Premenstrual dysphoric disorders (PMDD)
      e. Bulimia nervosa
   3. Adverse effects
      a. Nausea
      b. Nervousness
      c. Insomnia
      d. Headache
      e. Sexual dysfunction

Drugs with strong antagonism at H_1 histamine receptors in the brain are very sedating.

Drugs typically increasing QT_c: thioridazine, tricyclic antidepressants, Class 1A and III antiarrhythmics; risk of producing life-threatening torsade de pointes

TCAs produce conduction abnormalities: ECG is needed prior to therapy to rule out atrioventricular (AV) block or other abnormalities.

SSRIs used to treat depression, obsessive-compulsive disorder, panic disorders, premenstrual dysphoric disorders (PMDD), bulimia nervosa.

SSRIs usually do *not* cause weight gain as do TCAs.

SSRIs are noted for producing sexual dysfunction.

TABLE 10-5. **Pharmacologic Profile of Antidepressants**

DRUG	ANTIMUSCARINIC EFFECTS	SEDATIVE EFFECTS	AMINE PUMP BLOCKADE		
			SEROTONIN	NOREPINEPHRINE	DOPAMINE
Tricyclic Antidepressants					
Amitriptyline	+++	+++	+++	++	o
Clomipramine	++	+++	+++	+	o
Desipramine	+	+	o/+	+++	o
Imipramine	++	++	+	++	o
Nortriptyline	++	++	+	++	o
Selective Serotonin Reuptake Inhibitors (SSRI)					
Citalopram	o	o	+++	o	o
Escitalopram	o	o	+++	o	o
Fluoxetine	+	+	+++	o/ +	o/+
Fluvoxamine	o	o	+++	o	o
Paroxetine	o	o	+++	o	o
Sertraline	+	o	+++	o	o
Other Antidepressants					
Amoxapine	++	++	+	++	+
Atomoxetine (SNRI)	o	o	o	+++	o
Bupropion	o	o	+/ o	+/o	+
Desvenlafaxine (dual inhibitor)	o	o	++	+++	o/+
Duloxetine (dual inhibitor)	o	o	+++	++	o/+
Maprotiline (SNRI)	++	++	o	+++	o
Mirtazapine*	o	+++	o	o	o
Nefazodone	+++	++	+/ o	o	o
Trazodone	o	+++	++	o	o
Venlafaxine (dual inhibitor)	o	o	+++	++	o/+

*Blocks α_2-adrenoreceptors and $5\text{-}HT_2$ serotonin receptors.
o, None; +, slight; ++, moderate; +++, extensive.
SNRI, selective norepinephrine reuptake inhibitor.

D. Other antidepressants (see Box 10-2)

  1. Mechanism of action
- Greater selectivity than TCAs for either norepinephrine or serotonin

  2. Adverse effects
- Less cardiotoxicity and anticholinergic activity than TCAs

  3. Selected antidepressants

    a. Amoxapine

      (1) Use for depression in psychotic patients

      (2) Also has antipsychotic activity

    b. Bupropion

      (1) Structurally similar to amphetamine

      (2) Inhibits dopamine reuptake

      (3) Uses

        (a) Depression

        (b) Smoking cessation

        (c) Attention-deficit/hyperactivity disorders

      (4) Adverse effects

        (a) Seizures

        (b) Anorexia

        (c) Aggravation of psychosis

    c. Maprotiline
- Selective norepinephrine reuptake inhibitor (SNRI)

    d. Mirtazapine

      (1) Mechanism of action
- Blockade of $5-HT_2$ serotonin and α_2-adrenergic presynaptic receptors on adrenergic and serotonergic neurons

      (2) Uses

        (a) Treat depression in patients who do *not* tolerate SSRIs

        (b) Useful in treating depression with coexisting anxiety disorder

      (3) Adverse effects (reputed)

        (a) Weight gain

        (b) Sedation

    e. Trazodone

      (1) Mechanism of action

        (a) Inhibits serotonin reuptake into the presynaptic neurons

        (b) Has *no* anticholinergic activity

        (c) May cause cardiac arrhythmias and priapism

        (d) Very strong H_1 histamine receptor blocker

      (2) Uses

        (a) Depression

        (b) Insomnia (low doses, which causes sedation)

    f. Nefazodone
- Less sedating than trazodone

    g. Dual inhibitors

      (1) Examples

        (a) Venlafaxine

        (b) Desvenlafaxine

        (c) Duloxetine

      (2) Mechanism of action

        (a) Similar mechanism of action to the TCAs

        (b) *But* a better adverse effect profile, because they do *not* block
- α_1-adrenergic receptors
- Histamine H_1 receptors
- Muscarinic receptors

      (3) Uses

        (a) Depression

        (b) Duloxetine also useful for painful physical symptoms (e.g., back pain, shoulder pain) associated with depression and anxiety

E. Monoamine oxidase (MAO) inhibitors

  1. Pharmacokinetics

    a. Long-lasting effects due to irreversible inhibition of the enzyme

    b. Therapeutic effect develops after 2 to 4 weeks of treatment

---

Amoxapine is used to treat psychotic depression.

Bupropion is used for smoking cessation.

Maprotiline is an SNRI.

Mirtazapine is an α_2-adrenergic antagonist; increases synaptic levels of norepinephrine and serotonin by a different mechanism than uptake inhibitors.

Mirtazapine noted for causing weight gain.

Trazodone may cause priapism (prolonged, painful erection of the penis), which can lead to impotence.

Trazodone mostly used as a hospital hypnotic drug.

Venlafaxine, desvenlafaxine, and duloxetine "dual" uptake inhibitors.

2. Mechanism of action
   - Inhibition of MAO-A and B, thus increasing concentration of both norepinephrine and serotonin in the brain
3. Uses
   a. "Atypical" depression, characterized by attendant anxiety and phobic features
   b. Depression in patients refractory to TCAs
4. Adverse effects
   a. Postural hypotension
   b. CNS effects, such as restlessness and insomnia
   c. Hepatotoxicity
   d. Possible hypertensive crisis
5. Drug interactions
   a. Examples
      (1) Meperidine
      (2) TCAs
      (3) SSRIs
   b. Cause "serotonin syndrome" (marked increase in synaptic serotonin)
   c. Potentially very severe reactions, characterized by:
      (1) Excitation
      (2) Sweating
      (3) Myoclonus and muscle rigidity
      (4) Hypertension
      (5) Severe respiratory depression
      (6) Coma
      (7) Vascular collapse
      (8) Possibly resulting in death
   d. Treat with cyproheptadine

F. Therapeutic summary of selected antidepressant drugs: (Table 10-6)

III. Drug used as mood stabilizers (Box 10-3)

A. General:
1. Several drugs are used as mood stabilizers to treat *mood disorders* characterized by intense and sustained mood shifts.
2. A common mood disorder is *bipolar disorder* or manic depression.
3. Mood stabilizers suppress swings between *mania* and *depression*.
4. Both the intensity and frequency of mood swings are reduced.
5. Mood stabilizer drugs are also used to treat *borderline personality disorder*.

B. Drugs
1. Lithium
   - Used in the treatment of bipolar disorders because it decreases the severity of the manic phase and lengthens the time between manic phases
   a. Pharmacokinetics
      (1) Narrow range of therapeutic serum levels
      (2) Delayed onset of action (6–10 days)
   b. Mechanism of action
      (1) Mood stabilizing actions are unknown
      (2) *But* does modify
         (a) Ion fluxes
         (b) Neurotransmitter synthesis and turnover rates
         (c) Second messenger systems
            - Particularly the inositol phosphate (IP) pathway
   c. Uses
      (1) Bipolar disorders
         - Lithium is the preferred mood stabilizer for patients who are suicidal.
      (2) Nonpsychiatric uses
         (a) Neutropenia
         (b) Thyrotoxic crisis
         (c) Migraine and cluster headaches
         (d) Considered a last choice for syndrome of inappropriate antidiuretic hormone (SIADH) secretion
   d. Adverse effects at therapeutic serum concentrations
      (1) Symptoms and signs
         (a) Fine hand tremor

MAOIs for "Atypical" depression.

Ingestion of tyramine-containing foods (e.g., certain cheeses, wines, preserved meats) while taking MAO inhibitors may precipitate a hypertensive crisis.

Patients who are taking MAO inhibitors should *not* take meperidine, dextromethorphan, TCAs, or SSRIs: they produce "serotonin syndrome"

Mood stabilizers decrease both frequency and intensity of mood swings in patients with bipolar disorders.

Lithium has a narrow therapeutic index.

Lithium has a delayed onset of action.

Lithium affects the polyphosphoinositide (PI) pathway.

Lithium-induced tremors can be treated with propranolol.

TABLE 10-6. Therapeutic Summary of Selected Antidepressant Drugs

DRUGS	CLINICAL APPLICATIONS	ADVERSE EFFECTS	CONTRAINDICATIONS
Mechanism: *Therapeutic due to blocking NE and 5-HT reuptake at presynaptic neuron; many adverse effects associated with blocking α-adrenergic, muscarinic and histaminic receptors*			
Tricyclic Antidepressants Amitriptyline Clomipramine Desipramine Imipramine Nortriptyline	Endogenous depression Nocturnal enuresis in children (Imipramine) Amitriptyline (Analgesic for certain chronic and neuropathic pain; prophylaxis against migraine headaches) Obsessive-compulsive disorder (OCD) (Clomipramine)	Hypotension Anticholinergic effects Sedation Dangerous in overdose (arrhythmias and seizures)	Hypersensitivity Heart disease With MAO inhibitors can get serotonin syndrome Pregnancy
Mechanism: *Selective inhibitors of 5-HT reuptake at presynaptic neuron*			
SSRIs Citalopram Escitalopram Fluoxetine Fluvoxamine Paroxetine Sertraline	Major depressive disorder Anxiety disorders Binge-eating and vomiting in patients with moderate-to-severe bulimia nervosa (OCD) Premenstrual dysphoric disorder (PMDD) Panic disorder with or without agoraphobia	Generally safer than tricyclics Sexual dysfunction Nausea and vomiting Agitation Discontinuation syndrome	Hypersensitivity With MAO inhibitors can get serotonin syndrome
Mechanism: *Inhibition of MAO-A and B; MAO-A metabolizes NE and 5-HT; MAO-B metabolizes DA*			
MAO inhibitors Phenelzine Tranylcypromine	Symptomatic treatment of atypical, non-endogenous, or neurotic depression	Risk of hypertensive crisis with tyramine containing foods Dizziness Drowsiness Agitation	Hypersensitivity With other sympathomimetics Serotonin syndrome when used with other drugs that affect serotonin
Mechanism: *Dual inhibitors of NE and 5-HT reuptake at presynaptic neuron without blocking α-adrenergic, muscarinic and histaminic receptors*			
Desvenlafaxine Duloxetine Venlafaxine	Major depressive disorder (MDD) Generalized anxiety disorder (GAD) Management of pain associated with diabetic neuropathies Management of fibromyalgia	Somnolence Increase blood pressure Sexual dysfunction	Hypersensitivity Serotonin syndrome when used with other drugs that affect serotonin
Mechanism: *Blocks dopamine reuptake at presynaptic neurons.*			
Bupropion	Major depressive disorder Seasonal affective disorder (SAD) Adjunct in smoking cessation	Lowers seizure threshold Agitation Lowest incidence of sexual dysfunction	Hypersensitivity Seizure disorders
Mechanism: *Inhibits reuptake of serotonin and also significantly blocks histamine (H_1) and $α_1$-adrenergic receptors.*			
Trazodone	Hospital hypnotic	Very sedating	Hypersensitivity
Mechanism: *$α_2$-Adrenergic antagonist; results in increased release of norepinephrine and serotonin; also a potent antagonist of 5-HT_2 and 5-HT_3 serotonin receptors and H, histamine receptors*			
Mirtazapine	Depression Sleep aid	Very sedating Extensive weight gain	Hypersensitivity
Mechanism: *Inhibits the reuptake of serotonin and norepinephrine; a metabolite has significant dopamine receptor blocking activity similar to haloperidol.*			
Amoxapine	Depression Psychotic depression Depression accompanied by anxiety or agitation	Drowsiness Prolactin increase Extrapyramidal symptoms	Hypersensitivity

DA, dopamine; 5-HT, 5-hydroxytryptamine; NE, norepinephrine; MAO, monoamine oxidase.

Box 10-3 MOOD STABILIZER DRUGS

Carbamazepine
Clonazepam
Lamotrigine
Lithium
Olanzapine
Valproic acid

Use of lithium causes nephrogenic diabetes insipidus and hypothyroidism.

(b) Dry mouth
(c) Weight gain
(d) Mild nausea and vomiting
(e) Diarrhea
(f) Polydipsia and polyuria (lithium induced diabetes insipidus)
   • Treat with amiloride
(g) Hypothyroidism

        (h) Impotence and decreased libido
        (i) Nephrotic syndrome
        (j) Neutrophilic leukocytosis
          • Inhibits activation of neutrophil adhesion molecules
      (2) Electrocardiogram
        (a) Flattened or inverted T waves
        (b) Produced by the inhibition of potassium cellular reuptake
        (c) Leads to intracellular hypokalemia
  2. Alternatives to lithium use in bipolar disorders:
    a. Carbamazepine
    b. Clonazepam
    c. Valproic acid
    d. Lamotrigine
    e. Olanzapine
      • Preferred for patents whose dominant mood swing is manic

> Several anticonvulsants are used as alternative to lithium for treating mood disorders; less toxic.

  C. Therapeutic summary of selected mood stabilizer drugs: (Table 10-7)

IV. Attention-deficit/hyperactivity disorder (ADHD) Drugs (Box 10-4)
  A. April 2008: The American Heart Association (AHA) has issued a statement recommending that all children diagnosed with ADHD who may be candidates for stimulant medications have a thorough cardiovascular assessment prior to initiation of drug therapy.
  B. Stimulants used in treating ADHD.
    1. Amphetamines
      a. Examples
        (1) Amphetamine
        (2) Dextroamphetamine
        (3) Lysdexamphetamine
          • A prodrug converted to dextroamphetamine
      b. CNS stimulants
      c. Used for the treatment of
        (1) ADHD
        (2) Narcolepsy
        (3) Exogenous obesity
    2. Methylphenidate and dexmethylphenidate (more active, *d-threo*-enantiomer, of racemic methylphenidate)
      a. CNS stimulants similar to the amphetamines
      b. Used in the treatment of:
        (1) ADHD in children
        (2) Narcolepsy
          • Methylphenidate is available as a transdermal formulation

> Methylphenidate is most widely used to treat ADHD in children.

TABLE 10-7. Therapeutic Summary of Selected Mood Stabilizer Drugs

DRUGS	CLINICAL APPLICATIONS	ADVERSE EFFECTS	CONTRAINDICATIONS
Mechanism: *Alters cation transport across the cell membrane and influences reuptake of serotonin and/or norepinephrine; second messenger systems involving the phosphatidylinositol cycle are inhibited; postsynaptic D_2 receptor supersensitivity is inhibited.*			
Lithium	Management of bipolar disorders Treatment of mania in individuals with bipolar disorder Treatment of syndrome of inappropriate antidiuretic hormone (SIADH) secretion	Tremors (treat with propranolol) Fatigue Polyuria/polydipsia Cardiac arrhythmias Thyroid abnormalities Leucocytosis	Hypersensitivity Cardiac disease Renal disease Pregnancy
Mechanism: *Stabilize electrical activity in the brain*			
Anticonvulsants Carbamazepine Clonazepam Lamotrigine Valproic acid	Mood stabilizer Anticonvulsants	See Chapter 9 Less adverse effects than lithium	See Chapter 9
Mechanism: *Greater $5\text{-}HT_2$ than D_2 receptor blocking actions*			
Olanzapine	Preferred mood stabilizer for patents whose dominant mood swing is manic	Less extrapyramidal effects; less autonomic effects Strong sedation Weight gain	Hypersensitivity

Box 10-4	ATTENTION-DEFICIT/HYPERACTIVITY DISORDER (ADHD) DRUGS

Amphetamine
Atomoxetine
Bupropion
Dexmethylphenidate
Dextroamphetamine
Lysdexamphetamine
Methylphenidate
Modafinil

C. Bupropion

Bupropion inhibits dopamine reuptake.

1. An antidepressant that selectively inhibits dopamine reuptake
2. Used off-label for the treatment of:
   a. ADHD
   b. Neuropathic pain

D. Atomoxetine

Atomoxetine is an SNRI.

1. An SNRI (selective norepinephrine reuptake inhibitor)
2. First non-stimulant drug approved for ADHD

E. Modafinil

1. Acts on central adrenergic $_{1B}$ receptors but also affects GABAergic, glutaminergic, and serotonergic synapses

Modafinil used to treat ADHD and fatigue in MS.

2. Used to treat ADHD and fatigue in multiple sclerosis (MS) and other disorders

F. Therapeutic summary of selected ADHD drugs: (Table 10-8)

TABLE 10-8. **Therapeutic Summary of Selected Attention Deficit/Hyperactivity Disorder (ADHD) Drugs**

DRUGS	CLINICAL APPLICATIONS	ADVERSE EFFECTS	CONTRAINDICATIONS
Mechanism: *Mild CNS stimulants that affect the reuptake of norepinephrine and dopamine into presynaptic neurons*			
Amphetamine-like drugs Dexmethylphenidate Dextroamphetamine Lysdexamphetamine Methylphenidate	ADHD Narcolepsy	Insomnia Decreased appetite Abuse potential	Hypersensitivity Idiosyncratic reactions to sympathomimetic amines Cardiac disease
Mechanism: *Selectively inhibits the reuptake of norepinephrine*			
Atomoxetine	ADHD	Headache Hypertension Agitation	Hypersensitivity Narrow-angle glaucoma
Mechanism: *Blocks dopamine reuptake at presynaptic neurons.*			
Bupropion	Depression Smoking cessation ADHD	Tachycardia Headaches Anxiety Seizures	Hypersensitivity Seizure disorders
Mechanism: *Acts on central α_{1B} adrenergic receptors but also affects GABAergic, glutaminergic, and serotonergic synapses*			
Modafinil	ADHD Fatigue in multiple sclerosis	Headache Gastrointestinal upset	Hypersensitivity

CNS, central nervous system; GABA, γ aminobutyric acid.

CHAPTER 11

DRUGS USED IN THE TREATMENT OF PARKINSON'S DISEASE

I. General Considerations

A. Parkinsonism is associated with lesions in the basal ganglia, especially the substantia nigra and the globus pallidus (Fig. 11-1).

B. There is a reduction in the number of cells in the substantia nigra and a decrease in the dopamine content.

C. Activation of the 4 dopaminergic pathways (Table 11-1; also see Fig. 11-1) account for many of the beneficial as well as some of the adverse effects of drugs used in treating Parkinson's disease.

D. The lesions result in increased and improper modulation of motor activity by the extrapyramidal system, leading to a resting tremor, rigidity, and bradykinesia.

E. Therapy aims to increase the dopamine content through "replacement therapy" or reducing acetylcholine (ACh) activity, because proper function depends on the balance between the inhibitory neurotransmitter dopamine and the excitatory neurotransmitter ACh.

> Parkinson's disease: too little dopaminergic activity; too much cholinergic activity

II. Drugs Used to Treat Parkinson's disease (Box 11-1 and Fig. 11-2)

A. Levodopa (L-dopa)

1. Pharmacokinetics

   a. L-Dopa, the precursor to dopamine, has the ability to cross the blood-brain barrier (BBB) by facilitated diffusion.

   b. Dopamine *cannot* be used to treat Parkinson's disease, because this agent does *not* enter the brain after systemic administration.

   c. L-Dopa is rapidly metabolized, predominantly by decarboxylation (aromatic amino acid decarboxylase, AAAD) to dopamine, and excreted into the urine.

   d. L-Dopa is always given in combination with carbidopa or benserazide; peripheral dopa decarboxylase inhibitors.

2. Mechanism of action

   a. L-Dopa enters the brain

   b. Converted to dopamine

   c. Dopamine reacts with dopamine receptors in the central nervous system (CNS); see Figs. 11-1 and 11-2.

3. Adverse effects

   a. Due to stimulation of dopamine receptors

   b. Severe gastrointestinal problems

      (1) Nausea

      (2) Vomiting

      (3) Anorexia

      (4) Peptic ulcer

   c. Postural hypotension

   d. Arrhythmias

   e. Dyskinesia

      (1) Development of abnormal involuntary movements

      (2) Choreoathetosis, the most common presentation, involves the face and limbs

      (3) Effects resemble tardive dyskinesia induced by phenothiazines

   f. Psychosis

   g. Hypersexuality

> Dopamine is metabolized by monoamine oxidase (MAO) and catechol-*O*-methyltransferase (COMT) in endothelial cells of BBB.

> Use of carbidopa with L-dopa allows more L-dopa to enter the brain.

> The autoxidation of dopamine may contribute to destruction of dopaminergic neurons; this may limit the therapeutic time window to the effectiveness (3 to 5 years) of L-dopa therapy.

> Cardiovascular and gastrointestinal adverse effects occur early in therapy.

> CNS adverse effects occur late in therapy.

> Abnormal hypersexuality is a late occurring adverse effect of L-dopa.

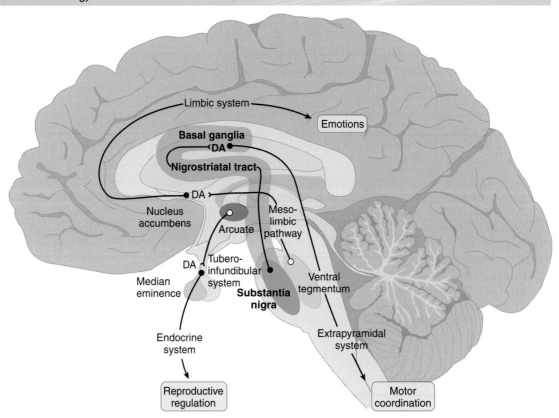

11-1: Dopaminergic (DA) pathways disrupted in Parkinson's disease. *(From Kester M, et al.: Elsevier's Integrated Pharmacology. Philadelphia, Mosby, 2007, Figure 13-7.)*

TABLE 11-1. **Central Dopamine Pathways**

DOPAMINE TRACT	ORIGIN	INNERVATION	BEHAVIORAL RESPONSE	AFFECT OF DOPAMINE AGONISTS
Nigrostriatal	Substantia nigra	Basal ganglia	Extrapyramidal symptoms Abnormal movements	Reduced symptoms of Parkinson's disease Dyskinesia
Mesolimbic	Ventral tegmental area	Limbic area Amygdala Olfactory tubercle	Memory Arousal Stimulus processing	Psychosis Hypersexuality Anxiety
Mesolimbic	Ventral tegmental area	Cingulated gyrus Septal nuclei	Motivational behavior	Psychosis
Mesocortical	Ventral tegmental area	Prefrontal and frontal cortex	Stress response Communication Cognition Social function	Psychosis Decreased mental acuity
Tuberoinfundibular	Arcuate nucleus of the hypothalamus	Anterior pituitary	Inhibition of prolactin release	Decreased prolactin release Increased libido

B. Other drugs used to treat Parkinson's disease

1. Bromocriptine

   a. Mechanism of action
      • Direct dopamine agonist that enters the CNS

   b. Uses
      (1) Lack of response to L-dopa or an unstable reaction to L-dopa
      (2) "On-off" symptoms, in which improved motility alternates with marked akinesia
      (3) Treatment of hyperprolactinemia associated with:

BOX 11-1   DRUGS USED TO TREAT PARKINSON'S DISEASE

Dopaminergic Drugs
Amantadine (increases synaptic dopamine)
Levodopa (prodrug to dopamine)

Dopamine Receptor Agonists
Apomorphine (used intravenously to treat acute symptoms)
Bromocriptine
Pergolide (withdrawn)
Pramipexole
Ropinirole

Peripheral Dopa Decarboxylase Inhibitors
Carbidopa (used with levodopa or levodopa and entacapone)
Benserazide (used with levodopa)

Catechol-*O*-methyl Transferase (COMT) Inhibitors
Entacapone
Tolcapone

Monoamine Oxidase Type B (MAO-B) Inhibitors
Rasagiline
Selegiline

Anticholinergics
Benztropine
Diphenhydramine
Orphenadrine
Procyclidine
Trihexyphenidyl

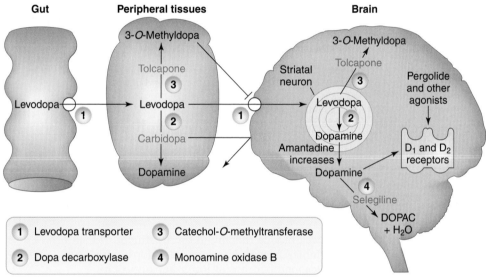

1   Levodopa transporter   3   Catechol-*O*-methyltransferase

2   Dopa decarboxylase   4   Monoamine oxidase B

11-2: Mechanisms of dopaminergic drugs used in the treatment of Parkinson's disease. Dopa decarboxylase is inhibited by carbidopa in the peripheral tissues but not in the brain, because carbidopa does not cross the blood-brain barrier. Catechol-*O*-methyltransferase is inhibited by tolcapone in both the peripheral tissues and the brain. Monoamine oxidase B is inhibited by selegiline. DOPAC, dihydroxyphenylacetic acid; D_1 and D_2, dopamine receptor subtypes.

       (a) Amenorrhea with or without galactorrhea
       (b) Infertility
       (c) Hypogonadism
       (d) Treatment of prolactin-secreting adenomas
       (e) Treatment of acromegaly
2. Pergolide (Withdrawn from U.S. market)
3. Pramipexole
    a. Mechanism of action
      • Agonist that binds to both the dopamine D_2 and D_3 receptors in the striatum and substantia nigra
    b. Uses
      (1) Delays the need for L-dopa when used as monotherapy
      (2) Reduce the "off" symptoms when added on to L-dopa therapy
4. Ropinirole
    a. Mechanism of action
      • Agonist that acts at both the dopamine D_2 and D_3 receptors
    b. Uses
      (1) Delays the need for L-dopa when used as monotherapy
      (2) Reduce the "off" symptoms when added on to L-dopa therapy
      (3) Also, for restless leg syndrome

Pergolide withdrawn from market because of association with valvular heart disease.

Pramipexole is now used as monotherapy for mild Parkinson's disease.

Ropinirole is now used as monotherapy for mild Parkinson's disease.

5. Amantadine
   a. Mechanism of action
      (1) Antiviral agent that releases dopamine
      (2) May block dopamine reuptake
      (3) Central cholinolytic effect
   b. Use
      (1) Early treatment of tremor, bradykinesia, rigidity associated with Parkinson's disease
      (2) Prophylaxis and treatment of influenza A viral infection
   c. Adverse effects
      (1) Blurred vision, constipation
      (2) Hallucinations, suicidal ideations
      (3) Livedo reticularis
6. Selegiline and Rasagiline
   a. Mechanism of action
      (1) Indirect dopamine agonists that selectively inhibit monoamine oxidase B
      (2) An enzyme that inactivates dopamine
      (3) Metabolized to methamphetamine
   b. Use
      (1) Most commonly given in conjunction with L-dopa
      (2) May be effective alone as a neuroprotectant due to its antioxidant and antiapoptotic effects
      (3) Selegiline is also available as a transdermal formulation
7. Tolcapone
   a. Mechanism of action
      (1) COMT inhibitor
      (2) Decreases the inactivation of L-dopa
      (3) Increases dopamine levels in the brain
   b. Use
      • Adjunct to L-dopa/carbidopa therapy
   c. Adverse effects
      • Hepatotoxicity
8. Entacapone
   a. A reversible inhibitor of peripheral COMT
   b. Use
      (1) Adjunct to L-dopa/carbidopa therapy in the treatment of Parkinson's disease
      (2) Available as a formulation with levodopa, carbidopa, entacapone
      (3) Preferred over tolcapone because of lower hepatotoxicity
9. Anticholinergic drugs
   a. Examples
      (1) Benztropine
      (2) Trihexyphenidyl
   b. Only those agents with anticholinergic activity that enter the CNS are prescribed.
   c. These drugs also decrease the tremor and symptoms produced by a dopamine D_2 receptor antagonist such as haloperidol.

III. Therapeutic summary of selected drugs used to treat Parkinson's disease: (Table 11-2)

Dopamine is metabolized by MAO-B; norepinephrine and serotonin are metabolized by MAO-A.

Selegiline, a selective MAO-B inhibitor, produces less interaction with tyramine than the nonselective MAO inhibitors.

Tolcapone causes hepatotoxicity.

Table 11-2. **Therapeutic Summary of Selected Drugs used to Treat Parkinson's Disease**

Drugs	Clinical Applications	Adverse Effects	Contraindications
Mechanism: *Increases synaptic dopamine in brain*			
Levodopa Amantadine	Parkinson's disease Influenza A prophylaxis (amantadine)	GI distress Orthostatic hypotension Arrhythmias Psychosis Dyskinesia	History of melanoma Narrow-angle glaucoma
Mechanism: *Dopaminergic agonists*			
Apomorphine (IV only) Bromocriptine Pergolide (withdrawn) Pramipexole Ropinirole	Parkinson's disease Restless leg syndrome (ropinirole)	Somnolence Orthostatic hypotension Arrhythmias Psychosis Dyskinesia	Concomitant use with other sedatives
Mechanism: *Inhibition of peripheral dopa decarboxylase*			
Carbidopa Benserazide	Used with levodopa or levodopa and entacapone in Parkinson's disease	Dominated by levodopa	History of melanoma Narrow-angle glaucoma
Mechanism: *Inhibition of catechol-O-methyl transferase (COMT)*			
Entacapone Tolcapone	Parkinson's disease	Somnolence Orthostatic hypotension Arrhythmias Psychosis Dyskinesia Hepatotoxicity (tolcapone)	Liver disease (tolcapone)
Mechanism: *Inhibition of monoamine oxidase type B (MAO-B)*			
Rasagiline Selegiline	Parkinson's disease	GI distress Orthostatic hypotension Arrhythmias Psychosis Dyskinesia	Concomitant use of other MAO inhibitors or sympathomimetics
Mechanism: *Inhibits central muscarinic receptors*			
Benztropine Orphenadrine Procyclidine Trihexyphenidyl	Parkinson's disease Treat extrapyramidal symptoms of neuroleptic drugs	Atropine-like; more sedation Dry mouth Blurred vision Urinary retention Constipation Tachycardia ↑ intraocular pressure Hyperthermia	Narrow angle glaucoma

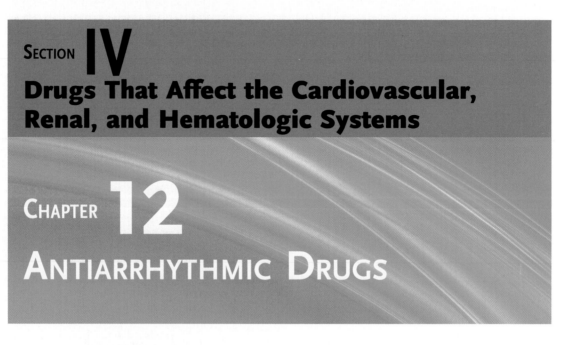

I. General Considerations

A. **Cardiac contraction** (Fig. 12-1): five-step process
1. Spontaneous development of the action potential in the sinoatrial (SA) node
2. Spread of the impulse through the atrium
3. Temporary delay of the impulse at the atrioventricular (AV) node
4. Rapid spread of the impulse along the two branches of the bundle of His and the Purkinje fibers
5. Spread of the impulse along the cardiac muscle fibers of the ventricles

B. **Electrophysiology of the heart**
1. Action potential (Fig. 12-2)
   a. The resting membrane potential of the myocardium (approximately –90 mV).
   b. Results from an unequal distribution of ions (high Na^+ outside, high K^+ inside).
2. Five phases of the action potential
   a. Rapid depolarization (phase 0)
      (1) Rapid inward movement of Na^+ due to the opening of voltage-gated sodium channels
      (2) Variation in resting membrane potential: –90mV to +15mV
   b. Initial rapid repolarization (phase 1)
      (1) Inactivation of sodium channels
      (2) Influx of Cl^-
   c. Plateau phase (phase 2)
      • Slow but prolonged opening of voltage-gated calcium channels
   d. Repolarization (phase 3)
      (1) Closure of calcium channels and K^+ efflux through potassium channels
      (2) Return of inactivated sodium channels to resting phase
   e. Diastole (phase 4)
      (1) Restoration of ionic concentrations by Na^+/K^+-activated ATPase (adenosine triphosphatase)
      (2) Restoration of resting potential
3. Important electrocardiographic (ECG) parameters (Fig. 12-3)
   a. P wave represents atrial depolarization
   b. PR interval equals the delay of conduction through the AV node
   c. QRS complex represents ventricular depolarization
   d. T wave represents ventricular repolarization
   e. QT interval equals duration of action potential in the ventricles

Know the five steps of the cardiac contraction.

Resting potential about –90 mV; high extracellular Na^+ and high intracellular K^+.

Na^+/K^+ activated ATPase (digoxin sensitive) maintains cell membranes resting potential.

Slowed AV node conduction increases PR interval; example vagal slowing of heart.

Delayed repolarization prolongs QT interval; example Class IA and III antiarrhythmic agents.

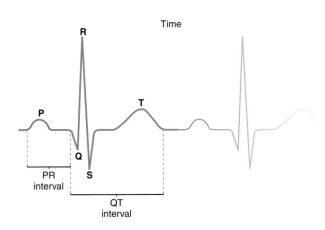

Superior vena cava

Sinoatrial node

Atrioventricular node

Bundle of His (common bundle)

Right atrium

Left atrium

Right ventricle

Left ventricle

Purkinje fibers

12-1: Schematic drawing of the heart.

Phase 0

SA node

Atrium

AV node

Phase 0

Purkinje fibers

Ventricle

Phase 0

Outside

Na⁺ Ca²⁺   Na⁺

Inside

K⁺ K⁺

12-2: Schematic representation of cardiac electrical activity in the sinoatrial (SA) node and Purkinje fibers as well as ion permeability changes and transport processes that occur during an action potential. AV, atrioventricular.

Time

R

P

Q   S

T

PR interval

QT interval

12-3: Schematic electrocardiogram (ECG) showing depolarization and repolarization of the heart. The P wave is produced by atrial depolarization, the QRS complex by ventricular polarization, and the T wave by ventricular repolarization. The PR interval measures the conduction time from atrium to ventricle, and the QT interval measures the duration of the ventricular action potential. The QRS complex measures the intraventricular conduction time.

II. Arrhythmias and Their Treatment
A. General
1. Arrhythmias are irregularities in heart rhythm
2. They result from disturbances in:
   a. Pulse generation
   b. Impulse conduction
   c. Or both
B. Antiarrhythmic drugs produce effects by altering one or more of the following factors:
1. Automaticity
2. Conduction velocity
3. Refractory period
4. Membrane responsiveness
C. These agents have varying effects on the electrophysiology of the heart (Table 12-1).

Disturbances in pulse generation or impulse conduction may result in arrhythmias.

Antiarrhythmic drugs target automaticity, conduction velocity, refractory period or membrane responsiveness.

TABLE 12-1. **Effects of Antiarrhythmic Drugs on the Electrophysiology of the Heart**

DRUG (CLASS)	SA NODE RATE	AV NODE REFRACTORY PERIOD	PR INTERVAL	QRS DURATION	QT INTERVAL
Quinidine (IA)	↑↓	↑↓	↑↓	↑↑↑	↑↑
Lidocaine (IB)	N	N	N	N	N
Propranolol (II)	↓↓	↑↑	↑↑	N	N
Sotalol (III)	↓↓	↑↑	↑↑	N	↑↑↑
Verapamil (IV)	↓↓	↑↑	↑↑	N	N

AV, atrioventricular; N, no major effect; SA, sinoatrial.

Class I drugs: sodium channel blockers

III. **Antiarrhythmic Drugs According to the Vaughn-Williams Classification** (Box 12-1)
    A. **Class I drugs: Sodium channel blockers**
        1. General
            a. All class I agents (Fig. 12-4)
                (1) Are also local anesthetics
                (2) Bind to open or inactivate sodium channels—use dependent binding
                (3) Inhibit phase 0 depolarization of the action potential
            b. Lidocaine is more effective in the treatment of ventricular arrhythmias
            c. Quinidine is more effective in the treatment of atrial arrhythmias

---

BOX 12-1   **ANTIARRHYTHMIC DRUGS**

CLASS IA (Binds to open sodium channels and extends ERP)
Disopyramide
Procainamide
Quinidine

CLASS IB (Binds to inactivated sodium channels and shortens ERP)
Lidocaine
Mexiletine
Tocainide

Class IC (Binds to all sodium channels; minimal effect on ERP)
Flecainide
Propafenone

Class II (Beta blockers)
Esmolol
Metoprolol
Propranolol

Class III (Potassium channel blockers; extend ERP)
Amiodarone
Dofetilide
Ibutilide
Sotalol

Class IV (Calcium channel blockers)
Diltiazem
Verapamil

Miscellaneous Antiarrhythmic Agents
Adenosine
Digoxin
Magnesium
Potassium

ERP, effective refractory period

12-4: Effects of class I antiarrhythmic drugs on the action potential and the electrocardiogram (ECG). ERP, effective refractory period.

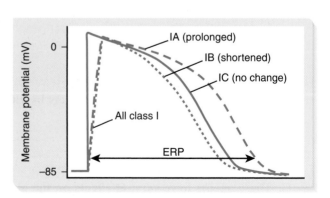

2. Class IA drugs
   - Block open or activated sodium channels, also block potassium channel; thus prolong action potential and effective refractory period (ERP)
     a. Examples
        (1) Quinidine
        (2) Procainamide
        (3) Disopyramide
     b. Quinidine
        (1) Mechanism of action
           (a) Inhibition of sodium channels, extending ERP, thereby decreasing myocardial conduction velocity, excitability, and contractility
           (b) Blockade of α-adrenergic receptors, producing vasodilation and leading to a reflex increase in the SA node rate
           (c) Blockade of I_K channels, prolonging duration of action potential
           (d) Blockade of muscarinic receptors, thereby decreasing vagal tone, thus increasing heart rate and enhancing conduction through AV node
        (2) Uses
           (a) Conversion to or maintenance of sinus rhythm in patients with atrial fibrillation, flutter, or ventricular tachycardia
           (b) Treatment of paroxysmal supraventricular tachycardia (PSVT)
           (c) Prevention of PSVT in patients with reentrant tachycardias Including Wolff-Parkinson-White syndrome
           (d) Also, has activity against *Plasmodium falciparum* malaria
        (3) Adverse effects
           (a) Torsades de pointes
              - Rapid, polymorphic ventricular tachycardia with a characteristic twist of the QRS complex
           (b) ECG changes
              Prolonged QRS complex
              Giant U wave
              - ST-segment depression
              - Flattened T wave
           (c) Diarrhea
           (d) Cinchonism
              - Giddiness
              - Lightheadedness
              - Ringing in the ears
              - Impaired hearing
              - Blurred vision
           (e) Thrombocytopenia
     c. Procainamide
        (1) This local anesthetic is equivalent to quinidine as an antiarrhythmic agent and has similar cardiac and toxic effects.
        (2) Additional adverse effect
           - Drug-induced lupus erythematosus (anti-histone antibodies)
        (3) The 2000 guidelines added intravenous procainamide to the cardiopulmonary resuscitation algorithm for refractory ventricular fibrillation/pulseless ventricular tachycardia.
3. Class IB drugs (see Fig. 12-4)
   a. Examples
      (1) Lidocaine
      (2) Tocainide
      (3) Mexiletine
   b. Mechanism of action
      (1) Bind to inactivated voltage gated sodium channels
      (2) Decrease the duration of the action potential and the effective refractory period
      (3) By inhibiting the slow Na^+ "window" current
   c. Lidocaine (also see Chapter 8)
      (1) Pharmacokinetics
         (a) Short-acting because of rapid hepatic metabolism (metabolic clearance)
         (b) Loading dose should be followed by continuous intravenous infusion.

Quinidine's block of α and muscarinic receptors is pro-arrhythmic by increasing heart rate and AV conduction.

Muscarinic receptor blocking activity: Disopyramide > quinidine > procainamide.

Quinidine *not* used much today clinically but often tested on Board Exams.

Class IA and III agents most likely to cause torsades de pointes; treat it with magnesium.

Quinidine may cause cinchonism.

About one third of patients who receive long-term procainamide therapy develop reversible lupus-related symptoms.

Procainamide is inactivated by N-acetyltransferase, longer effect in people who are slow acetylators

Quinidine and procainamide are effective against both atrial and ventricular arrhythmias.

Class I drugs and ERP: class IA, prolong ERP; class IB, reduce ERP; class IC, *no* change.

Lidocaine has a high "first pass" effect (metabolic clearance); parenteral only.

(2) Mechanism of action
    (a) Acts primarily on the Purkinje fibers
    (b) Depresses automaticity
    (c) Has a higher affinity for ischemic tissue
    (d) Suppresses spontaneous depolarizations in the ventricles
    (e) Breaks up reentry circuits

(3) Use

Lidocaine preferred agent to treat ventricular arrhythmias post-MI.

    (a) Considered the drug of choice for acute treatment of ventricular arrhythmias from myocardial infarction (MI), or cardiac manipulation.
    (b) The 2000 guidelines now consider lidocaine a second choice behind other alternative agents (e.g. amiodarone, procainamide) for the treatment of ventricular arrhythmias associated with cardiopulmonary resuscitation.
    (c) Also, used as a local anesthetic

(4) Adverse effects
    (a) Arrhythmias
    (b) Seizures (in elderly patients)

d. Tocainide and mexiletine
- Orally effective congeners of lidocaine
    (1) Pharmacokinetics
        (a) Resistant to first-pass hepatic metabolism
        (b) Half-life ($t_{1/2}$) of 8–20 hours

Mexiletine used to treat diabetic neuropathy.

    (2) Uses
        (a) Oral administration for treatment of ventricular arrhythmia
        (b) Treatment of diabetic neuropathy (mexiletine)
    (3) Adverse effects
        (a) Dizziness
        (b) Vertigo
        (c) Nausea
        (d) Vomiting
        (e) Arrhythmias

4. Class IC Drugs
  a. Examples
    (1) Flecainide
    (2) Propafenone
  b. Mechanism of action (see Fig. 12-4)
    (1) Bind to all sodium channels
    (2) Slow dissociation
    (3) Markedly slows phase 0 depolarization
    (4) *No* effect on the duration of the action potential

Class I drugs and ERP: class IA, prolong ERP; class IB, reduce ERP; class IC, no change.

Class IC agents increase mortality with chronic use.

  c. Uses
    (1) *Not* first choice agents because they are very pro-arrhythmogenic and increase mortality with chronic use
    (2) Used to treat life-threatening ventricular arrhythmias when other drugs fail

B. Class II drugs: β-Adrenergic receptor antagonists (see Chapter 5)

Class II drugs: β-adrenergic receptor antagonists.

  1. General
    a. Examples
      (1) Propranolol
      (2) Metoprolol
      (3) Esmolol (IV only)
    b. Class II drugs slow phase 4 depolarization in the SA node.

Class II agents slow phase 4 depolarization in SA node.

  2. Mechanism of action
    a. Blockade of β_1-receptors
    b. Reduce heart rate
    c. Reduce myocardial contractility
    d. Prolong AV conduction
    e. Prolong the AV refractory period

Propranolol is a nonselective beta blocker.

  3. Propranolol (see Chapter 5)
    a. Uses
      (1) Treatment and prophylaxis of PSVT and atrial fibrillation (orally effective)
      (2) Possible prevention of recurrent infarction in patients recovering from MI

(3) Also, used in the management of:
  (a) Hypertension
  (b) Angina pectoris
  (c) Pheochromocytoma
  (d) Essential tremor
  (e) Migraine prophylaxis
 b. Adverse effects
  (1) Sedation
  (2) Sleep disturbance
  (3) Sexual dysfunction
  (4) Cardiac disturbance
  (5) Asthma
4. Metoprolol
 a. Similar to propranolol but β_1-adrenergic selective
 b. Used to treat
  (1) Atrial fibrillation and atrial flutter
  (2) Angina pectoris
  (3) Hypertension
  (4) Hemodynamically-stable acute myocardial infarction
  (5) Ventricular arrhythmias associated with excess sympathetic activation
  (6) Atrial ectopy
  (7) Migraine prophylaxis
  (8) Essential tremor
  (9) Aggressive behavior
5. Esmolol
 a. Pharmacokinetics
  (1) Very short-acting ($t_{1/2} = 9$ min)
  (2) Administered by intravenous infusion
 b. Uses
  (1) Short-term control of supraventricular tachyarrhythmias, including sinus tachycardia and PSVT
  (2) Emergency control of ventricular rate in patients with atrial fibrillation or atrial flutter
 c. Adverse effects
  (1) AV block
  (2) Cardiac arrest
  (3) Hypotension

C. Class III: Potassium channel blockers
1. General
 a. Examples
  (1) Amiodarone
  (2) Dofetilide
  (3) Ibutilide
  (4) Sotalol
 b. Class III drugs increase the duration of the action potential because they block potassium channels (Fig. 12-5).
2. Mechanism of action (see Fig. 12-5)
 a. Prolong repolarization
 b. Increase the ERP
3. Amiodarone
 a. Pharmacokinetics
  (1) Long $t_{1/2}$ (13–103 days)
  (2) To achieve therapeutic levels requires a 15–30 days loading dose regimen
 b. Mechanism of action
  (1) Inhibits adrenergic stimulation; alpha- and beta-blocking properties
  (2) Blocks voltage gated sodium channels
  (3) Blocks potassium channels; reason for Class III designation
  (4) Blocks calcium channels
  (5) Prolongs the action potential and refractory period in myocardial tissue
  (6) Decreases AV conduction and sinus node function
  (7) Blocks adrenergic receptors (noncompetitive)

Margin notes:

Both propranolol and metoprolol are used to treat essential tremor.

Don't use propranolol in patients with asthma.

Both propranolol and metoprolol are used for migraine prophylaxis..

Esmolol has a very short half-life ($t_{1/2} = 9$ min).

Esmolol for emergency treatment; propranolol for prophylactic treatment of supraventricular arrhythmias

Class III drug: potassium channel blockers

Class IA and class III are most likely to cause torsades de pointes.

Amiodarone has very complex pharmacokinetics.

Amiodarone has properties of Class I, II, III, and IV antiarrhythmic agents.

12-5: Effects of class III antiarrhythmic drugs on the action potential and the electrocardiogram (ECG). ERP, effective refractory period.

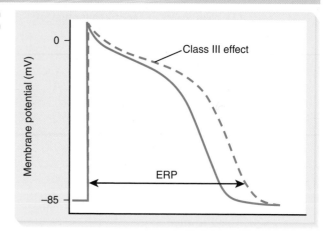

c. Uses
(1) Approved for atrial and ventricular arrhythmias
(2) The 2000 guidelines recommend that intravenous amiodarone be used prior to lidocaine in patients receiving life support for ventricular fibrillation/pulseless ventricular tachycardia.
(3) Amiodarone is very effective against both supraventricular (atrial fibrillation or flutter) tachycardia and ventricular arrhythmias, but its toxicity is worthy of consideration.

d. Adverse effects
(1) Cardiovascular effects
(a) Torsades de pointes
(b) ECG changes (prolonged QT interval and QRS complex)
(2) Liver effects
(a) Fatty change resembling alcoholic hepatitis
(b) Liver fibrosis
(3) Other effects
(a) Pulmonary reactions such as pneumonitis, fibrosis (most severe)
(b) Photodermatitis, paresthesias, tremor, ataxia, thyroid dysfunction, constipation
(c) Skin discoloration, corneal deposits

4. Sotalol
a. Mechanism of action
(1) An oral, nonselective β-adrenergic receptor antagonist
(2) Also blocks potassium channels
b. Uses
(1) Life-threatening sustained ventricular tachycardia
(2) Atrial fibrillation
c. Adverse effects
(1) Prolonged QT interval
(2) Torsades de pointes

5. Ibutilide (IV only)
a. Mechanism of action
(1) Blocks delayed rectifier potassium current
(2) Promotes the influx of sodium through slow inward sodium channels
(3) Converts atrial fibrillation or flutter to normal sinus rhythm without altering:
(a) Blood pressure
(b) Heart rate
(c) QRS duration
(d) PR interval
b. Use
• An intravenous Class III antiarrhythmic agent recommended for rapid conversion of atrial fibrillation or atrial flutter to normal sinus rhythm.

6. Dofetilide
a. Orally effective, class III antiarrhythmic agent
b. Used for the conversion and maintenance of normal sinus rhythm in atrial fibrillation/flutter in highly symptomatic patients

Amiodarone is very effective for treatment of acute arrhythmias *but* has numerous adverse effects when used long-term.

Amiodarone can produce life-threatening pulmonary fibrosis.

Sotalol blocks potassium channels and β-adrenergic receptors.

Intravenous ibutilide converts atrial fibrillation or flutter to normal sinus rhythm.

Oral dofetilide controls ventricular rate in antiarrhythmic drug-resistant patients with atrial fibrillation.

D. Class IV: Calcium channel blockers

 1. General

  a. Examples

   (1) Verapamil

   (2) Diltiazem

  b. Class IV drugs slow phase 4 depolarization in the SA node and decrease the heart rate (Fig. 12-6).

 2. Mechanism of action

  a. Blockade of calcium influx via a voltage-sensitive calcium channels (L-type)

  b. Effects on the myocardium

   (1) Reduce the rate of SA node discharge

   (2) Slow conduction through the AV node

   (3) Prolong the AV node refractory period (prolong the PR interval)

   (4) Decrease myocardial contractility

  c. Vasodilation

 3. Uses

  a. Acute and chronic management of PSVT

  b. Control of ventricular rate in atrial flutter or atrial fibrillation

   • Verapamil is more effective than digoxin

  c. Coronary artery vasodilator in Prinzmetal's angina

 4. Adverse effects

  a. Hypotension

  b. Dizziness

  c. Constipation (especially verapamil)

  d. Edema

  e. AV block

E. Miscellaneous antiarrhythmic drugs

 1. Adenosine

  a. Pharmacokinetics

   (1) In blood, $t_{1/2}$ about 10 seconds

   (2) Route of administration

    • Intravenous

  b. Mechanism of action

   (1) Enhances potassium conductance

   (2) Inhibits cyclic adenosine monophosphate (cAMP)–dependent calcium influx

  c. Uses

   (1) Drug of choice in the acute management of reentrant PSVTs

   (2) Including those associated with Wolff-Parkinson-White syndrome

 2. Digoxin (see Chapter 14); used to treat atrial fibrillation (decreases AV conduction) and heart failure

 3. Magnesium (intravenous)

  a. Mechanism of action

   (1) Unknown

   (2) But likely an anti-calcium effect

  b. Uses

   (1) Torsades de pointes

    • The 2000 guidelines conclude that intravenous magnesium during cardiopulmonary resuscitation is *only* effective for the treatment of patients with hypomagnesemic states or polymorphic ventricular tachycardia (torsades de pointes)

   (2) Digitalis-induced arrhythmias in patients who are in the hypomagnesemic state

Class IV drugs: calcium channel blockers

Verapamil has the strongest cardiac effects among the calcium channel blockers.

Verapamil is often used to control the ventricular rate of patients with atrial fibrillation.

Calcium channel blockers produce constipation and peripheral edema.

Adenosine is the drug of choice for prompt conversion of PSVT to sinus rhythm.

Digoxin is now used more to control ventricular rate than treat congestive heart failure.

Magnesium treats torsades de pointes.

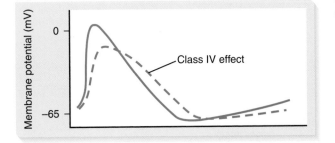

12-6: Effects of class IV antiarrhythmic drugs on the action potential.

Potassium treats digoxin cardiotoxicity.

Need to use oral anticoagulants (warfarin) in patients with atrial fibrillation.

    4. Potassium (intravenous)
      a. Treatment of hypokalemia
      b. Treatment of digoxin toxicity (arrhythmias or ECG changes) associated with hypokalemia

IV. Management of Atrial Fibrillation
    A. Consists of rate control and anticoagulation with warfarin (goal of international normalized ratio [INR] of 2-3)
      1. Rate control is defined as ventricular rate of 50–100 beats/minute with usual daily activities and *not* exceeding 120 beats/minute except with moderate to strenuous activity
      2. Recommended treatments
        a. Conventional rate control agents in young adults
          (1) Beta Blockers
          (2) Calcium channel blockers
          (3) Digoxin
        b. Rate control agents in patients with heart failure, coronary artery disease, or ongoing ischemia
          (1) Beta Blockers
          (2) Digoxin
        c. Amiodarone or others agents are useful:
          (1) When rate control with preferred agents fail
          (2) When cardioversion is anticipated.

V. Therapeutic summary of selected drugs used to treat arrhythmias: (Table 12-2)

TABLE 12-2. Therapeutic Summary of Selected Drugs used to Treat Arrhythmias

DRUGS	CLINICAL APPLICATIONS	ADVERSE EFFECTS	CONTRAINDICATIONS
Mechanism: *Bind to open sodium channels and also block potassium channels; prolong ERP*			
Class IA Disopyramide Procainamide Quinidine	Atrial arrhythmias Ventricular arrhythmias	Hypotension Syncope Anticholinergic Wide QRS complex Prolonged QT (Torasade de pointes) Cinchonism (quinidine) Thrompcytopenia (quinidine) SLE-like syndrome (procainamide)	Hypersensitivity With drugs that prolong QT Thrombocytopenia (quinidine)
Mechanism: *Bind to inactivated sodium channels; decrease ERP*			
Class IB Lidocaine (IV only) Mexiletine Tocainide	Ventricular arrhythmias from myocardial infarction Local anesthetic Neuropathic pain (mexiletine)	Many CNS effects Arrhythmias Seizures	Hypersensitivity Severe degrees of SA, AV, or intraventricular heart block
Mechanism: *Bind to all sodium channels; minimal effect on ERP*			
Class IC Flecainide Propafenone	Refractory ventricular arrhythmias	Increased mortality with chronic use Very pro-arrhythmogenic	Hypersensitivity Pre-existing second- or third-degree AV block Coronary artery disease
Mechanism: *β-Adrenergic receptor blockers*			
Class II Esmolol (IV only) Metoprolol Propranolol	Tachycardia Control ventricular rate in atrial fibrillation Intraoperative or postoperative arrhythmias (esmolol)	Bradycardia Hypotension Bronchoconstriction Hyperlipidemia Hyperkalemia Fatigue	Hypersensitivity Severe hyperactive airway disease Cardiogenic shock Severe sinus bradycardia Heart block
Mechanism: *Potassium channel blockers*			
Class III Amiodarone Dofetilide Ibutilide Sotalol	Life-threatening recurrent ventricular fibrillation Hemodynamically-unstable VT Heart rate control in patients with atrial fibrillation Conversion of atrial fibrillation to sinus rhythm (ibutilide)	Torsades de pointes Pulmonary toxicity (amiodarone) Bradycardia Arrhythmias Thyroid dysfunction (amiodarone)	Hypersensitivity Cardiogenic shock Pregnancy (amiodarone)

(Continued)

TABLE 12-2. **Therapeutic Summary of Selected Drugs used to Treat Arrhythmias—Cont'd**

DRUGS	CLINICAL APPLICATIONS	ADVERSE EFFECTS	CONTRAINDICATIONS
Mechanism: *Calcium channel blockers: slow action potential upstroke in SA and AV nodal tissue*			
Class IV Diltiazem Verapamil	Supraventricular tachyarrhythmias Control ventricular rate in atrial fibrillation Migraine (verapamil)	Constipation Bradycardia Hypotension	Hypersensitivity Second- or third-degree AV block Wolff-Parkinson-White syndrome Cardiogenic shock Congestive heart failure
Mechanism: *Slows conduction through AV node, interrupts re-entry pathways through the AV node, restores normal sinus rhythm*			
Adenosine	Conversion of PSVTs to normal sinus rhythm	Facial flushing Dyspnea Discomfort of neck, throat, jaw Headache	Hypersensitivity Second- or third-degree AV block or sick sinus syndrome
Mechanism: Unknown, but anti-calcium effect			
Magnesium	Torsade de pointes Prevention and treatment of seizures in severe pre-eclampsia or eclampsia Treatment of cardiac arrhythmias (VT/VF) caused by hypomagnesemia	Flushing Hypotension Diarrhea	Hypersensitivity Heart block Myocardial damage
Mechanism: *Suppression of the AV node conduction; increases effective refractory period; decreases conduction velocity; enhances vagal tone*			
Digoxin	Control ventricular rate in atrial fibrillation Congestive heart failure	All types of arrhythmias Gastrointestinal distress Visual disturbances (blurred or yellow vision)	Hypersensitivity Heart block Wolff-Parkinson-White syndrome
Mechanism: *Potassium, major cation; essential for the conduction of nerve impulses in heart, brain, and skeletal muscle; contraction of cardiac, skeletal and smooth muscles; maintenance of normal renal function, acid-base balance, carbohydrate metabolism, and gastric secretion*			
Potassium	Treatment or prevention of hypokalemia Treatment of digoxin cardiotoxicity	Hyperkalemia	Hyperkalemia

AV, atrioventricular; ERP, effective refractory period; PSVTs paroxysmal supraventricular tachycardias; SA, sinoatrial; SLE, systemic lupus erythematosus; VF, ventricular fibrillation; VT, ventricular tachycardia.

I. **General Considerations**

A. **Classification of blood pressure for adults aged 18 years or older** (Table 13-1).

B. **Treatment rationale**

1. Sustained hypertension leads to cardiovascular and renal damage, especially myocardial infarction (MI) and stroke.

2. Reducing blood pressure decreases risks of morbidity and death.

C. **Treatment methods**

1. First-line treatment
   • Diet and lifestyle changes
2. Second-line treatment
   • Pharmacologic intervention (Box 13-1)
   a. Without concomitant conditions, a thiazide-type diuretic should always be considered first
      (1) Effective
      (2) Well tolerated
      (3) Inexpensive
   b. Alternatives include
      (1) Angiotensin converting enzyme (ACE) inhibitors
      (2) Angiotensin receptor blockers (ARB)
      (3) β-adrenergic blockers
      (4) Calcium channel blockers (CCB)
      (5) Combination of the above
   c. Selection of pharmacologic treatment with concomitant conditions. Table 13-2 provides guidance.

II. **Diuretics** (see Chapter 15)

A. **General**

1. Diuretics decrease filling pressure of the heart (preload) and reduce peripheral resistance (decrease afterload).

2. Thiazides and thiazide-related diuretics are most often used because they have vasodilatory properties in addition to diuretic effects.

3. Thiazide-related compounds
   a. Chlorthalidone
   b. Indapamide
   c. Metolazone

4. Loop diuretics are only used in patients who *don't* respond or are allergic to thiazide diuretics (ethacrynic acid).

5. Potassium-sparing diuretics are usually used in combination with other diuretics to prevent loss of potassium.

B. **Use**

1. Hypertension (first-line therapy)

2. Thiazides are administered alone or in combination with other drugs.

C. **Adverse effects**

1. Hyponatremia

2. Hypokalemia (except with potassium-sparing diuretics)

3. Metabolic alkalosis

4. Hyperlipidemia

5. Hyperglycemia

Control of hypertension: decreased risk for stroke, myocardial infarction, renal failure

First line treatment: weight loss (most important), reduce sodium intake, stop smoking

Alternatives to thiazides for initial treatment of hypertension: ACEIs, ARBs, β-blockers, CCBs.

Diuretics decrease preload and afterload

Thiazide-related compounds: Chlorthalidone, indapamide, metolazone.

A thiazide or thiazide-like diuretic is a good medication to use first in treatment of hypertension.

Table 13-1. **Classification of Blood Pressure for Adults**

CATEGORY	SYSTOLIC, MM Hg	DIASTOLIC, MM Hg
Hypotensive	<90	or <60
Normal	**90–119**	**and 60–79**
Prehypertension	120–139	or 80–89
Stage 1 Hypertension	140–159	or 90–99
Stage 2 Hypertension	≥160	or ≥100

BOX 13-1   ANTIHYPERTENSIVE DRUGS

Diuretics
Loop diuretics
  Furosemide
Potassium-sparing diuretics
  Spironolactone
Thiazide diuretics
  Hydrochlorothiazide
Thiazide-like diuretics
  Chlorthalidone
  Indapamide
  Metolazone

Sympatholytics
β-Receptor Antagonists
  Atenolol
  Metoprolol
  Propranolol
α₁-Receptor Antagonists
  Doxazosin
  Prazosin
  Terazosin
α₂-Receptor Agonists
  Clonidine
  Methyldopa

Vasodilators
Calcium channel blockers
  Amlodipine
  Diltiazem
  Nifedipine
Others
  Hydralazine
  Minoxidil
  Sodium nitroprusside
  Fenoldopam

Renin/Angiotensin System Inhibitors
Angiotensin-converting Enzyme (ACE) Inhibitors
  Captopril
  Enalapril
  Lisinopril
  Ramipril
Angiotensin Receptor Blockers
  Losartan
  Valsartan
Renin Inhibitors
  Aliskiren

    6. Hyperuricemia
    7. Sexual dysfunction
  D. Contraindication
    • Patients with sulfonamide hypersensitivities
III. Sympatholytic Drugs
  A. β-Adrenergic receptor antagonists (see Chapter 5)
    1. Pharmacologic properties
      a. Mechanism of action
        • blockade of β receptors
          (1) Decrease heart rate and contractility
            • Decreases myocardial oxygen consumption
          (2) Decrease blood pressure
          (3) Decrease renin release
          (4) Decrease sympathetic outflow from the brain
      b. Use
        (1) A first-line drug therapy for hypertension
        (2) Especially in patients with heart failure or previous MI
      c. Adverse effects
        (1) Central nervous system (CNS) depression
        (2) Increased serum lipids
        (3) Hyperkalemia
        (4) Exacerbate asthma
        (5) Cardiac disturbances
        (6) Sexual dysfunction
    2. Selected drugs
      a. Propranolol (nonselective)
        • Inhibitor of both β₁ and β₂ receptors

Diuretics most commonly cause hyponatremia, hypokalemia, and metabolic alkalosis.

Loop diuretics, except ethacrynic acid, and all thiazide-type diuretics contain a sulfonamide structure and are contraindicated in patients with sulfonamide hypersensitivities.

Beta-blockers decrease sympathetic outflow from the brain via a different mechanism from the centrally-acting sympatholytics (clonidine).

Abrupt withdrawal of either beta blockers or clonidine leads to rebound hypertension.

Beta blockers all end in -olol (e.g., propranolol) except those that also block α receptors: labetalol, carvedilol.

106 Rapid Review Pharmacology

TABLE 13-2. Selection of Antihypertensive Drugs

PATIENT CHARACTERISTIC	MOST PREFERRED DRUGS	LEAST PREFERRED DRUGS
Demographic Traits		
African heritage	Calcium channel blocker, thiazide diuretic	—
Pregnancy	Methyldopa, hydralazine	ACE inhibitor, angiotensin receptor antagonist (ARB)
Lifestyle Traits		
Physically active	ACE inhibitor, calcium channel blocker, alpha blocker	Beta blocker
Noncompliance	Drug with once-daily dosage regimen; transdermal Clonidine (transdermal)	Oral centrally acting α-adrenoceptor agonist
Concomitant Conditions		
Angina pectoris	Beta blocker, diltiazem Verapamil	Hydralazine, minoxidil
Asthma, COPD	Calcium channel blocker, ACE inhibitor	Beta blocker
Benign prostatic hyperplasia	Alpha blocker	—
Collagen disease	ACE inhibitor (but not captopril), calcium channel blocker	Hydralazine, methyldopa
Depression	ACE inhibitor, calcium channel blocker	Centrally acting α-adrenoceptor agonist, beta blocker, reserpine
Diabetes mellitus	ACE inhibitor, calcium channel blocker, angiotensin receptor antagonist	Beta blocker, diuretic
Gout	—	Diuretic
Heart failure	ACE inhibitor, diuretic Hydralazine	Calcium channel blocker
Hypercholesterolemia	Alpha blocker, ACE inhibitor, calcium channel blocker	Beta blocker, thiazide
Migraine	Beta blocker, calcium channel blocker	—
Myocardial infarction	Beta blocker, ACE inhibitor, ARB	—
Osteoporosis	Thiazide	—
Peripheral vascular disease	ACE inhibitor, calcium channel blocker, alpha blocker	Beta blocker

ACE, angiotensin-converting enzyme; ARB, angiotensin receptor blocker; COPD, chronic obstructive pulmonary disease.

    b. Metoprolol (selective)
       (1) β_1-selective
       (2) Half-life ($t_{1/2}$) 3 to 4 hours
       (3) Extended release product available
    c. Atenolol (selective)
       (1) β_1-selective, with a longer half-life ($t_{1/2}$) of 6 to 9 hours
       (2) Better tolerated than propranolol in patients with asthma
       (3) Fewer CNS-related adverse effects than other β-adrenergic receptor antagonists (less lipid-soluble)

B. α_2-Adrenergic receptor agonists
    1. Methyldopa
      a. Mechanism of action
        • This centrally acting agent is converted to α-methylnorepinephrine, which stimulates α_2-adrenergic receptors in the CNS to decrease sympathetic outflow.
      b. Use
       (1) Methyldopa is the preferred drug to treat hypertension during pregnancy
       (2) Methyldopa is *not* considered a drug of choice in the elderly
      c. Adverse effects
       (1) Sedation
       (2) Dry mouth
       (3) Postural hypotension
       (4) Failure of ejaculation
       (5) Anemia
         (a) Triggers autoantibody production against red blood cell (RBC) Rh antigens (positive Coombs' test)
         (b) Causes warm (IgG-mediated) autoimmune hemolytic anemia

Methyldopa is the preferred antihypertensive during pregnancy.

Patients receiving methyldopa may have a positive Coombs' test; autoantibodies against Rh antigens

2. Clonidine
    a. Mechanism of action
        (1) Direct stimulation of central α_2-receptors
        (2) Decreases sympathetic and increases parasympathetic tone
        (3) Reduces:
            (a) Blood pressure
            (b) Heart rate
            (c) Renin secretion
    b. Use
        (1) Transdermal preparation should be considered for noncompliant patients.
        (2) Formulation for continuous epidural administration as adjunctive therapy with intraspinal opiates for treatment of cancer pain in patients tolerant to or unresponsive to intraspinal opiates
        (3) Unlabeled use for many CNS problems
            (a) Heroin or nicotine withdrawal
            (b) Severe pain
            (c) Dysmenorrhea
            (d) Vasomotor symptoms associated with menopause
            (e) Ethanol dependence
            (f) Prophylaxis of migraines
            (g) Glaucoma
            (h) Diabetes-associated diarrhea
            (i) Impulse control disorder
            (j) Attention-deficit/hyperactivity disorder (ADHD)
            (k) Clozapine-induced sialorrhea
    c. Adverse effects
        (1) Dry mouth
        (2) Sedation
        (3) Postural hypotension
        (4) Withdrawal from high-dose therapy may result in life-threatening hypertensive crises due to increased sympathetic activity.
C. **α_1-Adrenergic receptor antagonists** (see Chapter 5)
    1. Examples
        a. Prazosin
        b. Doxazosin
        c. Terazosin
    2. Mechanism of action
        a. α_1-Adrenergic receptor antagonists block α_1-receptors selectively on arterioles and venules, thus decreasing peripheral vascular resistance (afterload).
        b. These drugs relax the bladder neck and the prostate by blocking the α_1-adrenergic receptors located in smooth muscle.
    3. Uses
        a. Hypertension
        b. Benign prostatic hyperplasia (BPH)
    4. Adverse effects:
        a. Postural hypotension
            • First-dose effect, so start with half-dose and dose in evening
        b. Dizziness
        c. Decrease semen volume
        d. Must not be taken if patient is undergoing cataract surgery
IV. **Vasodilators**
A. **Overview**
    1. Directly relax vascular smooth muscles
    2. This leads to compensatory mechanisms and the need for the use of drug combinations to block these compensatory effects (Fig. 13-1)
B. **Hydralazine**
    1. Pharmacokinetics
        a. Oral bioavailability is dependent on the acetylation phenotype (*N*-acetyltransferase) of patients.
        b. About 50% of patients are *slow* acetylators and 50% are *fast* acetylators.
    2. Mechanism of action
        a. Relaxation of the vascular smooth muscle of the arterioles

Clonidine is the only antihypertensive agent available as a transdermal patch.

Clonidine has many non-labeled uses because of its CNS actions.

Clonidine causes dry mouth.

Withdrawal from clonidine should occur slowly (over 1 week) to avoid a hypertensive crisis.

Abrupt withdrawal of either beta blockers or clonidine leads to rebound hypertension.

All α_1-adrenergic receptor antagonists end in -zosin.

Tamsulosin and alfuzosin, selective for α_1-receptors in prostrate, treat BPH without producing orthostatic hypotension.

First-dose effect of alpha blockers can lead to profound hypotension.

Hydralazine is an arterial dilator.

13-1: Compensatory response to vasodilators when used to treat hypertension.

b. Causes reflex tachycardia and increased renin secretion
c. Which may be blocked by:
(1) Propranolol
(2) Centrally acting sympatholytics
3. Uses
a. Heart failure (with nitrates)
b. Hypertension (safe in pregnancy)
4. Adverse effects
a. Drug-induced systemic lupus erythematosus-like syndrome, which is reversible on drug withdrawal (10–20%)
b. Peripheral neuritis with paresthesias (numbness, pain, and tingling in the hands and feet)
• This effect can be prevented by the administration of pyridoxine.

C. Minoxidil
1. Pharmacokinetics
• A prodrug converted to minoxidil sulfate, an active metabolite
2. Mechanism of action
a. Induction of delay in the hydrolysis of cyclic adenosine monophosphate (cAMP) via inhibition of phosphodiesterase may contribute to vasodilatory action.
b. Increase in K^+ permeability leads to vasodilation.
c. A potent arteriolar dilator.
3. Uses
a. Hypertension
b. Facilitation of hair growth (topically)

Combination therapy with isosorbide dinitrate and hydralazine is especially effective in the African-American population.

Hydralazine and procainamide cause lupus-like adverse effects.

Minoxidil: antihypertensive that facilitates hair growth.

  4. Adverse effects
    a. Reflex tachyphylaxis
    b. Palpitations
    c. Hypertrichosis
 D. **Sodium nitroprusside**
  1. Pharmacokinetics
    a. Metabolic conversion to cyanide and thiocyanate may cause severe toxic reactions if the infusion of sodium nitroprusside is continued for several days.
    b. Arterial pressure may be titrated by intravenous administration because of its rapid action and short (minutes) half-life ($t_{1/2}$).
  2. Mechanism of action
    a. Occurs via the release of nitric oxide
    b. Involves relaxation of smooth muscle in both arterioles and venules
    c. Decreases both preload and afterload
  3. Uses
    a. Hypertensive emergencies
    b. Acute MI
    c. Aortic dissection
  4. Adverse effects:
    a. Hypotension
    b. Reflex tachycardia
    c. Cyanide toxicity
 E. **Calcium channel blockers** (see Chapter 12)
  1. Examples
    a. Amlodipine
    b. Diltiazem
    c. Nifedipine
    d. Verapamil
      • Extended-release or long-acting preparations are preferred for chronic use.
  2. Uses
    a. Control of elevated blood pressure by relaxation of smooth muscles
    b. Essential hypertension
    c. Chronic stable angina or angina from coronary artery spasm (Prinzmetal's angina)
    d. Atrial fibrillation or atrial flutter
  3. Adverse effects:
    a. Peripheral edema
    b. Frequent constipation (verapamil)
    c. Gingival hyperplasia ("-dipines")
 F. **Fenoldopam**
    • An intravenous dopamine DA_1 agonist used for the acute treatment of severe hypertension
V. **Drugs That Affect the Renin Angiotensin System (RAS)**
 A. **Angiotensin-converting enzyme (ACE) inhibitors**
  1. Examples
    a. Captopril
    b. Enalapril
    c. Lisinopril
    d. Ramipril
    e. There are many ACE inhibitors and all end in -pril
  2. Pharmacokinetics
    • Most, *except* captopril, are inactive prodrugs that are converted to the active metabolite (e.g., enalapril is converted to enalaprilate; ramipril is converted to ramiprilate)
  3. Mechanism of action
    a. Blockade of conversion of angiotensin I to angiotensin II by inhibiting ACE
    b. Inhibition of inactivation of bradykinin (cough, angioedema)
      • Bradykinin causes vasodilation and contributes to lowering of blood pressure
    c. Increased plasma renin due to decrease in angiotensin II and aldosterone
      • Angiotensin II has a negative feedback mechanism on renin secretion at the macula densa
    d. Decreases both preload and afterload

Nitroprusside: metabolic conversion to cyanide (systemic asphyxiant)

Nitroprusside: initial drug of choice in lowering blood pressure in aortic dissection.

All dihydropyridine calcium channel blockers end in -dipine: amlodipine, felodipine, isradipine, nicardipine, nisoldipine, nifedipine, nimodipine

Relative efficacy of calcium channel blockers as vasodilators: nifedipine > diltiazem > verapamil

Relative efficacy of calcium channel blockers in control of heart rate: verapamil > diltiazem > nifedipine

Calcium channel blockers are noted for causing hypotension and peripheral edema.

All ACE inhibitors end in -pril: benazepril, captopril, enalapril, fosinopril, lisinopril, moexipril, perindopril, quinapril, ramipril, trandolapril.

    e. Aldosterone-inhibitory effect is frequently lost over time
- Requires addition of aldosterone blocker

    f. Prevents vascular and cardiac hypertrophy and remodeling

4. Uses
    a. Hypertension
- Excellent choice in patients with diabetes mellitus

    b. Diabetic nephropathy
- Prevents progression of renal disease until patient gets better control of glucose levels

    c. Heart failure
    d. Post-MI

5. Adverse effects
    a. Dry hacking cough (bradykinin effect)
    b. Angioedema (life-threatening)
    c. Occasionally, acute renal failure in patients with bilateral renal artery stenosis
    d. Hyperkalemia

6. Contraindication
- Pregnancy

B. Angiotensin Receptor Blockers (ARBs)

1. Examples
    a. Losartan
    b. Candesartan
    c. Valsartan
    d. There are several and all end in -sartan

2. Mechanism of action
    a. Blockade of angiotensin II type 1 (AT_1) receptors
    b. More complete inhibition of angiotensin effects than ACE inhibitors
    c. *No* effect on bradykinin metabolism

3. Uses
    a. Hypertension
    b. Heart failure
    c. Diabetic nephropathy

4. Adverse effects
    a. Similar to those of the ACE inhibitors
    b. Usually *no* cough or angioedema; still can occur but very rarely
    c. Also, contraindicated during pregnancy
    d. Hyperkalemia

C. Renin Inhibitor
- Aliskiren

1. Pharmacokinetics
    a. Poor oral absorption
- Decreased by high-fat meal

    b. Aliskiren is a substrate of P-glycoprotein
- Concurrent use of P-glycoprotein inhibitors may increase absorption.

2. Mechanism of action
- A direct renin inhibitor

3. Use
- Treatment of hypertension, alone or in combination with other antihypertensive agents

4. Similar to ARBs

VI. Drugs Used in the Treatment of Hypertension Urgencies and Emergency (Box 13-2)

A. Hypertension urgency
- Goal is to relieve symptoms and bring blood pressure to reasonable level within 24 to 48 hours; aiming for optimal control over several weeks.

B. Hypertension emergency
- Goal is to reduce mean arterial pressure by 25% in 1 to 2 hours; then to reduce blood pressure to 160/100 mm Hg over next 6 to 12 hours.

V. Therapeutic summary of selected drugs used to treat hypertension: (Table 13-3)

BOX 13-2	DRUGS USED IN THE EMERGENCY TREATMENT OF HYPERTENSION

Intravenous Agents	Oral Agents
Diazoxide	Captopril
Enalaprilat	Clonidine
Esmolol	Nifedipine
Fenoldopam	
Hydralazine	
Labetalol	
Nicardipine	
Nitroglycerin, intravenous	
Sodium nitroprusside	

TABLE 13-3. : Therapeutic Summary of Selected Drugs used to Treat Hypertension

DRUGS	CLINICAL APPLICATIONS	ADVERSE EFFECTS	CONTRAINDICATIONS
Mechanism: *Inhibits sodium reabsorption in the distal tubules; increases excretion of sodium, water, potassium and hydrogen ions*			
Thiazide-type diuretics	Management of mild to moderate hypertension	Hyponatremia	Sulfonamide hypersensitivity
Hydrochlorothiazide	Treatment of edema in congestive	Hypokalemia (except with potassium-sparing diuretics)	Pregnancy
Chlorthalidone	heart failure and nephrotic		Anuria
Indapamide	syndrome	Hyperuricemia	
Metolazone		Sexual dysfunction	
		Hyperglycemia	
		Hyperlipidemia	
Mechanism: *β-Receptor antagonists*			
Atenolol	Hypertension	AV block	Lung disease
Metoprolol	Angina	Bronchospasm	Cardiogenic shock
Nadolol	Supraventricular arrhythmias	Sedation	Heart block
Propranolol	Migraine headache (propranolol)	Wheezing	
Timolol	Essential tremor	Mask hypoglycemia	
Releases nitric oxide	Glaucoma (timolol)		
Nebivolol			
Also block alpha receptors			
Labetalol			
Carvedilol			
Mechanism: *α₁-Receptor antagonists*			
Doxazosin	Hypertension	First-dose postural hypotension	Concurrent use with
Prazosin	Benign prostatic hyperplasia (BPH)	Nasal congestion	phosphodiesterase-5
Terazosin		Hepatotoxicity	(PDE-5) inhibitors such as
		Pancreatitis	sildenafil
Mechanism: *α₂-Receptor agonists; centrally acting*			
Clonidine	Hypertension	Bradycardia	Hypersensitivity
Methyldopa	CNS effects (clonidine)	Dry mouth	Hepatic disease (methyldopa)
		Constipation	
		Sedation	
		Autoimmune hemolytic anemia (methyldopa)	
Mechanism: *Calcium channel blockers*			
Amlodipine	Hypertension	Peripheral edema	Hypersensitivity
Diltiazem	Angina pectoris	Constipation	Heart failure
Nifedipine	Atrial fibrillation	Headache	
Verapamil	Atrial fluter		
Mechanism: *Angiotensin-converting enzyme (ACE) inhibitors; decrease preload afterload and cardiac remodeling*			
Benazepril	Hypertension	Dry hacking cough	Hypersensitivity
Captopril	Diabetic nephropathy	Angioedema	Pregnancy
Enalapril	Heart failure	Hyperkalemia	
Fosinopril	Post-MI	Hypotension	
Lisinopril			
Moexipril			
Perindopril			
Quinapril			
Ramipril			
Trandolapril			

(Continued)

TABLE 13-3. : **Therapeutic Summary of Selected Drugs used to Treat Hypertension—Cont'd**

DRUGS	CLINICAL APPLICATIONS	ADVERSE EFFECTS	CONTRAINDICATIONS
Mechanism: *Angiotensin receptor blockers (ARB) inhibitors; decrease preload afterload and cardiac remodeling*			
Candesartan Eprosartan Irbesartan Losartan Olmesartan Telmisartan Valsartan	Hypertension Diabetic nephropathy Heart failure Post-MI	Hyperkalemia Hypotension	Hypersensitivity Pregnancy
Mechanism: *Renin inhibitor; decrease preload afterload and cardiac remodeling*			
Aliskiren	Hypertension Diabetic nephropathy	Hyperkalemia Hypotension	Hypersensitivity Pregnancy
Mechanism: *Potent arteriolar dilators*			
Hydralazine Minoxidil	Hypertension Hypertension emergency Prevent hair loss (minoxidil)	Hypotension Reflex tachycardia Peripheral edema Hypertrichosis	Hypersensitivity
Mechanism: *Nitric oxide donor; arteriole and venule dilator*			
Sodium nitroprusside	Management of hypertensive crises; aortic dissection Congestive heart failure for controlled hypotension to reduce bleeding during surgery	Headache Hypotension Palpitation Increased cyanide	Hypersensitivity
Mechanism: *DA, agonist; vasodilation*			
Fenoldopam	Hypertension emergency	Angina Facial flushing Excessive hypotension Headache	Hypersensitivity

AV, atrioventricular; CNS, central nervous system; DA, dopamine; MI, myocardial infarction.

CHAPTER 14
OTHER CARDIOVASCULAR DRUGS

I. General Considerations
A. Goal of antianginal therapy
- Decrease oxygen demand of myocardial tissue or increase oxygen supply (Fig. 14-1).

B. Antianginal drugs
1. Used to treat angina pectoris caused by myocardial ischemia (Box 14-1).
2. Vasodilator action on the coronary, cerebral, and peripheral vascular beds

C. Coronary blood flow
1. Depends on:
   a. Aortic diastolic pressure
   b. Duration of diastole
   c. Resistance of the coronary vascular bed

D. Metabolic modulators
1. Myocardium generates energy from metabolism of fatty acids.
2. Use of pFOX inhibitors (e.g., trimetazidine) shifts metabolism to glucose metabolism, which is more efficient in generating adenosine triphosphate (ATP) in the ischemic heart.
3. Ranolazine initially assigned to pFOX inhibitor group; now believed to block a late sodium current that facilitates calcium entry via the sodium-calcium exchanger.

II. Antianginal Drugs
A. Nitrites and nitrates
1. Pharmacokinetics
   - Classification is primarily based on duration of action.
     a. Rapid-acting agents
        (1) Amyl nitrite (inhalation)
        (2) Nitroglycerin (intravenous, sublingual)
     b. Long-acting agents
        (1) Isosorbide dinitrate (regular oral, sustained-release oral, sublingual)
        (2) Nitroglycerin (transdermal, ointment, sustained-release oral)
        (3) Isosorbide dinitrate (regular oral, sustained-release oral)
2. Mechanism of action
   a. Vasorelaxation mechanism
      (1) Release of the nitrite ion
      (2) Nitrite metabolized to nitric oxide (NO)
      (3) NO activates guanylyl cyclase
         - Increases cyclic guanosine monophosphate (cGMP) levels
      (4) cGMP relaxes vascular smooth muscle
   b. Nitrates do *not* increase total coronary blood flow in patients with ischemia
      (1) But, they redistribute blood to ischemic areas by dilating large supply epicardial arteries
      (2) Thus, correcting the myocardial oxygen imbalance (see Fig. 14-1).
   c. Effects of nitrate-induced vasodilation
      (1) Increases venous capacitance (reducing preload)
      (2) Decreases arteriole resistance (decreases afterload)
      (3) Preload is affected more greatly (decreased return of blood to right heart) than afterload.
      (4) Reduction of preload and afterload lowers oxygen demand.

Objective of antianginal therapy: to balance O_2 demand with O_2 supply in myocardial tissue.

Ischemic heart preferentially uses fatty acid oxidation rather than glucose oxidation to generate ATP.

Both sodium nitroprusside and organic nitrates increase cGMP levels via a nitric oxide-dependent mechanism.

Nitrate-induced vasodilation results in

Nitrates redistribute blood to ischemic areas but do *not* increase overall coronary blood flow.

Nitrates reduce preload more than afterload because they dilate large veins.

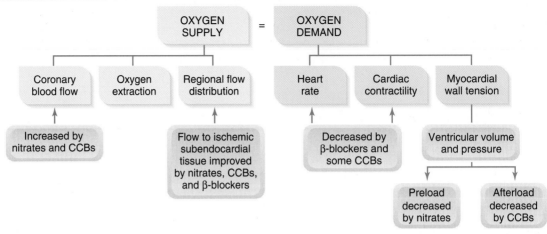

14-1: Effects of nitrates, calcium channel blockers (CCBs), and beta blockers on myocardial oxygen supply and demand.

BOX 14-1 ANTIANGINAL DRUGS	
Nitrites and Nitrates	**Calcium Channel Blockers**
Amyl nitrite	Amlodipine
Isosorbide dinitrate	Diltiazem
Isosorbide mononitrate	Nifedipine
Nitroglycerin	Verapamil
β-Adrenergic Receptor Antagonists	**Metabolic Modulators**
Atenolol	Ranolazine
Metoprolol	
Propranolol	

d. Drugs used to treat erectile dysfunction (ED)
  (1) Discussed with the nitrates because:
    (a) Nitrates increase the formation of cGMP
    (b) ED drugs, selectively inhibit the breakdown of cGMP
       Inhibit phosphodiesterase type 5 (PDE-5) in the corpus cavernosum
  (2) Drugs include:
    (a) Sildenafil; duration 2 to 4 hours
    (b) Tadalafil; duration up to 36 hours
    (c) Vardenafil; duration 2 to 6 hours
  (3) Should *not* be given concomitantly with other vasodilators, including nitrates
  (4) Should stop taking these drugs with either vision or hearing loss
  (5) Sildenafil is *also* used to treat pulmonary arterial hypertension
3. Uses of nitrates
  a. Treatment of acute angina pectoris
  b. Prophylaxis of angina attacks
  c. Treatment of heart failure (with hydralazine)
  d. Treatment of hypertensive emergencies, control of perioperative hypertension
4. Adverse effects
  a. Headaches (usually transient)
  b. Dizziness
  c. Hypotension
  d. Flushing
  e. Reflex tachycardia
  f. Methemoglobinemia (nitrites)
    (1) Methemoglobin contains oxidized iron (ferric)
    (2) Methemoglobin *cannot* bind to oxygen
5. Tolerance
  a. Develops and disappears rapidly (2–3 days)
    • Headaches disappear as tolerance develops
  b. Limits the usefulness of nitrates in continuous prophylaxis
    • To counter tolerance, patches are usually removed between 10 PM and 6 AM.

ED drugs inhibit phosphodiesterase; hence increasing cGMP.

Don't use sildenafil type ED drugs with organic nitrates.

"Monday disease": Industrial workers had severe headaches on Monday from organic nitrates in the workplace; each day the headache was less due to tolerance. The tolerance was reversed over the weekend and the cycle started again on Monday.

B. **β-Adrenergic receptor antagonists** (see Chapter 5)
1. Mechanism of action
   a. β-Adrenergic receptor antagonists inhibit the reflex tachycardia produced by nitrates.
   b. Myocardial oxygen requirements are reduced due to decreases in:
      (1) Heart rate
      (2) Myocardial contractility
      (3) Blood pressure
2. Uses
   a. Angina (in combination with other drugs, such as nitrates)
   b. Other uses described in Chapter 5

> Beta blockers reduce heart rate and blood pressure, leading to relief of angina and improved exercise tolerance in patients with severe angina.
>
> Beta blockers are *not* effective in treating Prinzmetal's angina.

C. **Calcium channel blockers** (see Chapter 12)
1. Mechanism of action
   a. Block calcium movement into cells, inhibiting excitation-contraction coupling in myocardial and smooth muscle cells
   b. Reduced:
      (1) Heart rate
      (2) Blood pressure
      (3) Contractility
2. Uses
   a. Ischemic coronary artery disease
   b. Prinzmetal's or variant angina
   c. Also, used to treat hypertension and arrhythmias

> Calcium channel blockers are effective in the treatment of Prinzmetal's angina.

3. Adverse effects
   a. Flushing
   b. Edema
   c. Dizziness
   d. Constipation

D. **Metabolic Modulator**
- Ranolazine
  1. Mechanism of action
     a. Ranolazine was first reported as a pFOX inhibitor
     b. Inhibits fatty acid oxidation shifting myocardial metabolism to glucose
     c. Leads to more efficient production of ATP in ischemic tissue
     d. Now believed to inhibit the late phase of the inward sodium channel (late I_{Na}) in ischemic cells during cardiac repolarization reducing intracellular sodium concentrations; this leads to:
        (1) Reduced calcium influx via Na^+/Ca^{2+} exchange
        (2) Decreased intracellular calcium
        (3) Reduced ventricular tension and myocardial oxygen consumption

> pFOX inhibitor: inhibits fatty acid oxidation; shifts metabolism to glucose for energy.

  2. Use
     - Treatment of refractory chronic angina in combination with amlodipine, beta blockers, or nitrates

E. **Therapeutic summary of selected drugs used to treat angina:** (Table 14-1)

III. **Drugs That Affect Cholesterol and Lipid Metabolism**
A. **General considerations**
1. Hyperlipidemia is defined as high levels of serum lipids.
   a. Primary hyperlipidemia is caused by genetic predisposition.
   b. Secondary hyperlipidemia arises as a complication of disease states, such as:
      (1) Diabetes
      (2) Hypothyroidism
      (3) Cushing's disease
      (4) Acromegaly
2. Atherosclerosis may result from the following contributing factors:
   a. High levels of plasma lipids (particularly low density lipoprotein)
   b. Metabolic syndrome (hyperinsulinemia)
   c. Inflammation
3. Therapy
   a. First-line treatment
      - Control by diet and lifestyle modifications
   b. Second-line treatment
      - Pharmacologic intervention (Box 14-2; Table 14-2)
   c. The metabolism of lipoproteins and the mechanism of action of some antihyperlipidemic drugs are summarized in Fig. 14-2.

> Diet and lifestyle changes are first-line and drug second-line therapy for hyperlipidemias.

TABLE 14-1. **Therapeutic Summary of Selected Drugs used to Treat Angina**

DRUGS	CLINICAL APPLICATIONS	ADVERSE EFFECTS	CONTRAINDICATIONS
Mechanism: *Metabolized to nitric oxide that activates guanylyl cyclase, increasing cyclic guanosine monophosphate (cGMP) levels, which in turn relaxes vascular smooth muscle*			
Amyl nitrite Isosorbide dinitrate Isosorbide mononitrate Nitroglycerin	Treatment of acute angina pectoris Prophylaxis of angina attacks Treatment of heart failure (with hydralazine) Treatment of hypertensive emergencies Control of perioperative hypertension	Headaches Dizziness Hypotension Peripheral edema Reflex tachycardia	Hypersensitivity Head trauma Concurrent use with phosphodiesterase-5 inhibitors (sildenafil, tadalafil, or vardenafil) Angle-closure glaucoma
Mechanism: *β-Adrenergic receptor antagonists*			
Atenolol Metoprolol Propranolol	Angina Hypertension Essential tremor Arrhythmias Migraine prophylaxis	AV block Bronchospasm Sedation Wheezing Mask hypoglycemia	Lung disease Cardiogenic shock Heart block
Mechanism: *Calcium channel blockers: Decrease cardiac work load and vasodilation (especially dihydropyridines)*			
Amlodipine Diltiazem Nifedipine Verapamil	Angina Supraventricular tachyarrhythmias Control ventricular rate in atrial fibrillation Migraine (verapamil)	Constipation Bradycardia Hypotension	Hypersensitivity Second- or third-degree AV block Wolff-Parkinson-White syndrome Cardiogenic shock Congestive heart failure

AV, atrioventricular.

BOX 14-2   DRUGS USED IN THE TREATMENT OF HYPERCHOLESTEROLEMIA

Bile Acid-Binding Resins
Cholestyramine
Colestipol
Colesevelam

HMG-CoA Reductase Inhibitors
Atorvastatin
Fluvastatin
Lovastatin
Pravastatin
Rosuvastatin
Simvastatin

Lipoprotein Lipase Stimulators
Gemfibrozil
Fenofibrate
Niacin

Inhibitors of Cholesterol Absorption
Ezetimibe

HMG-CoA, 3-hydroxy-3-methylglutaryl coenzyme A

Table 14-2. **Effects of Drug Therapy on Serum Lipid Concentrations**

DRUG OR CLASS EFFECTS	LDL CONCENTRATION (%)	HDL CONCENTRATION (%)	TOTAL DECREASE IN TRIGLYCERIDE CONCENTRATION (%)	OTHER
HMG-CoA reductase inhibitors	↓ 10–15	↑ 10	↓ 10–20	Increase in hepatic LDL receptors
Bile acid-binding resins	↓ 20–40	↑ 0–2	↑ 0–5	Increase in hepatic LDL receptors
Gemfibrozil	↓ 10	↑ 10–25	↓ 40–50	Activation of lipoprotein lipase
Niacin (nicotinic acid)	↓ 10	↑ 20–80	↓ 10–15	Decrease in lipolysis and lipoprotein levels

HDL, high-density lipoprotein; HMG-CoA, 3-hydroxy-3-methylglutaryl coenzyme A, LDL, low-density lipoprotein.

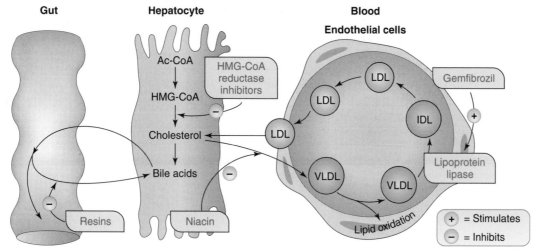

14-2: Sites of action and mechanisms of drugs used in the treatment of hyperlipidemia. The bile acid resins decrease the reabsorption of bile acids from the gut. The 3-hydroxy-3-methylglutaryl coenzyme A(HMG-CoA) reductase inhibitors block the rate-limiting step of cholesterol synthesis. Niacin affects lipid metabolism, transport, and clearance. Gemfibrozil stimulates lipoprotein lipase. IDL, intermediate-density lipoprotein; LDL, low-density lipoprotein; VLDL, very low density lipoprotein; Ac-CoA, acetyl-coenzyme A.

B. Bile acid-binding resins (see Box 14-2)
  1. Examples
     a. Cholestyramine
     b. Colestipol
     c. Colesevelam
  2. Mechanism of action
     a. Resins bind bile acids in the intestine to form an insoluble, nonabsorbable complex that is excreted in the feces along with the unchanged resin.
     b. This action causes:
        (1) Increase in the conversion of plasma cholesterol (CH) to bile acids
        (2) Increased expression of low-density lipoprotein (LDL) receptors, thus decreasing plasma cholesterol levels
  3. Uses
     • Should be administered with each meal
     a. Elevated LDL level (in combination with other drugs)
     b. Heterozygous familial hypercholesterolemia (but not effective in the homozygous form)
     c. Reduction of itching (pruritus) in cholestasis
     d. Binding of toxicological agents such as digoxin
     e. Adjunctive treatment of pseudomembranous colitis (binds *Clostridium difficile* toxin)
  4. Adverse effects
     a. Nausea
     b. Malabsorption of fat-soluble vitamins (e.g., vitamin K) and other drugs, such as digoxin, iron salts, tetracycline, and warfarin in the intestine due to the binding of these drugs to the resin
     c. Constipation
C. HMG-CoA (3-hydroxy-3-methylglutaryl coenzyme A) reductase inhibitors (see Box 14-2)
  1. Examples ("Statins")
     a. Atorvastatin
     b. Fluvastatin
     c. Lovastatin
     d. Pravastatin
     e. Rosuvastatin
     f. Simvastatin
  2. Mechanism of action
     a. The "statins" inhibit HMG-CoA reductase (the rate-limiting step in cholesterol synthesis), thereby decreasing cholesterol levels

Bile acid binding resins decrease bile acid uptake, thus more CH is converted to bile acids lowering CH levels and upregulating liver LDL receptors.

Bile acid binding sequestrants disrupt enterohepatic cycle.

Resins are *not* effective in homozygous familial hyperlipidemia; they do *not* express LDL receptors.

All these drug names end in -statin: atorvastatin, fluvastatin, lovastatin, pravastatin, rosuvastatin, simvastatin.

Statins inhibit HMG-CoA reductase (rate limiting enzyme of cholesterol synthesis)

b. The resulting increase in synthesis of LDL cholesterol receptors (up-regulation) in liver cells decreases plasma cholesterol.

c. May exert other beneficial effects as well, they:

    (1) Decrease C-reactive protein (CRP) in patients with CHD

        (a) CRP is increased in atherosclerotic plaques that are breaking down in the coronary artery (called inflammatory plaques)

        (b) Inflammatory plaques serve as the nidus for platelet thrombus formation in the coronary artery

        (c) Statin drugs stabilize inflammatory plaques, decreasing the risk for developing a coronary artery thrombosis

    (2) Enhance the endothelial production of NO

    (3) Increase plaque stability (see above)

    (4) Reduce lipoprotein oxidation

      • Oxidized low density lipoprotein is a free radical that enhances the formation of atherosclerotic plaques.

    (5) Decrease platelet aggregation

3. Uses

    a. Primary prevention of cardiovascular disease (CVD).

      • Reduces the risk of myocardial infarction (MI) or stroke in patients without evidence of heart disease who have multiple CVD risk factors or type 2 diabetes

    b. Secondary prevention of CVD

      • Reduce the risk of MI, stroke, revascularization procedures, and angina in patients with evidence of heart disease

    c. Treatment of dyslipidemias

      • Reduces elevations in total cholesterol, LDL-C, apolipoprotein B, and triglycerides in patients with elevations of one or more components, and/or to increase high-density lipoprotein-C (HDL-C) as present in type IIa, IIb, III, and IV hyperlipidemias

    d. Treatment of primary dysbetalipoproteinemia, homozygous familial hypercholesterolemia

    e. Treatment of heterozygous familial hypercholesterolemia

      • In adolescent patients (10–17 years of age, females >1 year postmenarche) having LDL-C of 190 mg/dL or LDL-C of 160 mg/dL with positive family history of premature CVD or with two or more CVD risk factors.

4. Adverse effects

    a. Elevated hepatic enzymes

    b. Skeletal muscle toxicity (elevated creatine kinase), myositis, rhabdomyolysis

      • Some studies show that HMG-CoA reductase inhibitors may decrease synthesis of coenzyme Q, which is a component in the oxidative phosphorylation pathway; hence, decreasing synthesis of ATP in muscle.

D. Lipoprotein lipase stimulators (see Box 14-2)

1. Fibric acid derivatives

    a. Examples

      (1) Gemfibrozil

      (2) Fenofibrate

    b. Mechanism of action

      (1) Ligands for the peroxisome proliferators-activated receptor-alpha (PPARα) protein

        • A receptor that regulates transcription of many genes involved in lipid metabolism

      (2) Activates lipoprotein lipase, promoting delivery of triglycerides to adipose tissue

      (3) Decreases hepatic triglyceride production

      (4) Interferes with the formation of very low density lipoprotein (VLDL) in the liver

    c. Uses

      • Treatment of hypertriglyceridemia in patients with hyperlipidemia (types IV and V) who are at greater risk for pancreatitis and who have *not* responded to dietary intervention

    d. Adverse effects

      (1) Myalgias

      (2) Cholelithiasis

      (3) Contraindicated in patients with pre-existing gallbladder disease

      (4) May increase LDL in patients with hypertriglyceridemia

---

Margin notes:

Statins should be given in the evening since most cholesterol synthesis occurs at night time.

Monitor liver functional enzymes (LFE) and muscle enzymes (creatine kinase) with -statins.

Fibric acid derivatives are best for lowering serum triglyceride levels.

Fibric acid drugs may aggravate gallbladder disease.

2. Niacin (nicotinic acid)
   a. Mechanism of action
     (1) Reduces hepatic VLDL secretion (like gemfibrozil)
     (2) Enhances VLDL clearance by activating lipoprotein lipase (like gemfibrozil)
     (3) Decreases LDL and triglycerides and increases HDLs
   b. Uses
     (1) Adjunctive treatment of dyslipidemias
       • Lowers the risk of recurrent MI and/or slow progression of coronary artery disease
     (2) Often used in combination therapy with other antidyslipidemic agents when additional triglyceride (TG)-lowering or HDL-increasing effects are desired
     (3) Treatment of hypertriglyceridemia in patients at risk of pancreatitis
     (4) Treatment of peripheral vascular disease and circulatory disorder
     (5) Treatment of pellagra
     (6) Dietary supplement
   c. Adverse effects
     (1) Generalized pruritus as a result of peripheral vasodilation, characterized by flushing, warmth, and burning or tingling of the skin, especially of the face or neck; reduced by:
       (a) Taking after meals
       (b) Taking aspirin 30 minutes prior to dose
       (c) Using extended-release formulations
     (2) Increased hepatic enzymes
     (3) Acanthosis nigricans
     (4) Leg cramps
     (5) Myalgia
     (6) Gout
     (7) Worsen type 2 diabetes
E. Drugs that prevent cholesterol absorption (see Box 14-2)
  • Ezetimibe
   1. The U.S. Food and Drug Administration (FDA) has communicated that, to date, *no* advantage has been found by using the ezetimibe/simvastatin combination, even though it lowered LDL cholesterol more effectively compared to simvastatin alone, there was *no* difference seen in mean change in carotid intima-media thickness; adverse events were similar between both groups.
   2. Selectively blocks the intestinal absorption of cholesterol and phytosterols
   3. Used as monotherapy or in combination with HMG-CoA reductase inhibitors (-statins) for the treatment of hypercholesterolemia
F. Therapeutic summary of selected drugs used to lower lipids: (Table 14-3)
IV. Inotropic Agents and Treatment of Heart Failure (Box 14-3)
  A. Drugs that should be considered in the treatment of heart failure (Fig. 14-3)
    1. Angiotensin-converting enzyme (ACE) inhibitors and angiotensin receptor blockers (ARBs)
     a. Decrease afterload
     b. Decrease preload
     c. Decrease remodeling
    2. β-adrenergic receptor antagonists (bisoprolol, carvedilol, metoprolol)
     a. Decrease heart work load
     b. Decrease remodeling
    3. Diuretics (especially loops)
    4. Vasodilators
     a. Nitrates
     b. Hydralazine
     c. Nesiritide
     d. Bosentan
    5. Positive inotropes (increase force of contraction)
     a. Digoxin
     b. Dobutamine
     c. Inamrinone
     d. Milrinone
  B. Digoxin (also, see Chapter 12)
    1. General
     a. Digoxin has a positive inotropic and various electrophysiologic effects on the heart

---

Fibric acid drugs and niacin lower VLDL levels.

Niacin is best for raising HDL; the good cholesterol.

Nicotinic acid: cheapest lipid-lowering drug; decreased CH and TG; increased HDL-CH.

Peripheral vasodilation occurs frequently with niacin; pretreatment with aspirin prevents this development.

Ezetimibe: selectively block intestinal reabsorption of CH

Drugs that inhibit the renin-angiotensin system decrease afterload, preload and remodeling.

Beta blockers are beneficial but calcium channel blockers are detrimental in patients with heart failure.

Digoxin: positive inotropic effect.

TABLE 14-3. **Therapeutic Summary of Selected Drugs used to Lower Lipids**

DRUGS	CLINICAL APPLICATIONS	ADVERSE EFFECTS	CONTRAINDICATIONS
Mechanism: *Binds with bile acids to form an insoluble complex that is eliminated in feces; thereby increases the fecal loss of bile acid-bound low-density lipoprotein cholesterol*			

Cholestyramine
Colestipol
Colesevelam
	Adjunct in management of
	  primary hypercholesterolemia
	Relief of pruritus associated with
	  elevated levels of bile acids
		Constipation
		Abdominal pain and distention, belching,
		  flatulence, nausea, vomiting, diarrhea
			Hypersensitivity

Mechanism: *Inhibiting of 3-hydroxy-3-methylglutaryl-coenzyme A (HMG-CoA) reductase; the rate-limiting step in cholesterol biosynthesis*			
Atorvastatin Fluvastatin Lovastatin Pravastatin Rosuvastatin Simvastatin	Primary prevention of cardiovascular disease Treatment of dyslipidemias	Elevated hepatic enzymes Skeletal muscle toxicity (↑creatine kinase) Myositis Rhabdomyolysis	Pregnancy Hypersensitivity Liver disease Breast feeding
Mechanism: *Ligands for the peroxisome proliferators-activated receptor-alpha (PPARα) protein, a receptor that regulates transcription of genes involved in lipid metabolism*			
Gemfibrozil Fenofibrate	Hypertriglyceridemia	Dyspepsia Myalgias Cholelithiasis	Hypersensitivity Liver disease Renal disease Pre-existing gallbladder disease
Mechanism: *Reduces hepatic VLDL secretion; enhances VLDL clearance by activating lipoprotein lipase, decreases LDL and triglycerides and increases HDLs*			

Niacin
  (nicotinic
  acid)
	Adjunctive treatment of
	  dyslipidemias
	Treatment of
	  hypertriglyceridemia
	Treatment of pellagra
	Dietary supplement
		Facial flushing
		Acanthosis nigricans
		Leg cramps
		Myalgia
		Gout
		Worsen diabetes
			Hypersensitivity
			Liver disease
			Active peptic ulcers

Mechanism: *Inhibits absorption of cholesterol at the brush border of the small intestine via the sterol transporter*			
Ezetimibe	Primary hypercholesterolemia; Usually in combination with other drugs	Diarrhea Transaminases increased Arthralgia	Pregnancy Hypersensitivity Liver disease Breast feeding

HDL, high-density lipoprotein; LDL, low-density lipoprotein; VLDL, very low-density lipoprotein.

BOX 14-3 **DRUGS USED IN THE TREATMENT OF HEART FAILURE**

Digitalis Glycosides
Digoxin

Other Inotropic Agents
β-Adrenergics
Dobutamine
Dopamine
Phosphodiesterase Inhibitors
Inamrinone
Milrinone

Vasodilators
Bosentan
Hydralazine
Nesiritide
Nitrates
Sodium nitroprusside

Diuretics
Loop
Furosemide

Potassium-sparing
Eplerenone
Spironolactone
Thiazide
Hydrochlorothiazide

Angiotensin-converting Enzyme (ACE) Inhibitors
Captopril
Enalapril
Lisinopril

Angiotensin Receptor Blockers (ARBs)
Losartan
Valsartan

β-Adrenergic Receptor Antagonists
Bisoprolol
Carvedilol
Metoprolol

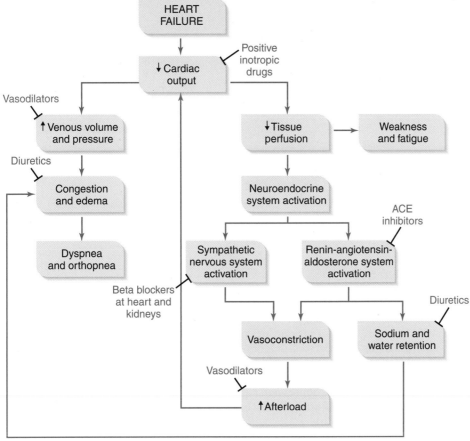

14-3: Algorithm of the pathogenesis and treatment of heart failure, indicating the sites where certain drugs may interfere with the development of heart failure. ACE, angiotensin-converting enzyme.

TABLE 14-4. Pharmacokinetic Parameters of Digitalis Glycosides

PARAMETER	DIGOXIN
Route of administration	Oral, intravenous
Oral bioavailability (%)	75
Time to peak effect (hr)	3–6
Volume of distribution (L/kg)	6.3*
Plasma protein binding (%)	20–40
Half-life (hr)	40
Elimination	Renal

*The large volume of distribution of digoxin is due to tissue protein binding; it is displaced by quinidine.

    b. It is derived from the leaves of the plant *Digitalis purpurea* (foxglove) or *D. lanata*

2. Pharmacokinetics (Table 14-4)
3. Mechanism of action (Fig. 14-4)
    a. Inhibition of Na^+/K^+-activated adenosine triphosphatase (ATPase), thus increasing the force of myocardial contraction by increasing available intracellular calcium
    b. Increase vagal stimulation, leading to decreased heart rate
    c. Slow conduction through the atrioventricular (AV) node
4. Uses
    a. Treatment of congestive heart failure
    b. To slow ventricular rate in tachyarrhythmias such as:
       (1) Atrial fibrillation
       (2) Atrial flutter
       (3) Supraventricular tachycardia (paroxysmal atrial tachycardia)
    c. Cardiogenic shock

Quinidine increases digoxin levels by interfering with tissue protein binding and renal excretion of digoxin.

Na^+/K^+-activated ATPase is the digoxin receptor.

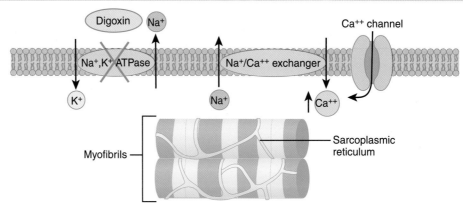

14-4: Mechanism of digoxin. *(From Kester M, et al.: Elsevier's Integrated Pharmacology. Philadelphia, Mosby, 2007, Figure 8-11.)*

    5. Adverse effects
      a. Toxicity
        (1) Nausea and vomiting (earliest signs of toxicity)
        (2) Mental status changes
        (3) Changes in color vision (green or yellow halos)
        (4) Changes on electrocardiogram
          (a) Decreased QT interval
          (b) Increased PR interval
          (c) ST-segment depression
          (d) All types of arrhythmias (most serious signs of intoxication)
      b. Treatment of toxicity
        (1) Discontinue medication
        (2) Correct either potassium or magnesium deficiency
        (3) Give digoxin antibody (digoxin immune Fab, or Digibind) for severe toxicity
    6. Precautions
      • The hypokalemia that often occurs with diuretic therapy increases the toxicity associated with digoxin therapy.
C. Diuretics (see Chapter 15)
    1. Decrease edema
    2. Loop diuretics are preferred for congestive heart failure (CHF) or pulmonary edema
    3. Thiazide diuretics are preferred for hypertension
D. Angiotensin-converting enzyme (ACE) inhibitors and angiotensin receptor blockers (ARBs) (see Chapter 13)
    1. Decrease peripheral resistance
    2. Decrease salt and water retention
    3. Decrease tissue remodeling
E. β-Adrenergic receptor antagonists (see Chapter 5)
    1. Increase life expectancy in patients with mild and moderate congestive heart failure
    2. Decrease workload on heart and accompanying remodeling
    3. Alpha/beta blocker (carvedilol) also effective in extending the life expectancy of CHF patients
F. Beta agonists in severe heart failure (see Chapter 5)
    1. Examples
      a. Dobutamine
      b. Dopamine
    2. Stimulate β_1 receptors in heart
    3. Positive inotropic agents that should be used for acute treatment only
G. Phosphodiesterase inhibitors
    1. Examples
      a. Inamrinone
      b. Milrinone

Toxicity: nausea and vomiting earliest sign of toxicity.

Digoxin has a low therapeutic index.

Potassium wasting diuretics increase the toxicity of digoxin.

ACE inhibitors all end in -pril.

ARBs all end in -sartan.

Metoprolol, bisoprolol, and carvedilol are the beta blockers that have been shown to prolong life expectancy in patients with heart failure.

Dobutamine and dopamine (β₁ receptor stimulants) are useful positive inotropes for acute heart failure.

2. Cyclic adenosine monophosphate (cAMP)-dependent inotropes and vasodilators, which are given intravenously for the short-term management of congestive heart failure

3. Long-term use is associated with increased morbidity and mortality rates.

   H. Vasodilators

     1. Hydralazine and organic nitrates (see Chapter 13)
- Decrease afterload and/or preload

     2. Nesiritide

       a. An intravenous recombinant form of a human brain natriuretic peptide (BNP), a naturally occurring hormone produced in the ventricles of the heart

       b. Indicated for the acute treatment of decompensated congestive heart failure (CHF)

     3. Bosentan

       a. An endothelin-receptor antagonist

       b. Indicated for use in primary pulmonary hypertension

I. Therapeutic summary of selected drugs used to treat heart failure (Table 14-5)

Inamrinone and milrinone inhibit phosphodiesterase-type 3 (increase cAMP); sildenafil type drugs inhibit phosphodiesterase-type-5 (increase cGMP).

Isosorbide dinitrate plus hydralazine is the preferred treatment of heart failure, as adjunct to standard therapy, in self-identified African-Americans.

Nesiritide, a BNP analogue, is used to treat decompensated CHF.

Bosentan, an endothelin-receptor antagonist, is used to treat primary pulmonary hypertension.

TABLE 14-5. Therapeutic Summary of Selected Drugs used to Treat Heart Failure

DRUGS	CLINICAL APPLICATIONS	ADVERSE EFFECTS	CONTRAINDICATIONS
Mechanism: *Inhibition of Na$^+$/K$^+$-activated ATPase*			
Digoxin	Congestive heart failure To slow the ventricular rate	All types of arrhythmias Gastrointestinal distress Visual disturbances (blurred or yellow vision)	Hypersensitivity Heart block Wolff-Parkinson-White syndrome
Mechanism: *β-Adrenergic agonist used as positive inotropes*			
Dobutamine Dopamine	Short-term management of patients with cardiac decompensation	Tachycardia Hypertension Thrombocytopenia	Hypersensitivity Idiopathic hypertrophic subaortic stenosis
Mechanism: *Positive inotrope that inhibits myocardial cyclic adenosine monophosphate (cAMP) phosphodiesterase activity and increases cellular levels of cAMP*			
Inamrinone Milrinone	Short-term therapy in patients with intractable heart failure	Arrhythmias Hypotension Thrombocytopenia	Hypersensitivity Severe aortic or pulmonic valvular disease
Mechanism: *Angiotensin-converting enzyme (ACE) inhibitors; decrease preload, afterload, and cardiac remodeling*			
Benazepril Captopril Enalapril Fosinopril Lisinopril Moexipril Perindopril Quinapril Ramipril Trandolapril	Hypertension Diabetic nephropathy Heart failure Post-MI	Dry hacking cough Angioedema Hyperkalemia Hypotension	Hypersensitivity Pregnancy
Mechanism: *Angiotensin receptor blockers (ARB) inhibitors; decrease preload, afterload, and cardiac remodeling*			
Candesartan Eprosartan Irbesartan Losartan Olmesartan Telmisartan Valsartan	Hypertension Diabetic nephropathy Heart failure Post-MI	Hyperkalemia Hypotension	Hypersensitivity Pregnancy
Mechanism: *Reduce preload and edema (see Chapter 15)*			

Diuretics
Loop
  Furosemide
Potassium-sparing
  Eplerenone
  Spironolactone
Thiazide
  Hydrochlorothiazide
	Congestive heart failure
	See Chapter 15
		See Chapter 15	Hypersensitivity
			See Chapter 15

(Continued)

TABLE 14-5. **Therapeutic Summary of Selected Drugs used to Treat Heart Failure—Cont'd**

DRUGS	CLINICAL APPLICATIONS	ADVERSE EFFECTS	CONTRAINDICATIONS
Mechanism: *Reduce afterload and/or preload by various mechanisms of vasodilatation*			
Vasodilators	Congestive heart failure	Hypotension	Hypersensitivity
Bosentan	Pulmonary artery hypertension	Reflex tachycardia	
Hydralazine		Severe headache	
Nesiritide			
Nitrates			
Sodium nitroprusside			
Mechanism: *Beta blockers known to decrease morbidity and mortality in patients with heart failure*			
Bisoprolol	Heart failure	AV block	Lung disease
Carvedilol	Hypertension	Bronchospasm	Cardiogenic shock
Metoprolol	Essential tremor	Sedation	Heart block
	Arrhythmias	Wheezing	
	Migraine prophylaxis	Mask hypoglycemia	

ATPase, adenosine triphosphatase, AV, atrioventricular; MI, myocardial infarction.

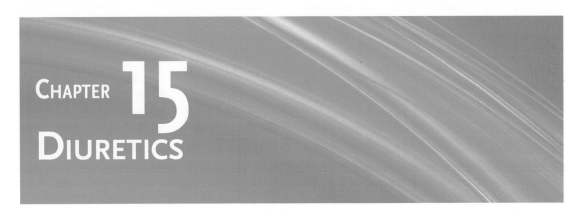

CHAPTER 15
DIURETICS

I. General Considerations
A. Role of the kidney
1. The kidney is the most important organ in maintaining body fluid composition.
2. It is the chief means of excreting most drugs and nonvolatile metabolic waste products.
3. It plays a fundamental role in maintaining pH, controlling levels of electrolytes and water, and conserving substances such as glucose and amino acids.

B. Functions of the renal nephrons
1. Glomerular filtration
   a. Blood is forced into the glomerulus and filtered through capillaries into the glomerular capsule.
      • The glomerular filtration rate (GFR) is 120 mL/min.
   b. Plasma filtrate is composed of fluids and soluble constituents.
   c. Substances normally *not* filtered include cells, plasma proteins and substances bound to them, lipids, and other macromolecules.
      • Approximately 99% of the filtrate is reabsorbed.
2. Tubular secretion
   a. This process involves the movement of substances from the blood into the renal tubular lumen.
   b. Many drugs are actively secreted by anion (e.g., penicillins and most other β-lactam drugs, glucuronide conjugates of drugs) or cation (e.g., protonated forms of weak bases and quaternary ammonium compounds) transport systems.
   c. Probenecid blocks anion transport and N-methylnicotinamide blocks cation transport in the kidney.

C. Review Chapter 2: Electrolyte and Acid-Base Disorders
Rapid Review: Laboratory Testing in Clinical Medicine

II. Diuretics
• Classification is based on sites (Fig. 15-1) and mechanisms of action (Table 15-1).

A. Carbonic anhydrase inhibitors (Box 15-1)
1. Examples
   a. Acetazolamide
   b. Brinzolamide
   c. Dorzolamide
2. Carbonic anhydrase inhibitors act in the proximal renal tubules (Fig. 15-2).
   a. Carbonic anhydrase is located in the brush border and cytosol of the proximal renal tubule (PRT) cells.
   (1) H$^+$ ions in the PRT are exchanged for filtered sodium (step 1).
   (2) H$^+$ ions combine with filtered bicarbonate in the brush border of the PRT to produce carbonic acid (H$_2$CO$_3$; step 2).
   (3) Carbonic anhydrase (c.a.) in the brush border dissociates H$_2$CO$_3$ to CO$_2$ and water, which are reabsorbed into the PRT (step 3).
   (4) In the PRT cytosol, c.a. reforms H$_2$CO$_3$, which dissociates into H$^+$ and bicarbonate (step 4).
   (5) Bicarbonate is reabsorbed into the blood and H$^+$ ions are exchanged for filtered sodium to repeat the cycle (step 5).
   (6) A Na$^+$/K$^+$-ATPase (adenosine triphosphatase) moves sodium into the blood (step 6).

GFR is 120 mL/min

Probenecid blocks renal anion transport

Carbonic anhydrase inhibitors: proximal tubule diuretic

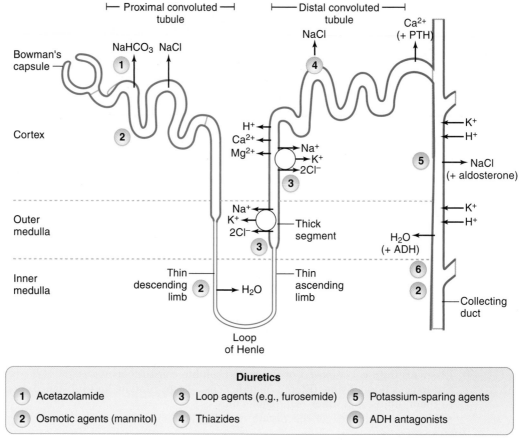

15-1: Tubule transport systems and sites of action of diuretics. ADH, antidiuretic hormone; PTH, parathyroid hormone.

TABLE 15-1. **Diuretics Mechanisms, Uses, and Adverse Effects**

DRUG CLASS (AGENT)	MECHANISM	USES	ADVERSE EFFECTS
Carbonic anhydrase inhibitors (acetazolamide)	Inhibit carbonic anhydrase in proximal tubule, changing composition of urine	Glaucoma Urinary alkalinization Acute mountain sickness Pseudotumor cerebri	Hyperchloremic normal anion gap metabolic acidosis
Loop diuretics (furosemide)	Inhibit $Na^+/K^+/2Cl^-$ symport along thick ascending limb of loop of Henle	Acute pulmonary edema Refractory edema Hypertension Hyperkalemia Ascites Hypercalcemia	Hyperglycemia Hyperuricemia Hypocalcemia Hypomagnesemia Volume depletion Hypokalemia Hyponatremia Metabolic alkalosis
Loop diuretics (ethacrynic acid)	Inhibit sulfhydryl-catalyzed enzyme systems responsible for reabsorption of sodium and chloride in proximal and distal tubules	Edema Sulfonamide sensitivity	Ototoxicity
Thiazide diuretics (hydrochlorothiazide)	Inhibit Na^+/Cl^- symport in early distal convoluted tubule	Hypertension Heart failure Nephrolithiasis Nephrogenic diabetes insipidus	Hypokalemic metabolic alkalosis Hypomagnesemia Hypercalcemia Hyperlipidemia Hyponatremia Hyperglycemia Hyperuricemia

Continued

TABLE 15-1. **Diuretics Mechanisms, Uses, and Adverse Effects—cont'd**

DRUG CLASS (AGENT)	MECHANISM	USES	ADVERSE EFFECTS
Potassium-sparing diuretics (amiloride)	Inhibit Na^+/K^+ ion exchange in late distal tubule and collecting duct	Adjunctive treatment of edema/hypertension in combination with thiazides or loop diuretics Antagonize potassium loss associated with other diuretics	Cardiac arrhythmias from hyperkalemia Hyperchloremic normal anion gap metabolic acidosis
Potassium-sparing diuretics (spironolactone)	Block binding of aldosterone to receptors in cells of late distal renal tubules	Diagnose primary hyperaldosteronism Treat polycystic ovary syndrome, hirsutism, ascites, and heart failure	Gynecomastia Impotence
Osmotic diuretics (mannitol)	Increase osmotic gradient between blood and tissues and remove water because diuretic is filtered and not reabsorbed	Maintain urine flow in acute renal failure Treat acute oliguria Reduce intracranial pressure and cerebral edema Treat acute glaucoma	Electrolyte imbalances Expansion of extracellular fluid

---

BOX 15-1   DIURETICS

Carbonic Anhydrase Inhibitors
Acetazolamide (oral)
Brinzolamide (eye drops)
Dorzolamide (eye drops)

Loop Diuretics
Bumetanide
Ethacrynic acid
Furosemide
Torsemide

Thiazide and Thiazide-like Diuretics
Chlorthalidone
Hydrochlorothiazide
Indapamide
Metolazone

Potassium-sparing Diuretics:
Aldosterone antagonists
Eplerenone
Spironolactone

Sodium-Potassium Exchange Inhibitors
Amiloride
Triamterene

Osmotic Diuretics
Glycerol
Mannitol

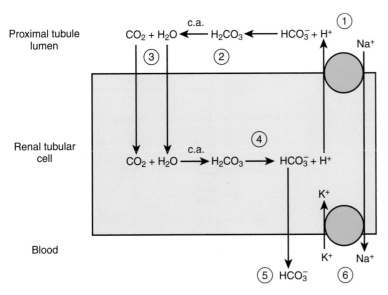

15-2: Reclamation of bicarbonate in the proximal tubule. See text for explanation. c.a., carbonic anhydrase *(From Goljan EF and Sloka KI: Rapid Review Laboratory Testing in Clinical Medicine. Philadelphia, Mosby, 2008, Figure 2-5.)*

b. Carbonic anhydrase inhibitors decrease the sodium/H^+ exchange by decreasing H^+ production in the PRT.

c. This changes the composition of urine by increasing bicarbonate, sodium, and potassium excretion (this effect lasts only 3 to 4 days).

d. Increased loss of bicarbonate alkalinizes the urine and produces a mild hyperchloremic normal anion gap metabolic acidosis (type II proximal renal tubular acidosis)

3. Uses

a. Glaucoma (chronic simple open-angle, secondary glaucoma, preoperatively in acute angle-closure)
   • Carbonic anhydrase inhibitors decreases production of aqueous humor; hence, lowering intraocular pressure.

b. Acute mountain sickness

c. Absence (petit mal) epilepsy

d. To produce urinary alkalosis

e. To treat drug-induced edema or edema due to congestive heart failure (adjunctive therapy)

4. Contraindications

a. Hepatic cirrhosis (decreased ammonia excretion)

b. May lead to hepatic encephalopathy

B. Loop (high-ceiling) diuretics (see Box 15-1)

1. General considerations

a. Examples

   (1) Bumetanide

   (2) Ethacrynic acid

   (3) Furosemide

   (4) Torsemide

b. Loop diuretics cause a profound diuresis (much greater than that produced by thiazides) and a decreased preload to the heart.

c. These drugs inhibit reabsorption of sodium and chloride in the thick ascending limb in the medullary segment of the loop of Henle (Fig. 15-3)

   (1) Increase excretion of obligated water (water attached to sodium, potassium, etc.), sodium, chloride, magnesium, and calcium (step 1)

   (2) Interfere with the chloride-binding cotransport system (step 2)

   (3) A Na^+/K^+-ATPase moves reabsorbed sodium into the interstitium (step 3)

   (4) Reabsorbed Cl^- and K^+ diffuse through channels into the interstitium (step 4)

d. These drugs are useful in patients with renal impairment because they retain their effectiveness when creatinine clearance is less than 30 mL/min (normal is 120 mL/min).

e. Loop diuretics up-regulate cyclooxygenase activity, thereby increasing prostaglandin E_2 (PGE_2) and prostaglandin I_2 (PGI_2) synthesis, resulting in increased renal blood flow.

2. Ethacrynic acid

a. Mechanism of action
   • Inhibition of a sulfhydryl-catalyzed enzyme system that is responsible for reabsorption of sodium and chloride in the proximal and distal tubules.

Carbonic anhydrase inhibitors: most common cause of proximal renal tubular acidosis; hyperchloremic normal anion gap metabolic acidosis.

Carbonic anhydrase inhibitors are contraindicated in hepatic cirrhosis; ammonium is not excreted, so serum ammonia accumulates, crosses into brain and leads to hepatic encephalopathy.

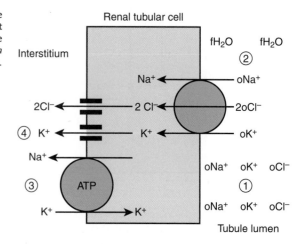

15-3: Sodium, potassium, chloride cotransported in the medullary segment of the thick ascending limb. See text for description. ATP, adenosine triphosphate; fH$_2$O, free water: oH$_2$O, obligated water. (From Goljan EF and Sloka KI: Rapid Review Laboratory Testing in Clinical Medicine. Philadelphia, Mosby, 2008, Figure 2-6.)

b. Uses
(1) In patients who are hypersensitive to sulfonamide drugs such as thiazides and furosemide (the most commonly used loop diuretic)
(2) Edema related to heart failure or cirrhosis
c. Adverse effects
- Ototoxicity, leading to hearing loss and tinnitus
3. Furosemide
- This drug is structurally related to thiazides and has many of the properties of those diuretics.
    a. Mechanism of action (see Fig. 15-3).
      - Inhibition of reabsorption of sodium and chloride by attaching to the chloride-binding site of the $Na^+/K^+/2Cl^-$ ($NKCC_2$) cotransporter in the thick ascending limb in the medullary segment of the loop of Henle
    b. Uses
      (1) Hypertension
      (2) Heart failure
      (3) Ascites
        - Must be careful; loop diuretic-induced metabolic alkalosis leads to increased reabsorption of ammonia (NH_3) from the bowel with the potential for precipitating hepatic encephalopathy.
      (4) Hypercalcemia
      (5) Pulmonary edema
    c. Adverse effects
      (1) Volume depletion
      (2) Hypokalemia
      (3) Hyperglycemia
        (a) Potassium levels in blood have a direct relationship with insulin secretion.
        (b) Hypokalemia leads to decreased insulin secretion resulting in hyperglycemia
        (c) Hyperkalemia increases insulin secretion, which drives potassium and glucose into adipose tissue and muscle.
      (4) Hypomagnesemia leading to hypocalcemia and tetany
        (a) Magnesium is a cofactor for adenylate cyclase.
        (b) Cyclic adenosine monophosphate (cAMP) is required for parathyroid hormone activation.
        (c) Hence, hypoparathyroidism produced leading to hypocalcemia and tetany.
      (5) Hyperuricemia
        - Volume depletion increases net reabsorption of uric acid in the PRT.
      (6) Metabolic alkalosis
      (7) Hyponatremia
4. Bumetanide and torsemide are similar but more potent and have a longer duration of action than furosemide.

C. Thiazide diuretics
1. General considerations
    a. These diuretics differ from each other only in potency and duration of action.
    b. The most commonly used thiazide diuretic is hydrochlorothiazide.
    c. Thiazide diuretics are used in much lower doses to treat hypertension than those needed to treat edema.
    d. Thiazides lower blood pressure by depleting sodium and reducing blood volume.
      - Chronic retention of sodium leads to vasoconstriction of peripheral resistance arterioles causing an increase in diastolic blood pressure.
    e. The Seventh Report of the Joint National Committee on Prevention, Detection, Evaluation, and Treatment of High Blood Pressure states that thiazide-type diuretics should be used in drug treatment for most patients with uncomplicated hypertension, either alone or combined with drugs from other classes.
2. Mechanism of action (Fig. 15-4)
    a. Inhibit sodium and chloride reabsorption by attaching to the chloride site of the $Na^+–Cl^-$ cotransporter (NCC cotransporter) in the early distal convoluted tubules causing increased excretion of sodium, chloride, and water (step 1).
    b. A Na^+/K^+-ATPase moves sodium into the blood (step 2).
      (1) Increased delivery of sodium to the aldosterone-enhanced sodium-potassium channels in the late distal and collecting tubules (Fig. 15-5) leads to increased

Persons with sulfonamide allergies *cannot* take many drugs including all thiazide-related diuretics, carbonic anhydrase inhibitors and all loop diuretics except ethacrynic acid.

Ethacrynic acid noted for causing ototoxicity.

Loop and thiazide diuretics produce many of the same responses with most effects being more pronounced with loop diuretics; a notable difference is on calcium, where loops promote and thiazides reduce calcium excretion.

Metabolic alkalosis increases the absorption of ammonia from the bowel; detrimental in hepatic encephalopathy

Loop diuretics and thiazides cause hypokalemia; administer them in combination with a potassium-sparing diuretic or potassium supplements.

Thiazide diuretics continue to be considered the first drug to use in managing hypertension despite the fact that they worsen the lipid profile and diabetes, two, contributing factors in the cause of hypertension.

15-4: Sodium-chloride cotransporter in the early distal tubule. See text for description. ATP, adenosine triphosphate *(From Goljan EF and Sloka KI: Rapid Review Laboratory Testing in Clinical Medicine. Philadelphia, Mosby, 2008, Figure 2-7.)*

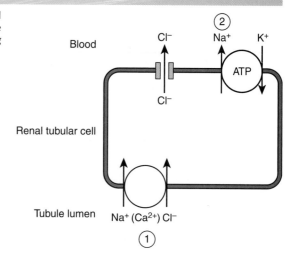

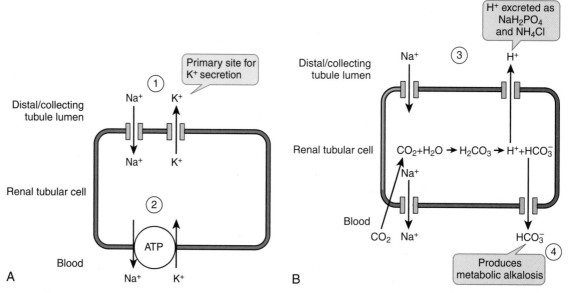

15-5: Sodium-potassium channels **A,** and sodium-hydrogen ion channels **B,** in the late distal tubule and collecting duct. See text for description. ATP, adenosine triphosphate *(From Goljan EF and Sloka KI: Rapid Review Laboratory Testing in Clinical Medicine. Philadelphia, Mosby, 2008, Figure 2-8.)*

exchange of sodium for potassium resulting in potassium loss in the urine (potential for hypokalemia) (step 2).

(2) Sodium then exchanges with H^+ ions, leading to a loss of H^+ in the urine and increased reabsorption of bicarbonate into the blood (step 3) (potential for metabolic alkalosis).

(3) The enhanced sodium-potassium/H^+ exchange also applies to the loop diuretics (see above).

- This explains why loop diuretics and thiazide diuretics are the most common cause of hyponatremia, hypokalemia, and metabolic acidosis and emphasizes the importance of potassium supplements or potassium-sparing drugs when taking the above diuretics.

c. Increase calcium reabsorption (*no* advantage in osteoporosis *but* useful in decreasing calcium excretion in calcium stone formers)

d. Reduction in plasma volume, which increases plasma renin activity and aldosterone excretion, resulting in a decrease in renal blood flow and GFR

3. Uses
   a. Hypertension
   b. Heart failure
   c. Edema

Loop diuretics and thiazides are the most common cause of hyponatremia, hypokalemia, and metabolic alkalosis.

Thiazides decrease calcium excretion into the urine in calcium stone formers.

    d. Renal calculi (decreased calcium excretion)
- The majority of calcium stone formers reabsorb more calcium from their gastrointestinal tracts (called absorptive hypercalciuria) leading to hypercalciuria and increased risk for calcium stone formation.

    e. Nephrogenic diabetes insipidus
- Volume depletion decreases urine volume; hence, decreasing the amount of times the patient has to void.

  4. Adverse effects
    a. Hypokalemia
    b. Hyponatremia
    c. Metabolic alkalosis
    d. Hyperlipidemia
    e. Hyperuricemia (see loop diuretic discussion)
    f. Hypomagnesemia
    g. Decreased glucose tolerance (see loop diuretic discussion)
    h. Hypercalcemia
- The rule of thumb is that if hypercalcemia develops while a patient is taking a thiazide, he or she most likely has primary hyperparathyroidism, since calcium reabsorption in the Na^+/Cl^- cotransporter is parathyroid hormone mediated.

  5. Numerous others with different potencies; end in -thiazide; often found in fixed formulations with other drugs to treat hypertension.

  6. Thiazide-related drugs used in the treatment of hypertension include:
    a. Chlorthalidone
    b. Indapamide
    c. Metolazone

D. Potassium-sparing diuretics (see Box 15-1)
- These drugs are used in combination with other diuretics to protect against hypokalemia.

  1. Aldosterone antagonists
    a. Examples
      (1) Spironolactone
      (2) Eplerenone
    b. Mechanism of action (see Fig. 15-4)
- Competitive inhibition of the aldosterone receptor; eplerenone is more specific

    c. Uses
      (1) Diagnosis of primary hyperaldosteronism
      (2) Treatment of heart failure
      (3) Adjunct with thiazides or loop diuretics to prevent hypokalemia
      (4) Drug of choice for treatment of hirsutism (e.g., polycystic ovarian syndrome)
        (a) Spironolactone binds to androgen receptors in hair follicles; hence, preventing growth of hair follicles
        (b) Reduction in 5-alpha reductase activity, which normally converts testosterone to the more potent, hair follicle stimulating hormone, dihydrotestosterone (DHT).
      (5) Treatment of acne and hair loss in women
      (6) Topical treatment of male baldness
      (7) Treatment of ascites in cirrhosis
    d. Adverse effects
      (1) Antiandrogenic effects with spironolactone, such as impotence and gynecomastia in males
- Spironolactone binds to androgen receptors producing an anti-androgen effect, while leaving estrogen unopposed.
      (2) Hyperkalemia
- Blocks the aldosterone-enhanced sodium-potassium channel; the primary channel for potassium excretion.

  2. Sodium-potassium ion exchange inhibitors
    a. Examples
      (1) Triamterene
      (2) Amiloride
    b. Mechanism of action (see Fig. 15-5)

Use thiazide diuretics in patients who form calcium calculi because these drugs decrease calcium excretion, thus preventing calculi formation.

Loop diuretics and thiazides cause hypokalemia; administer them in combination with a potassium-sparing diuretic.

Use thiazide diuretics cautiously in patients with diabetes mellitus, gout, and hyperlipidemia, as well as those who are receiving digitalis glycosides.

Thiazide-like diuretics used to treat hypertension: chlorthalidone, indapamide, metolazone.

Spironolactone is the drug of choice in treating hirsutism.

Spironolactone may produce impotence and gynecomastia

Renin-angiotensin system inhibitors may increase hyperkalemia when using potassium-sparing diuretics.

(1) Inhibits sodium reabsorption (blocks ENaC; epithelial sodium channel) in the late distal tubule, cortical collecting tubule, and collecting duct subsequently reducing both potassium and hydrogen excretion resulting in weak natriuretic, diuretic, and antihypertensive activity

(2) Increases sodium loss

(3) Increases potassium retention

(4) Decreases calcium excretion

(5) Decreases magnesium loss

c. When potassium loss is minimal, sodium-potassium ion exchange inhibition causes only a slight reduction in potassium excretion.

d. When sodium renal clearance is increased by loop diuretics or mineralocorticoids, these drugs cause a significant decrease in potassium excretion.

e. Uses

(1) Adjunct with thiazides or loop diuretics to prevent hypokalemia

(2) Treatment for lithium-induced nephrogenic diabetes insipidus (amiloride)

f. Adverse effect

- Hyperkalemia

E. Osmotic diuretics (Box 15-1)

- Agents that are filtered and not completely reabsorbed

1. Examples

a. Mannitol

b. Glycerol

2. Mechanism of action

- Rise in blood osmolality increases the osmotic gradient

a. Mannitol given intravenously increases the osmotic gradient between blood and tissues.

b. This facilitates the flow of fluid out of the tissues (including the brain and the eye) and into the interstitial fluid.

c. This expands extracellular fluid; thus, contraindicated in:

(1) Congestive heart failure (CHF)

(2) Pulmonary edema

d. Finally, mannitol is filtered via glomerular filtration without reabsorption so water and electrolytes follow, leading to increased urinary output.

3. Uses

a. Treats increased intracranial pressure associated with cerebral edema

b. Promotion of diuresis in the prevention and/or treatment of oliguria or anuria due to acute renal failure

c. Decreases intraocular pressure in glaucoma

d. Removal of water-soluble toxins

e. Genitourinary irrigant in transurethral prostatic resection or other transurethral surgical procedures

4. Adverse effects

a. Circulatory overload

b. Pulmonary edema

F. Therapeutic summary of selected diuretic drugs (Table 15-2)

III. Agents That Affect Water Excretion

A. Vasopressin (antidiuretic hormone, or ADH)

1. General considerations

a. ADH is a peptide hormone synthesized in and secreted by the supraoptic and paraventricular nuclei in the hypothalamus and stored in and released from the posterior pituitary.

b. Its antidiuretic effects are due to increased reabsorption of free water (water without attached electrolytes) in the renal collecting ducts.

c. A disorder characterized by an absence of ADH is central diabetes insipidus (CDI).

- Produces polyuria, polydipsia, and hypernatremia

d. The synthetic analogue is desmopressin (preferred for treating CDI).

e. A disorder characterized by an excess of ADH is syndrome of inappropriate antidiuretic hormone (SIADH).

- Produces water retention, severe hyponatremia (usually <120 mEq/L), and cerebral edema

---

Side notes (left margin):

Amiloride inhibits the reabsorption of lithium therefore decreases the uncoupling of vasopressin (V_2) receptors from adenylyl cyclase

Mannitol given IV is an osmotic diuretic; when given orally is an osmotic cathartic.

Osmotic diuretics are absolutely contraindicated in pulmonary edema or CHF.

Use desmopressin to treat CDI.

TABLE 15-2. Therapeutic Summary of Selected Diuretic Drugs

DRUGS	CLINICAL APPLICATIONS	ADVERSE EFFECTS	CONTRAINDICATIONS
Mechanism: _Carbonic anhydrase inhibitors_			
Acetazolamide Brinzolamide Dichlorphenamide Dorzolamide Methazolamide	Glaucoma Urinary alkalinization Acute mountain sickness Pseudotumor cerebri	Hyperchloremic metabolic acidosis	Hypersensitivity Sulfonamide allergies Hepatic disease Severe renal disease Severe pulmonary obstruction
Mechanism: _Inhibits reabsorption of sodium and chloride in the ascending loop of Henle_			
Bumetanide Ethacrynic acid Furosemide Torsemide	Acute pulmonary edema Refractory edema Hypertension Hyperkalemia Ascites Ethacrynic acid (the preferred diuretic in patients with sulfonamide allergies)	Hyponatremia Hyperglycemia Hyperuricemia Hypocalcemia Volume depletion Hypokalemia Metabolic alkalosis Ototoxicity (especially ethacrynic acid)	Hypersensitivity Sulfonamide allergies (except ethacrynic acid) Severe electrolyte depletion
Mechanism: _Inhibits reabsorption of sodium and chloride in the distal convoluted tubule_			
Thiazide and Thiazide- like Diuretics Chlorthalidone Hydrochlorothiazide Indapamide Metolazone	Management of hypertension alone or in combination with other drugs Nephrolithiasis Nephrogenic diabetes insipidus	Hyponatremia Hyperglycemia Hyperuricemia Hypercalcemia Hypokalemia Metabolic alkalosis Hyperlipidemia	Hypersensitivity Sulfonamide allergies Anuria Renal decompensation Pregnancy
Mechanism: _Potassium sparing diuretic; aldosterone antagonist_			
Eplerenone Spironolactone	Management of edema associated with excessive aldosterone excretion Hypertension Congestive heart failure Primary hyperaldosteronism Hypokalemia Cirrhosis of liver accompanied by edema or ascites	Hyperchloremic metabolic acidosis Hyperkalemia Hirsutism Gynecomastia (spironolactone)	Hypersensitivity Renal dysfunction Hyperkalemia Pregnancy
Mechanism: _Potassium sparing diuretic; blocks ENaC (epithelial sodium channel)_			
Amiloride Triamterene	Counteracts potassium loss produced by other diuretics in the treatment of hypertension or edematous conditions including congestive heart failure, hepatic cirrhosis, and hypoaldosteronism Usually used in conjunction with more potent diuretics such as thiazides or loop diuretics Lithium induced diabetes insipidus (amiloride)	Hyperkalemia Metabolic acidosis	Hypersensitivity Renal dysfunction Hyperkalemia
Mechanism: _Osmotic diuretics: increase the osmotic pressure of the glomerular filtrate, thus inhibits tubular reabsorption of water and electrolytes_			
Glycerol Mannitol	Glaucoma Cerebral edema Promote diuresis Toxin removal	Electrolyte imbalances Expansion of extracellular fluid	Hypersensitivity Severe renal disease Congestive heart failure Pulmonary edema

  2. Mechanism of action
    a. Modulates renal tubular reabsorption of water, increasing permeability of the distal tubule and collecting ducts to water
      • This effect is mediated by an increase in cAMP associated with stimulation of the vasopressin-2 (V_2) receptor.
    b. This leads to increased urine osmolality, with maintenance of serum osmolality within an acceptable physiologic range (275–295 mOsm/kg)
    c. At high concentrations, causes vasoconstriction (helps maintain blood pressure during hemorrhage).
      • This effect occurs via the stimulation of the vasopressin-1 (V_1) receptor coupled to the polyphosphoinositide pathway.
  3. Uses
    a. Central (neurogenic) diabetes insipidus (CDI)

ADH activation of the V_2 receptor increases cAMP production that leads to insertion of water channels (aquaporin 2) in renal collecting ducts.

ADH activation of the V_1 receptor stimulates the polyphosphoinositide pathway in vascular smooth muscle resulting in vasoconstriction.

Vasopressin: treatment CDI; severe bleeding disorders.

- Caused by hypothalamic dysfunction, pituitary stalk transection, or destruction of the posterior pituitary gland.
  b. Adjunct in treatment of esophageal varices, hemorrhage, upper gastrointestinal bleeding, variceal bleeding (vasoconstrictor effect)
4. Adverse effect
  - Water intoxication (overhydration)

B. Desmopressin

Desmopressin: treatment of CDI; hemophilia A; von Willebrand's disease (VWD)

1. It has 4000:1 antidiuretic-to-vasopressor activity
2. Injection
   a. Treatment of CDI
   b. Treatment of mild hemophilia A and **von Willebrand's disease** (VWD) with factor VIII coagulant activity >5%
     - Increases the release of von Willebrand's factor and factor VIII coagulant from endothelial cells
3. Nasal solutions to treat CDI.
4. Nasal spray to treat hemophilia A and VWD.
5. Tablet to treat CDI, primary nocturnal enuresis
6. Unlabeled use
   a. To treat uremic bleeding associated with acute or chronic renal failure
   b. Prevention of surgical bleeding in patients with uremia.

C. ADH antagonists

CDI: treat with desmopressin; nephrogenic diabetes insipidus: treat with a thiazide diuretic; Li$^+$ induced diabetes insipidus: treat with amiloride

- Inhibit effects of ADH at the collecting tubule producing nephrogenic diabetes insipidus (NDI)
1. Lithium salts
   a. Mechanism of action
     - Reduction in V$_2$ receptor-mediated stimulation of adenylyl cyclase in the medullary collecting tubule of the nephron, thus decreasing Aquaporin 2 expression and increasing water loss
   b. Use
     - SIADH secretion; last choice for treatment
   c. Adverse effects
     - Li$^+$ induced NDI; produces polyuria that is usually, but *not* always, reversible

Lithium and demeclocycline used to treat SIADH.

2. Demeclocycline
   a. Mechanism of action
     - Reduced formation of cAMP, limiting the actions of ADH in the distal portion of the convoluted tubules and collecting ducts of the kidneys
   b. Use
     - SIADH secretion, particularly when caused by a small cell carcinoma of the lung
   c. Adverse effects
     (1) NDI (treated with thiazide diuretics)
     (2) Renal failure
3. Conivaptan
   a. Intravenous synthetic vasopressin antagonist
   b. Mechanism of action
     - An arginine vasopressin (AVP) receptor antagonist with affinity for both subtypes (V$_{1A}$ and V$_2$) of the AVP receptor.

Conivaptan is a vasopressin antagonist.

   c. Use
     (1) Treatment of euvolemic and hypervolemic hyponatremia in hospitalized patients
     (2) Euvolemic hyponatremia is a dilutional hyponatremia due to an increase in total body water, without evidence of pitting edema (e.g., SIADH)
     (3) Hypervolemic hyponatremia is a dilutional hyponatremia due to an increase in both total body water and sodium to a lesser degree with clinical evidence of pitting edema (e.g., CHF)
       - Only indicated in CHF if the expected benefit outweighs the increased risk for adverse effects.
   d. Adverse effects
     (1) Orthostatic hypotension
     (2) Fever
     (3) Hypokalemia
     (4) Headache

D. Therapeutic summary of selected drugs that affect antidiuretic hormone actions (Table 15-3)

TABLE 15-3. Therapeutic Summary of Selected Drugs that affect Antidiuretic Hormone (ADH) Actions

DRUGS	CLINICAL APPLICATIONS	ADVERSE EFFECTS	CONTRAINDICATIONS
Mechanism: *An ADH analogue with high antidiuretic-to-vasopressor activity*			
Desmopressin	Treatment of central diabetes insipidus Treatment of von Willebrand's disease, mild hemophilia A Treatment of primary nocturnal enuresis	Water intoxication (overhydration)	Hypersensitivity Severe renal disease
Mechanism: *Reduction in vasopressin (V₂) receptor–mediated stimulation of adenylyl cyclase in the medullary collecting tubule of the nephron*			
Lithium	Treatment of syndrome of inappropriate antidiuretic hormone (SIADH) secretion Management of bipolar disorders Treatment of mania in individuals with bipolar disorder	Tremors (treat with propranolol) Fatigue Polyuria/polydipsia Cardiac arrhythmias Thyroid abnormalities Neutrophil leukocytosis	Hypersensitivity Cardiac disease Renal disease Pregnancy
Mechanism: *Reduced formation of cAMP, limiting the actions of ADH in the distal portion of the convoluted tubules and collecting ducts*			
Demeclocycline (a tetracycline antibiotic)	SIADH Treatment of susceptible bacterial infections (acne, gonorrhea, pertussis and urinary tract infections)	GI distress Teeth discoloration (children <8 years)	Hypersensitivity Children <8 years of age Pregnancy
Mechanism: *An arginine vasopressin (AVP) receptor antagonist with affinity for both subtypes (V₁ₐ and V₂) of the AVP receptor*			
Conivaptan	Treatment of euvolemic and hypervolemic hyponatremia	Orthostatic hypotension Fever Hypokalemia	Hypersensitivity Concurrent use with strong CYP3A4 inhibitors

cAMP, cyclic adenosine monophosphate; GI, gastrointestinal.

CHAPTER 16
DRUGS USED IN THE TREATMENT OF COAGULATION DISORDERS

I. General Considerations

A. Clot formation at the tissue level results from complex interactions (Fig. 16-1).

1. Enzymatic pathway for clot formation (Fig. 16-2)

   a. Intrinsic pathway

   (1) All required factors (XII, XI, IX, VIII) are present in blood and coagulation is initiated by collagen from damaged blood vessel.

   (2) Factors II, VII, IX, and X in the final common pathway are *not* limiting.

   (3) This system is slow in producing a clot.

   (4) Measured by partial thromboplastin time (PTT)

   (5) Used to monitor heparin therapy

   b. Extrinsic pathway

   (1) Requires tissue factor (tissue thromboplastin, factor III) which activates factor VII

   (2) Factors II, VII, IX, and X in the final common pathway are limiting.

   (3) This system is fast in producing a clot

   (4) Measured by prothrombin time (PT) or international normalized ratio (INR), if using warfarin therapy

   (5) Used to monitor warfarin therapy

B. Hematologic drugs

- These agents have various clinical indications (Table 16-1).

1. Drugs used to reduce the formation of thrombi or increase the destruction of thrombi

   a. Antithrombotic drugs

   b. Anticoagulant drugs

   c. Fibrinolytic drugs

2. Hemostatic drugs used to prevent bleeding from small vessels (arterioles, capillaries, venules)

II. Antithrombotic Drugs (Antiplatelet Drugs)

- Interfere with platelet adhesion, aggregation, or synthesis (Box 16-1; Fig. 16-3).

A. Aspirin

- Nonsteroidal anti-inflammatory drug (NSAID); also used as an analgesic and as an antipyretic (see Chapter 18).

1. Mechanism of action

   a. Aspirin inhibits synthesis of thromboxane A_2 (TXA_2), a potent platelet aggregator and vasoconstrictor, by irreversible acetylation of cyclooxygenase (COX-1) in platelets.

   (1) COX is important in the production of prostaglandins, prostacyclins, and thromboxanes.

   (2) COX-1 is present in most tissues; functions include:

   (a) Maintenance of the bicarbonate-rich mucous barrier in the stomach

   (b) Vasodilation of afferent arterioles in the kidneys

   (c) Vasoconstriction and enhanced platelet aggregation (TXA_2 in platelets)

   (3) COX-2 is present at the sites of acute and chronic inflammation as well as in endothelial cells.

   - Vasodilation and inhibition of platelet aggregation (prostacyclin in endothelial cells)

   (4) Aspirin is non-selective and inhibits both COX-1 and COX-2

Intrinsic pathway: coagulation factors XII, XI, IX, VIII

Extrinsic pathway: coagulation factor VII; activated by tissue thromboplastin.

COX produces prostaglandins, prostacyclins, and thromboxanes.

COX-1 is in platelets and is inhibited by low-dose aspirin.

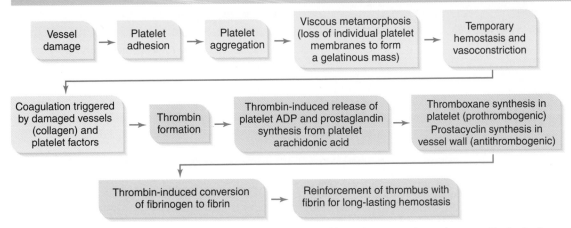

16-1: Events occurring after vessel damage that lead to the formation of fibrin clots. Note the involvement of both platelets and the coagulation pathway. ADP, adenosine diphosphate.

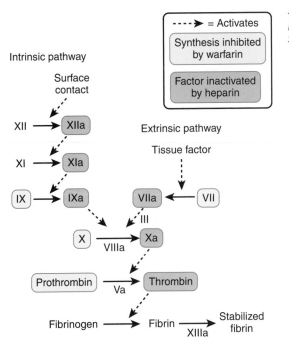

16-2: Intrinsic and extrinsic pathways of coagulation. *(From Brenner G and Stevens C: Pharmacology, 3rd ed. Philadelphia, Saunders, 2010, Figure 16-2.)*

TABLE 16-1. Clinical Uses of Anticoagulant, Antiplatelet, and Fibrinolytic Drugs

CLINICAL USE	PRIMARY DRUG*	SECONDARY DRUG*
Acute thrombotic stroke	Fibrinolytic drug	—
Artificial heart valve	Warfarin or aspirin	Dipyridamole
Atrial fibrillation	Heparin, warfarin, or LMWH	Aspirin
Deep vein thrombosis		
Treatment	Heparin, warfarin, or LMWH	—
Surgical prophylaxis	LMWH	Heparin
Heparin-induced thrombocytopenia (HIT)	"-rudins"	Argatroban
Myocardial infarction		
Treatment	Fibrinolytic drug, heparin, aspirin, or abciximab	—
Prevention	Aspirin	Clopidogrel
Percutaneous transluminal coronary angioplasty	Abciximab, heparin, aspirin, or clopidogrel	—
Pulmonary embolism	Fibrinolytic drug, heparin, warfarin, or LMWH	—
Stroke	Aspirin, clopidogrel, or warfarin	—
Transient ischemic attacks	Aspirin	Warfarin
Unstable angina	Aspirin, abciximab, heparin, or LMWH	—

*If aspirin is contraindicated or not tolerated, ticlopidine may be used. If warfarin is contraindicated or not tolerated, another oral anticoagulant may be used.
LMWH, low-molecular-weight heparin.

BOX 16-1 ANTITHROMBOTIC DRUGS

Platelet Inhibitors
Aspirin
Anagrelide
Cilostazol
Clopidogrel
Dipyridamole
Ticlopidine

Platelet-Receptor Glycoprotein Inhibitors
Abciximab
Eptifibatide
Tirofiban

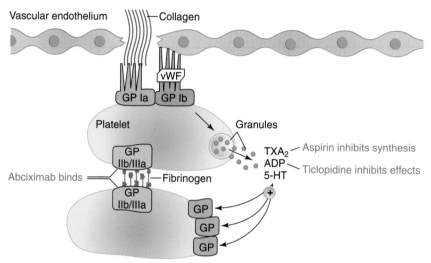

16-3: Platelet aggregation and sites of drug action. ADP, adenosine diphosphate; GP, glycoprotein; 5-HT, 5-hydroxytryptamine; TXA₂, thromboxane A₂; VWF, von Willebrand's factor.

COX-2 is in endothelial cells and is inhibited by high-dose aspirin and selective COX-2 inhibitors (celecoxib, rofecoxib).

TXA₂ stimulates platelet aggregation and causes vasoconstriction; PGI₂ inhibits platelet aggregation and causes vasodilation.

Use low-dose aspirin to prevent thrombus formation.

    b. TXA_2 increases the PIP_2 (phosphatidylinositol biphosphate pathway) in platelets, causing aggregation (reduced by aspirin).
    c. Low-dose aspirin therapy (1 baby [81 mg] or 1 adult [325 mg] tablet per day) primarily inhibits COX-1 to prevent synthesis of TXA_2 without decreasing the synthesis of prostacyclin (PGI_2) in endothelial cells, which inhibits platelet aggregation.
    d. Higher doses of aspirin (2 or more adult tablets per day) inhibit synthesis of both TXA_2 and PGI_2.
  2. Uses (see Table 16-1)
  3. Adverse effects
    a. Gastrointestinal (GI) irritation and bleeding
    b. Tinnitus, respiratory alkalosis followed by metabolic acidosis (high doses)

B. Platelet inhibitors (see Fig. 16-3)
  1. Ticlopidine and clopidogrel
    a. Mechanism of action
      (1) Interferes with adenosine diphosphate (ADP)-induced binding of fibrinogen to platelet membrane at specific receptor sites (GpIIb/IIIa)
      (2) Inhibits platelet aggregation and platelet-platelet interactions that produce platelet thrombi (e.g., coronary artery thrombosis)
    b. Uses
      (1) Prevents thrombotic stroke (initial or recurrent) in patients who are intolerant or unresponsive to aspirin
      (2) Prevents thrombus formation in patients with cardiac stents and in treatment of acute coronary syndromes (in combination with aspirin)

    c. Adverse effects
        (1) Severe bone marrow toxicity, including agranulocytosis (neutropenia), aplastic anemia (pancytopenia; rare); occurs mostly with ticlopidine
        (2) Thrombotic thrombocytopenic purpura
           • Platelet consumption syndrome associated with thrombocytopenia and hemolytic anemia
        (3) Clopidogrel is associated with a lower incidence of adverse cutaneous, GI, and hematologic reactions than ticlopidine.
        (4) Clopidogrel causes some drug-drug interactions (inhibits cytochrome P-450 enzymes); inhibits metabolism of:
           (a) Fluvastatin
           (b) Phenytoin
           (c) Tamoxifen
           (d) Tolbutamide
           (e) Warfarin
  2. Dipyridamole (vasodilator)
    a. Mechanism of action
        (1) Decreases platelet adhesion
        (2) Potentiates action of PGI_2, which is coupled to a cyclic adenosine monophosphate (cAMP)-generating system in platelets and vasculature, causing decreased platelet aggregation and vasodilation, respectively
    b. Uses
        (1) Given with warfarin to decrease thrombosis after artificial heart valve replacement
        (2) Prevention of thrombotic stroke (in combination with aspirin)
        (3) As vasodilator during myocardial perfusion scans (cardiac stress test)
  3. Abciximab (see Fig. 16-3): platelet-receptor glycoprotein inhibitor
    a. Eptifibatide and tirofiban are newer glycoprotein IIb/IIIa inhibitors.
    b. Mechanism of action
        • Binds to the glycoprotein receptors IIb/IIIa on activated platelets
        (1) Abciximab prevents binding of fibrinogen, von Willebrand factor, and other adhesive molecules to the glycoprotein receptor.
        (2) When given intravenously, the drug produces rapid inhibition of platelet aggregation.
    c. Uses
        (1) Acute coronary syndromes
        (2) Percutaneous transluminal coronary angioplasty
    d. Adverse effects
        (1) Bleeding
        (2) Thrombocytopenia
  4. Cilostazol
    a. Mechanism of action
        (1) Antithrombotic, antiplatelet and vasodilatory actions
        (2) Inhibits phosphodiesterase type III, and thereby, increases cAMP levels
    b. Uses
        (1) Intermittent claudication
        (2) Peripheral vascular disease
  5. Anagrelide
    a. Mechanism of action
        (1) Reduces elevated platelet counts in patients with essential thrombosis (too many platelets)
        (2) Inhibits megakaryocyte development in late postmitotic stage
    b. Used for treatment of thrombocytosis secondary to myeloproliferative disorders
  C. Therapeutic summary of selected antiplatelet drugs: (Table 16-2)

III. Anticoagulants (Box 16-2)
  • Pharmacologic properties of most common used agents (Tables 16-3 and 16-4).
  A. Standard unfractionated heparin (UFH)
    1. Mechanism of action
        • Heparin accelerates the action of antithrombin III (ATIII) to neutralize thrombin (factor IIa) and to a lesser extent other activated clotting factors that are serine proteases (e.g., XIIa, XIa, IXa, Xa).
    2. Uses (see Table 16-1)

Margin notes:

Because of the risk of bone marrow toxicity, patients who are receiving ticlopidine must have frequent complete blood counts (CBCs) with white blood cell differential count.

Ticlopidine is more toxic than clopidogrel.

Clopidogrel causes more drug-drug interactions than ticlopidine.

Dipyridamole enhances action of prostacyclin.

Warfarin plus dipyridamole for patients with artificial heart valve.

Abciximab prevents platelet aggregation during invasive procedures to the heart.

Cilostazol for treatment of intermittent claudication.

Anagrelide for treatment of too many platelets.

Heparin: enhances ATIII activity

Activated PTT (1.5-2 times control): basis for calculation of the heparin dose

Table 16-2. **Therapeutic Summary of Selected Antiplatelet Drugs**

DRUGS	CLINICAL APPLICATIONS	ADVERSE EFFECTS	CONTRAINDICATIONS
Mechanism: *Prevents formation of platelet thromboxane A$_2$; inhibits platelet aggregation*			
Aspirin	Prophylaxis of myocardial infarction Prophylaxis of stroke Analgesic Antipyretic Antiinflammatory	Bleeding Tinnitus Respiratory alkalosis followed by metabolic acidosis in overdose	Hypersensitivity Bleeding disorders In children (<16 years of age) for viral infections Pregnancy (especially 3rd trimester)
Mechanism: *Platelet ADP antagonist*			
Clopidogrel Ticlopidine	Reduces atherothrombotic events (myocardial infarction, stroke, vascular deaths) Treat unstable angina and non-ST-segment elevation myocardial infarction Patients with stents Ticlopidine should be reserved for patients who are intolerant to aspirin	Cutaneous Gastrointestinal problems Hematologic (all worse with ticlopidine)	Hypersensitivity Pathological bleeding; peptic ulcers or intracranial hemorrhage Coagulation disorders
Mechanism: *Inhibits phosphodiesterase and increases cAMP; decreases platelet aggregation and vasodilate*			
Dipyridamole	Used with warfarin to decrease thrombosis after artificial heart valve replacement Diagnostic in coronary artery disease	Hypotension Rash	Hypersensitivity
Mechanism: *Binds to the glycoprotein receptors IIb and IIIa on activated platelets; inhibits platelet aggregation*			
Abciximab Eptifibatide Tirofiban	Percutaneous coronary intervention	Hypotension Bleeding	Hypersensitivity Bleeding disorders
Mechanism: *Inhibitor of phosphodiesterase III; thus, increasing cAMP leading to inhibition of platelet aggregation, vasodilation, and inhibition of vascular smooth muscle cell proliferation*			
Cilostazol	Intermittent claudication Peripheral vascular disease	Bleeding Hypotension	Hypersensitivity Bleeding disorders Heart failure
Mechanism: *Inhibits megakaryocyte development in late postmitotic stage*			
Anagrelide	Treat thrombocythemia associated with myeloproliferative disorders	Palpitations Headache Thrombocytopenia	Hepatic disease

cAMP, cyclic adenosine monophosphate.

BOX 16-2   ANTICOAGULANTS

Heparin-Related Compounds
Fondaparinux
Heparin (UFH)
Low-molecular-weight heparins (LMWHs)
  Dalteparin
  Enoxaparin
  Nadroparin
  Tinzaparin

Direct Thrombin Inhibitors
The -rudins: hirudin, bivalirudin, lepirudin
Argatroban

Oral Anticoagulant
Warfarin

TABLE 16-3. **Comparison Between Unfractionated Heparin and Low-Molecular-Weight Heparins**

PROPERTY	HEPARIN	LMWH
Anti-Xa versus anti-IIa activity	1:1	2:1–4:1
PTT monitoring	Required	Not required
Inhibition of platelet function	++++	++
Endothelial cell protein binding	Extensive	Minimal
Dose-dependent clearance	Yes	No
Elimination half-life	Short (50–90 minutes)	Long (2–5 times longer)

LMWH, low-molecular-weight heparin; PTT, partial thromboplastin time; +, magnitude of effect.

3. Adverse effects
   a. Bleeding
   b. Hyperkalemia
      • Heparin blocks an enzymatic step in the synthesis of aldosterone
        producing hypoaldosteronism, which leads to reduced potassium secretion in
        the kidneys.

TABLE 16-4. **Comparison of the Properties of Heparin and Warfarin**

PROPERTY	HEPARIN	WARFARIN
Route of administration	Parenteral/subcutaneous	Oral
Site of action	Blood (*in vivo* and *in vitro*)	Liver
Onset of action	Immediate	Delayed; depends on half-lives of factors being replaced
Duration of action	4 hours	2–5 days
Mechanism of action	Accelerates action of antithrombin III to neutralize thrombin	Inhibits epoxide reductase, thus preventing activation of vitamin K
Laboratory control of dose	PTT	PT, INR (standardizes the PT)
Antidote	Protamine sulfate	Vitamin K (phytonadione), fresh frozen plasma
Safety in pregnancy	Yes	No (fetal warfarin syndrome)

INR, international normalized ratio; PT, prothrombin time; PTT, partial thromboplastin time.

     c. Thrombocytopenia
       (1) Heparin binds to platelets and an IgG antibody directed against heparin binds to the drug.
       (2) Splenic macrophages phagocytose and destroy the platelet.

> Heparin: most common cause of thrombocytopenia in a hospitalized patients.

B. Low-molecular-weight heparins (LMWHs)
  1. Examples
    a. Dalteparin
    b. Enoxaparin
    c. Nadroparin
    d. Tinzaparin
  2. Mechanism of action
    • Antifactor Xa (mostly) and antifactor IIa activity
  3. Uses
    a. Primary prevention of deep vein thrombosis (DVT) after hip replacement
    b. Other thrombolytic diseases (see Table 16-1)
    c. LMWHs have pharmacokinetic, pharmacodynamic, and safety advantages over UFH (see Table 16-3).
    d. A disadvantage of LMWHs is that they are *not* readily reversed with protamine sulfate.
    e. Anticoagulation during pregnancy
    f. When needed, monitored by evaluating anti-Xa activity
  4. Adverse effects
    a. Bleeding
    b. Allergic reactions

> LMWHs are *not* readily reversed by protamine sulfate.

C. Fondaparinux
  1. Synthetic pentasaccharide anticoagulant
  2. General considerations
    a. Antithrombotic activity as a result of ATIII-mediated selective inhibition of factor Xa
    b. Elimination half-life of 18 hours; allows for once a day dosing.
  3. Uses
    a. Venous thromboembolism prophylaxis following orthopedic surgery
    b. Pulmonary embolism (PE)
    c. Deep vein thrombosis (DVT)

D. Direct thrombin inhibitors
  1. Most are derivatives of hirudin (referred to as rudins), a peptide found in leeches.
  2. Examples
    a. Lepirudin
    b. Bivalirudin
    c. Argatroban
  3. Used for anticoagulation in patients with heparin-induced thrombocytopenia (HIT)

E. Oral anticoagulants (warfarin)
  1. Warfarin is a synthetic derivative of *coumarin*, which is found in certain plants.
  2. Mechanism of action
    a. Inhibits epoxide reductase in the liver, which normally activates vitamin K that is produced by bacteria or absorbed from the diet.

> Coumarin derivatives are used as rat poison.

> Warfarin inhibits epoxide reductase, which prevents activation of vitamin K.

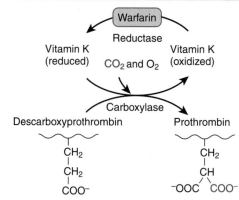

16-4: Mechanism of action of warfarin. (From Brenner G and Stevens C: Pharmacology, 3rd ed. Philadelphia, Saunders, 2010, Figure 16-3.)

Procoagulant vitamin K–dependent factors include II, VII, IX, and X.

Anticoagulant vitamin K–dependent factors also include protein C and S, which degrade factors V and VIII.

If bleeding is life-threatening, fresh frozen plasma is the treatment of choice.

PT is the basis for calculation of the warfarin dose.

Warfarin can cause fetal hemorrhage and skeletal malformations (fetal warfarin syndrome).

b. Activated vitamin K γ-carboxylates the procoagulant vitamin K-dependent factors II (prothrombin), VII, IX, X and the anticoagulant vitamin K-dependent factors protein C and S (Fig. 16-4).
(1) All of the vitamin K–dependent factors are synthesized in the liver and are non-functional until they are γ-carboxylated.
(2) Protein C and S inactivate factors V and VIII and enhance fibrinolysis.
c. Calcium binds to the γ-carboxylation sites on these factors, so that they can perform their functions in producing a fibrin clot or degrading coagulation factors.
3. Genetic factors increase patient sensitivity to warfarin
a. Genetic variations in the proteins CYP2C9 and VKORC1
(1) CYP2C9 deficiency is responsible for the lack of warfarin's metabolism requiring reduced dosing to prevent increased bleeding
(2) Mutations in VKORC1 require very high doses of warfarin to provide adequate anticoagulation
b. A genotyping test is available to provide important guidance on initiation of anticoagulant therapy.
4. Uses (see Table 16-1)
5. Adverse effects
• Bleeding
6. Monitoring
a. Target is a 1.5 to 3.5 fold increase in PT if human tissue thromboplastin is used (basis of the INR [international normalized ratio of test/control])
• INR standardizes the PT, regardless of the reagents or instrumentation used in measuring the PT.
b. Low-intensity anticoagulation (INR 1.5-2); long-term
c. Moderate-intensity anticoagulation (INR 2-3); used initially
d. High-intensity anticoagulation (INR 2.5-3.5); used for mechanical prosthetic heart valves
7. Comparison of the properties of warfarin to those of heparin (see Table 16-4)
8. Contraindications
a. Pregnancy
• Teratogenic effects—nasal hypoplasia, agenesis corpus callosum, fetal bleeding and death
b. Bleeding disorders
9. Drug interactions (many)
• Most relate to the cytochrome P450 system (Table 16-5).
F. Therapeutic summary of selected anticoagulant drugs (Table 16-6)
IV. Fibrinolytic (Thrombolytic) Drugs (Box 16-3)
    A. Basis of therapy
        1. Mechanism of action
          a. When coagulation begins, plasminogen is converted to plasmin, a protease that limits the spread of new clots and dissolves the fibrin in established fibrin clots (Fig. 16-5).
          b. Presence in the serum of D-dimers (cross-linked fibrin strands), indicates that plasmin is breaking down the fibrin clot.

TABLE 16-5. **Drugs That Interact with Warfarin**

DRUG	MECHANISM OF INTERACTION
Enhanced Response	
Allopurinol	Inhibits metabolism
Cimetidine	Inhibits metabolism
Ciprofloxacin	Inhibits metabolism
Co-trimoxazole	Inhibits metabolism
Erythromycin	Inhibits metabolism
Fluconazole	Inhibits metabolism
Metronidazole	Inhibits metabolism
Broad-spectrum antibiotics	Reduces availability of vitamin K
Sulfonamides	Displace from plasma albumin
Vitamin E toxicity	Prevents synthesis of vitamin K-dependent coagulation factors
Diminished Response	
Barbiturates	Induces hepatic microsomal enzymes
Carbamazepine	Induces hepatic microsomal enzymes
Primidone	Induces hepatic microsomal enzymes
Rifampin	Induces hepatic microsomal enzymes
Cholestyramine	Inhibits absorption
Estrogens	Stimulates synthesis of clotting factors
Vitamin K	Competes with warfarin

TABLE 16-6. **Therapeutic Summary of Selected Anticoagulant Drugs**

DRUGS	CLINICAL APPLICATIONS	ADVERSE EFFECTS	CONTRAINDICATIONS
Mechanism: *Accelerates the action of antithrombin III to neutralize thrombin (factor IIa); lesser extent other activated clotting factors*			
Heparin	Prophylaxis and treatment of thromboembolic disorders Maintain patency of IV devices Anticoagulation during pregnancy	Bleeding Heparin-induced thrombocytopenia (HIT)	Hypersensitivity Bleeding disorders HIT
Mechanism: *Accelerates the action of antithrombin III to neutralize mainly factor Xa; lesser extent thrombin (factor IIa)*			
Low-molecular-weight heparins (LMWHs) Dalteparin Enoxaparin Nadroparin Tinzaparin	Acute coronary syndromes Prevention and treatment of deep vein thrombosis Pulmonary embolism Anticoagulation during pregnancy	Bleeding HIT Effects not readily reversed by protamine sulfate	Hypersensitivity Bleeding disorders HIT
Mechanism: *Accelerates the action of antithrombin III to selectively neutralize factor Xa*			
Fondaparinux	Prevention and treatment of deep vein thrombosis Pulmonary embolism	Bleeding	Hypersensitivity Bleeding disorders HIT
Mechanism: *Direct thrombin inhibitors*			
Hirudin (leeches) Bivalirudin Lepirudin Argatroban	Anticoagulation in patients with HIT	Bleeding	Hypersensitivity Bleeding disorders
Mechanism: *Inhibits epoxide reductase in the liver, which prevents activation of vitamin K and subsequent γ-carboxylation of factors II, VII, IX, and X, as well as proteins C and S*			
Warfarin	Prophylaxis and treatment of thromboembolic disorders To prevent embolic complications from atrial fibrillation or cardiac valve replacement Adjunct to reduce risk of systemic embolism (e.g., recurrent myocardial infarction [MI], stroke) after MI	Bleeding Teratogenic	Hypersensitivity Bleeding disorders Pregnancy

---

BOX 16-3   FIBRINOLYTIC DRUGS

Forms of Recombinant Tissue Plasminogen Activator (tPA)
Alteplase
Reteplase
Tenecteplase

Other Fibrinolytic Agents
Urokinase

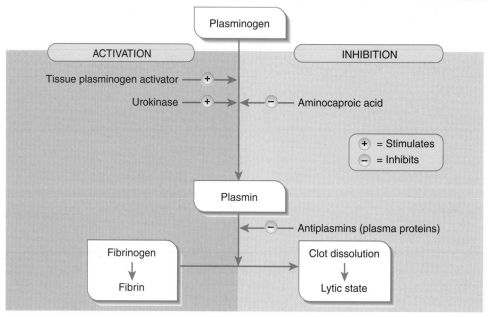

16-5: Site of action of drugs acting on the fibrinolytic system. Fibrinolytic drugs accelerate the conversion of plasminogen to plasmin, which is a protease that breaks down fibrinogen and fibrin to degradation products.

Thrombolytic agents are contraindicated if there is an increased risk of bleeding.

2. Uses (see Table 16-1)
   • Thrombolytic drugs must be given within 6 to 12 hours of a myocardial infarction (MI) to limit cardiac damage, and within 3 hours of a stroke.
3. Contraindication to thrombolytic therapy
   a. Surgery within 10 days
   b. Serious GI bleeding within 3 months
   c. History of hypertension (diastolic pressure >110 mmHg)
   d. Active bleeding or hemorrhagic disorder
   e. Previous cerebrovascular accident or active intracranial process
   f. Aortic dissection
   g. Acute pericarditis
4. Antidote
   a. Aminocaproic acid or tranexamic acid
   b. Competitively blocks plasminogen activation

B. Drugs used in thrombolytic therapy

Recombinant forms of human tPA most commonly used for thrombolytic therapy.

1. Recombinant forms of human tissue plasminogen activator (tPA)
   a. Alteplase
   b. Reteplase
   c. Tenecteplase
2. Mechanism of action
   a. These drugs cause a direct cleavage of the bond in plasminogen.
   b. These thrombolytic drugs selectively work within the thrombi.
3. Uses

Administer alteplase within 3 hours of symptoms of ischemic stroke.

   a. Management of acute myocardial infarction for the lysis of thrombi in coronary arteries
   b. Management of non-hemorrhagic acute ischemic stroke
   c. Acute myocardial infarction
      • Chest pain for longer than 20 minutes, less than 12 to 24 hours; S-T elevation greater than 0.1 mV in at least two electrocardiogram (ECG) leads
   d. Acute pulmonary embolism (age younger than 75 years)
      • Documented massive pulmonary embolism by pulmonary angiography or echocardiography or high probability lung scan with clinical shock
4. Alternative
   a. Urokinase
      • An enzyme derived from cultured human kidney cells is still used as a thrombolytic agent for the lysis of acute massive pulmonary emboli or pulmonary emboli with unstable hemodynamics.

b. Streptokinase
(1) Nonenzymatic protein isolated from streptococci
(2) Use discontinued in the Unites States because of hypersensitivity reactions
C. **Therapeutic summary of selected fibrinolytic drugs** (Table 16-7)
V. **Hemostatic Drugs and Blood Products** (Box 16-4)
A. **Vitamin K**
1. General information
a. This fat-soluble vitamin is found in leafy green vegetables.
b. It is produced by bacteria that colonize the human intestine and needs bile salts for absorption.
c. It is required for γ-carboxylation of glutamate residues in prothrombin (factor II) and factors XII, IX, and X, as well as anticoagulant factors protein C and protein S (see section III).
2. Uses
a. Prevention of hemorrhagic disease of the newborn (intramuscular or subcutaneous)
(1) Newborn bowel lacks bacterial colonization
(2) Requires up to 5 days for colonization and *de novo* synthesis of vitamin K
b. Treatment of dietary vitamin K deficiencies and reversal of the effect of warfarin (oral or parenteral)
• Fresh frozen plasma is required to correct life-threatening bleeding by over-anticoagulation by warfarin.
3. Adverse effects
a. Hemolysis
b. Jaundice
c. Hyperbilirubinemia occasionally occurs in newborns.
B. **Protamine sulfate**
1. Mechanism of action
a. Chemical antagonist of heparin
b. Less effective against LMWHs

> Most common cause of vitamin K deficiency in a hospital is use of broad spectrum antibiotics that kill colonic bacteria

> Newborns are always given an injection of vitamin K.

TABLE 16-7. **Therapeutic Summary of Selected Anticoagulant Drugs**

DRUGS	CLINICAL APPLICATIONS	ADVERSE EFFECTS	CONTRAINDICATIONS
Mechanism: *Recombinant tissue plasminogen activators that initiate local fibrinolysis by binding to fibrin in a thrombus*			
Alteplase	Acute myocardial infarction	Bleeding	Hypersensitivity
Reteplase	Acute pulmonary embolism	Hypotension	Bleeding disorders
Tenecteplase	Management of acute ischemic stroke		Intracranial bleeding
			Pregnancy
Mechanism: *Directly activates plasminogen to plasmin, which degrades fibrin, fibrinogen, and other procoagulant plasma proteins*			
Urokinase	Thrombolytic agent for the lysis of acute massive pulmonary emboli	Bleeding	Hypersensitivity
		Hypotension	Bleeding disorders
			Intracranial bleeding

BOX 16-4   HEMOSTATIC DRUGS AND BLOOD PRODUCTS

Fibrinolytic inhibitor
  Aminocaproic acid
Others
  Protamine sulfate
  Vitamin K
  Phytonadione
Blood product derivatives
  Antihemophilic Factor (Human)
  Antihemophilic Factor/von Willebrand Factor Complex (Human)
  Anti-inhibitor Coagulant Complex
  Antithrombin III
  Aprotinin
  Factor IX
  Factor IX Complex (Human)
  Plasma Protein Fraction
  Protein C Concentrate (Human)

2. Use
- Hemorrhage associated with heparin overdose

C. Aminocaproic acid:
1. Mechanism of action
- Fibrinolytic inhibitor (competitively inhibits plasminogen)
2. Use
- Treatment of hemorrhage caused by hyperfibrinolysis (as in aplastic anemia, abruptio placentae, hepatic cirrhosis)

Aminocaproic acid stops hyperfibrinolysis.

D. Desmopressin
1. Used in the maintenance of hemostasis and control of bleeding in mild hemophilia A and von Willebrand's disease.
2. Increases release of factor VIII coagulant and von Willebrand's factor from the endothelial cells (see Chapter 15)

E. Blood Product derivative
1. Antihemophilic Factor (Human)
- Used in the prevention and treatment of hemorrhagic episodes in patients with hemophilia A
2. Antihemophilic Factor/von Willebrand Factor Complex (Human) is used for:
   a. Prevention and treatment of hemorrhagic episodes in patients with hemophilia A or acquired factor VIII deficiency
   b. Prophylaxis with surgical and/or invasive procedures in patients with von Willebrand's disease (VWD) when desmopressin is either ineffective or contraindicated

Today blood products are mostly human derived.

   c. Treatment of spontaneous or trauma-induced bleeding, as well as prevention of excessive bleeding during and after surgery, in patients with VWD where use of desmopressin is known or suspected to be inadequate
3. Antithrombin III
- Used for the treatment of hereditary antithrombin III deficiency
4. Aprotinin
- Was used during cardiopulmonary bypass in coronary artery bypass graft surgery *but* removed from U.S. market May 2008.
5. Factor IX
- Used to control bleeding in patients with factor IX deficiency; also known as hemophilia B or Christmas disease
6. Factor IX Complex (Human)
- Used to control bleeding in patients with factor IX deficiency; also known as hemophilia B or Christmas disease
7. Plasma protein fraction
- Used as a plasma volume expander and in the maintenance of cardiac output in the treatment of certain types of shock
8. Protein C concentrate (human)
- Used in replacement therapy for severe congenital protein C deficiency

CHAPTER 17
HEMATOPOIETIC DRUGS

I. General Considerations
A. Causes of anemia
1. Failure to produce sufficient red blood cells (RBCs)
2. Inadequate synthesis of hemoglobin
3. Destruction of RBCs
4. Bleeding

B. Classification by mean corpuscular volume (MCV)
1. Different conditions may lead to the development of the various types of anemia (Table 17-1)
2. Microcytic
   a. Smaller than normal RBCs and decreased MCV ($<80\ \mu m^3$)
   b. Iron deficiency, anemia of chronic disease, and thalassemia (α and β) result in small RBCs with insufficient hemoglobin (microcytic hypochromic anemia)
3. Macrocytic
   a. Larger than normal RBCs and increased MCV ($>100\ \mu m^3$)
   b. Both folic acid deficiency and vitamin B_{12} deficiency cause impaired production and nuclear maturation of erythroid precursors (macrocytic hyperchromic or megaloblastic anemia).
   • Problems also occur with nuclear maturation of other hematopoietic elements (e.g., neutrophils).
4. Normocytic
   a. Normal sized RBCs and normal MCV ($80–100\ \mu m^3$)
   b. Causes include:
      (1) Renal failure
         • Decreased synthesis of erythropoietin (EPO)
      (2) Aplastic anemia
         • Suppression of hematopoiesis
      (3) Acute/chronic blood loss
      (4) Hemolytic anemia
         • Destruction of RBCs
      (5) Early stages of iron deficiency and anemia of chronic disease
         • Both are normocytic before they are microcytic

C. Agents used to treat anemia (Box 17-1)

II. Minerals
• Iron
A. Role of iron
1. Requirement for the synthesis of hemoglobin and myoglobin
2. Cofactor in many enzymes (e.g., cytochromes in the liver)

B. Causes of iron deficiency (see Table 17-2)

C. Clinical use
1. Treatment and prevention of iron deficiency anemia
2. Preparations
   a. Oral preparations
      • Preferred
         (1) Ferrous fumarate
         (2) Ferrous gluconate
         (3) Ferrous sulfate
         (4) Polysaccharide-iron complex

Iron deficiency due to bleeding is the most common cause of anemia

Microcytic anemia; MCV less than 80 μm^3

Microcytic anemia is most commonly due to iron deficiency.

Macrocytic anemia; MCV greater than 100 μm^3

Macrocytic anemia due to folic acid and/or vitamin B_{12} deficiency.

Normocytic anemia due to: decreased EPO; aplastic anemia; blood loss; hemolytic anemia.

Oral preparations of iron are preferred to treat iron deficiency anemia.

Table 17-1. **Etiology of Anemia**

TYPES OF ANEMIA	SPECIFIC CAUSE/PATHOPHYSIOLOGY
Microcytic Anemia	
Iron deficiency anemia	Increased need (e.g., growth, pregnancy, menstruation) Blood loss (e.g., gastrointestinal bleeding) Inadequate dietary intake Malabsorption
Anemia of chronic disease	Chronic infection, cancer, or liver disease Failure of increase in red blood cell production due to sequestration of iron in reticuloendothelial system in the bone marrow
Thalassemia	Hereditary disorder characterized by decreased globin chain production
Megaloblastic Anemia	
Folic acid deficiency anemia	Inadequate dietary intake Increased need during pregnancy Interference with utilization by other drugs (phenytoin, primidone, and phenobarbital; oral contraceptives; isoniazid) Malabsorption syndromes (e.g., high rates of cell turnover as in hemolytic anemia or alcoholism, or poor liver function)
Vitamin B_{12} deficiency anemia	Pernicious anemia (lack of intrinsic factor [IF]), which may occur following gastrectomy Lack of receptors for IF-vitamin B_{12} complex in ileum Fish tapeworm infestations Crohn's disease/ileotomy
Normocytic Anemia	
Anemia due to bone marrow failure	Myelofibrosis and multiple myeloma: direct effects Myelosuppressive chemotherapy Deficiency of hematopoietic growth factors and hormones (as in chronic renal failure) Aplastic anemia

---

BOX 17-1   HEMATOPOIETIC DRUGS

Minerals
Oral iron preparations
  Ferrous fumarate
  Ferrous gluconate
  Ferrous sulfate
  Polysaccharide-iron complex
Parenteral preparations
  Ferric gluconate
  Iron dextran complex
  Iron sucrose

Vitamins
Folate preparations
  Folic acid
  Leucovorin

Vitamin B_{12} preparations
  Cyanocobalamin
  Hydroxocobalamin

Hematopoietic Growth Factors
Darbepoetin alfa
Epoetin alfa
Filgrastim
Oprelvekin
Pegfilgrastim
Sargramostim

TABLE 17-2. **Causes of Iron Deficiency Anemia**

CLASSIFICATION	CAUSES	DISCUSSION
Blood loss	Gastrointestinal loss	Meckel's diverticulum (older children) PUD (most common cause adult men) Gastritis (e.g., NSAID) Hookworm infestation Polyps/colorectal cancer (most common cause in adults >50-yrs-old); positive stool for blood.
	Menorrhagia	Most common cause in women <50-yrs-old
Increased utilization	Pregnancy/lactation	Daily iron requirement in pregnancy is 3.4 mg and 2.5-3.0 mg in lactation Net loss of 500 mg of iron if not on iron supplements
	Infants/children	Iron required for tissue growth and expansion of blood volume
Decreased intake	Prematurity Infants/children	Loss of iron each day fetus is not in utero Blood loss from phlebotomy Most common cause of iron deficiency in young children
	Elderly	Restricted diets with little meat (lack of heme iron)
Decreased absorption	Celiac sprue	Absence of villous surface in the duodenum
Intravascular hemolysis	Microangiopathic hemolytic anemia	Chronic loss of Hb in urine leads to iron deficiency

Hb, hemoglobin; NSAID, non-steroidal anti-inflammatory drug; PUD, peptic ulcer disease. *(Modified from Goljan EF: Rapid Review Pathology, 3rd ed. Philadelphia, Mosby, 2010, Table 11-1.)*

b. Parenteral preparations
  • Required for very severe iron deficiency
    (1) Ferric gluconate
    (2) Iron dextran complex
    (3) Iron sucrose
D. Adverse effects
  1. Acute toxicity (when given orally); signs include:
    a. Diarrhea with bleeding
    b. Gastrointestinal (GI) irritation with bleeding
    c. Nausea
    d. Hematemesis
    e. Green, tarry stools
    f. Hepatic failure
    g. Metabolic acidosis
      • Iron tablets are radiopaque; therefore, an abdominal x-ray is useful in detecting undigested iron tablets.
  2. In children, acute iron toxicity is one of the leading causes of acute poisoning.
    • Antidote is intravenous deferoxamine
  3. Chronic toxicity
    a. Hemochromatosis
      • Autosomal recessive disease in which all the iron is reabsorbed in the small intestine
    b. Hemosiderosis
      • Acquired iron overload most often due to excessive blood transfusions (e.g., sickle cell disease)
  4. Boxed warning
    • Deaths associated with parenteral administration following anaphylactic-type reactions have been reported, especially with iron dextran complex.

Iron tablets radiopaque; abdominal radiograph useful in diagnosis and treatment

Acute iron toxicity requires treatment with intravenous deferoxamine, an iron chelating drug.

Hemochromatosis and hemosiderosis are iron-overload diseases

III. Vitamins
  • Folic acid and vitamin B_{12}
  A. General considerations:
  1. Both folic acid and/or vitamin B_{12} deficiency can lead to hematologic impairment and show hypersegmented polymorphonuclear neutrophils as well as a macrocytic anemia on blood smear.
  2. Functions of folic acid (Fig. 17-1)
    a. Tetrahydrofolate (FH_4) receives a methylene group ($-CH_2-$), a one-carbon transfer reaction, from serine to produce N^5,N^{10}-methylene-tetrahydrofolate.
      (1) The methylene group is then transferred by thymidylate synthase to dUMP (deoxyuridine monophosphate) to produce dTMP (deoxythymidine monophosphate) for DNA synthesis.
      (2) 5-Fluorouracil irreversibly inhibits thymidylate synthase.
    b. Two hydrogens from FH_4 are utilized in the formation of dTMP, resulting in the formation of dihydrofolate (FH_2).
    c. FH_2 is reduced to FH_4 by dihydrofolate reductase; some chemotherapeutic drugs target this enzyme and cause macrocytic anemia as an adverse effect.
      (1) Methotrexate

5-Fluorouracil inhibits thymidylate synthase.

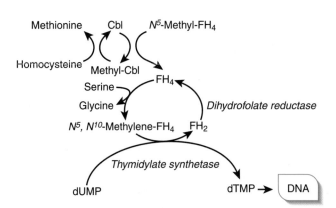

17-1: Vitamin B_{12} (cobalamin) and folic acid in DNA synthesis. Cobalamin (Cbl) is important in the demethylation of N^5-methyltetrahydrofolate (N^5-methyl-FH_4) and methylation of homocysteine to form methionine. Tetrahydrofolate (FH_4) receives a methylene group ($-CH_2-$) from serine to produce N^5,N^{10}-methylene-FH_4, which transfers the methylene group to deoxyuridine monophosphate (dUMP) to produce deoxythymidine monophosphate (dTMP). *(From Pelley JW and Goljan EF: Rapid Review Biochemistry, 2nd ed. Philadelphia, Mosby, 2007, Figure 4-3.)*

- A nonselective inhibitor of dihydrofolate reductase used as an anticancer agent, immunosuppressive agent, and widely used to treat rheumatoid arthritis

  (2) Trimethoprim
  - Highest affinity for bacterial dihydrofolate reductase

  (3) Pyrimethamine
  - Highest affinity for protozoan dihydrofolate reductase

3. Dietary folate
   a. Dietary polyglutamate forms of 5-methyltetrahydrofolate are converted by intestinal conjugase to the monoglutamate form, which is actively absorbed in the jejunum.
      (1) Intestinal conjugase is inhibited by phenytoin.
      (2) Monoglutamate reabsorption in the jejunum is inhibited by alcohol and oral contraceptive pills (OCPs).
   b. 5-Methyltetrahydrofolate requires vitamin B_{12} to be converted into the functional forms of tetrahydrofolate (See Fig. 17-1)
      (1) Vitamin B_{12} removes the methyl group and transfers it to homocysteine, which, in turn, transfers it to methionine.
      (2) Deficiency of either vitamin B_{12} or folate leads to an increase in homocysteine, which damages endothelial cells leading to vessel thrombosis.

4. Causes of folate deficiency (Table 17-3)

5. Tests for folate deficiency
   - Serum and RBC folate are the best tests.

6. Functions of vitamin B_{12}
   - Essential for normal synthesis of DNA and for maintenance of myelin throughout the nervous system; required by three key biochemical reactions
   a. DNA synthesis
      (1) Vitamin B_{12} is required to convert 5-CH_3-FH_4 (the dietary form) to FH_4.
      (2) FH_4 (more specifically its derivative 5,10-CH_2-FH_4) is required to convert dUMP to dTMP (see above).
   b. Odd chain fatty acid metabolism
      (1) Vitamin B_{12} is a cofactor in methylmalonyl CoA mutase, which is required to convert methylmalonyl-CoA to succinyl-CoA in odd-chain fatty acid metabolism.
      (2) Vitamin B_{12} deficiency causes an increase in propionyl and methylmalonyl CoA and their corresponding acids, which are proximal to the enzyme block.
      - Propionyl CoA replaces acetyl CoA in neuronal membranes, resulting in demyelination.
      (3) Demyelination syndromes associated with vitamin B_{12} deficiency include:
         (a) Subacute combined degeneration of the spinal cord (posterior columns and lateral corticospinal tract)

Methotrexate, trimethoprim, pyrimethamine inhibit dihydrofolate reductase.

Phenytoin inhibits intestinal conjugase; alcohol and OCPs inhibit reabsorption of monoglutamate.

Folic acid deficiency responsible for spina bifida.

Vitamin B_{12} required for dietary folates to support DNA synthesis.

Vitamin B_{12} required for myelin synthesis.

Table 17-3. **Causes of Folate Deficiency**

CLASSIFICATION	CAUSES	COMMENT AND ASSOCIATED FACTORS
Decreased intake	Malnutrition Infants/elderly Chronic alcoholics Goat's milk	Decreased intake most common cause of folate deficiency
Malabsorption	Celiac disease Bacterial overgrowth	Deficiency usually occurs in association with other vitamin deficiencies (fat and water soluble)
Drug inhibition	5-Fluorouracil	Inhibits thymidylate synthase
	Methotrexate Trimethoptime/ sulfamethoxazole	Inhibit dihydrofolate reductase
	Phenytoin	Inhibits intestinal conjugase
	Oral contraceptives	Inhibit uptake of monoglutamate in jejunum
	Alcohol	Alcohol also inhibits the release of folate from the liver
Increased utilization	Pregnancy/lactation Disseminated malignancy Severe hemolytic anemia	Increased utilization of folate in DNA synthesis
Increased loss	Renal dialysis	Sometimes mixed anemia; also erythropoietin deficient

(Modified from Goljan EF: Rapid Review Pathology, 3rd ed. Philadelphia, Mosby, 2010, Table 11-4.)

         (b) Peripheral neuropathies
         (c) Dementia
     c. Amino acid synthesis
        (1) Vitamin B_{12} and folate are required to convert homocysteine to methionine (see above discussion).
        (2) Deficiency of either vitamin B_{12} or folate leads to an increase in serum homocysteine, which damages endothelial cells leading to vessel thrombosis (e.g., coronary artery thrombosis).

> Vitamin B_{12} required for methionine synthesis.

  7. Dietary vitamin B_{12}
     a. Vitamin B_{12} binds to R factor in the mouth or esophagus to form a complex
       • R factor prevents destruction of vitamin B_{12} by gastric acid.
     b. Absorption of vitamin B_{12} requires intrinsic factor (IF):
        (1) IF is a glycoprotein synthesized by parietal cells located in the body and fundus of the stomach.
        (2) Before IF binds to vitamin B_{12} in the duodenum, pancreatic enzymes must cleave off R factor so that IF can combine with the vitamin to form a complex that is reabsorbed in the terminal ileum
        (3) Intrinsic factor is *not* used as a drug.

> Intrinsic factor is produced by parietal cells.

     c. Distribution
        (1) Once reabsorbed, vitamin B_{12} is transported via transcobalamin II, a plasma glycoprotein.
        (2) Excess vitamin is stored in liver
           (a) It takes 6 to 9 years to deplete stores from body.
           (b) Since it has long half-life, it is only given once a month in patients who *cannot* absorb it from diet

> Pernicious anemia is an autoimmune disease that destroys parietal cells.

  8. Causes of vitamin B_{12} deficiency (Table 17-4)
  9. Tests for vitamin B_{12} deficiency
     a. Schilling test
       • Uses radioactive cobalt to test the body's ability to take up vitamin B_{12} from the GI tract
     b. Measurement of urinary methylmalonate levels
       • Increased levels in deficiency

> Achlorhydria (lack of gastric acidity) is associated with lack of intrinsic factor.

     c. It is very important to diagnose the cause of megaloblastic anemia so that corrective therapy can be initiated appropriately with either vitamin B_{12} or folic acid, since folic acid can reverse the hematological damage due to vitamin B_{12} deficiency but *not* the neurological changes.

> Neurologic changes may result from vitamin B_{12} deficiency but *not* folate deficiency

B. Folate preparations
  1. Folic acid
     a. Treatment of megaloblastic and macrocytic anemias due to folate deficiency
     b. Dietary supplement to prevent neural tube defects
  2. Leucovorin (folinic acid)
     a. A reduced form of folic acid beyond the step blocked by dihydrofolate reductase inhibitors
     b. Uses
        (1) Antidote for folic acid antagonists (methotrexate, trimethoprim, pyrimethamine)

> Supplemental folate, unlike dietary folate does *not* require vitamin B_{12} to support hematopoiesis.

Table 17-4. **Causes of Vitamin B_{12} Deficiency**

CLASSIFICATION	CAUSES	ASSOCIATED FACTORS
Decreased intake	Pure vegan diet	Breast-fed infants of pure vegans may develop deficiency
Malnutrition		May occur in elderly patients
Malabsorption	↓ Intrinsic factor	Autoimmune destruction of parietal cells (i.e., pernicious anemia)
	↓ Gastric acid	Cannot activate pepsinogen to release vitamin B_{12}
	↓ Intestinal reabsorption	Crohn's disease or celiac disease involving terminal ileum (destruction of absorptive cells) Bacterial overgrowth (bacterial utilization of available vitamin B_{12}) Fish tapeworm Chronic pancreatitis (cannot cleave off R-binder)
Increased utilization	Pregnancy/lactation	Deficiency is more likely in a pure vegan

(Modified from Goljan EF: Rapid Review Pathology, 3rd ed. Philadelphia, Mosby, 2010, Table 11-3.)

Leucovorin (folinic acid) is used to reverse methotrexate and potentiate fluorouracil cytotoxicity.

(2) Rescue therapy following high-dose methotrexate

(3) Given with fluorouracil in the treatment of colon cancer

(4) Treatment of megaloblastic anemias when folate is deficient as in infancy, sprue, pregnancy

(5) Nutritional deficiency when oral folate therapy is *not* possible.

C. **Vitamin B$_{12}$ preparations**

1. Cyanocobalamin: uses
   a. Treatment of pernicious anemia
   b. Treatment of increased utilization of vitamin B$_{12}$ (e.g., during neoplastic treatment)
   c. Increased B$_{12}$ requirements due to:
      (1) Pregnancy
      (2) Thyrotoxicosis
      (3) Hemorrhage
      (4) Malignancy
      (5) Liver or kidney disease

Cyanocobalamin is the preferred Vitamin B$_{12}$ preparation for long-term use.

2. Hydroxocobalamin
   a. Treatment of pernicious anemia
   b. Diagnostic agent for Schilling test
   c. Treatment of cyanide poisoning
      • Hydroxocobalamin binds cyanide to form vitamin B$_{12a}$ cyanocobalamin, which is eliminated in the urine.

IV. **Hematopoietic Growth Factors**

A. **Role of hematopoietic growth factors**
   • These growth factors control the proliferation and differentiation of pluripotent stem cells.

B. **Causes of bone marrow failure** (see Table 17-1)

C. **Drugs used to treat bone marrow failure**

1. Epoetin alfa and darbepoetin alfa (erythropoietin)
   a. A glycoprotein that stimulates RBC production
      • Erythropoietin is produced in the kidney
   b. Used in patients with chronic renal failure, those with cancer who are receiving chemotherapy, and those with acquired immunodeficiency syndrome (AIDS)
   c. Used illegally by athletes for its performance-enhancing properties

Erythropoietin produced by the kidney supports erythropoiesis.

2. Sargramostim
   a. It is a recombinant granulocyte-macrophage colony-stimulating factor (GM-CSF)
   b. Promotes myeloid recovery in patients with non-Hodgkin's lymphoma, acute lymphoblastic leukemia, and Hodgkin's disease who are undergoing bone marrow transplantation
   c. Promotes myeloid recovery after standard-dose chemotherapy
   d. Treats drug-induced bone marrow toxicity or neutropenia associated with AIDS

GM-CSF promotes myelopoiesis.

3. Filgrastim and pegfilgrastim
   a. Granulocyte colony-stimulating factor (G-CSF)
   b. Prevents and treats chemotherapy-related febrile neutropenia
   c. Promotes myeloid recovery in patients undergoing bone marrow transplantation
   d. Pegfilgrastim has a prolonged duration of effect relative to filgrastim and a reduced renal clearance.

G-CSF promotes granulopoiesis.

4. Oprelvekin
   a. It is a recombinant human interleukin 11 (IL-11).
   b. Promotes the proliferation of hematopoietic stem cells and megakaryocyte progenitor cells; induces megakaryocyte maturation resulting in increased platelet production
   c. Prevents and treats chemotherapy-induced thrombocytopenia
   d. Reduces the need for platelet transfusions following myelosuppressive chemotherapy for nonmyeloid malignancies

IL-11 promotes megakaryopoiesis.

V. **Therapeutic summary of selected hematopoietic drugs** (Table 17-5)

TABLE 17-5. **Therapeutic Summary of Selected Hematopoietic Drugs**

DRUGS	CLINICAL APPLICATIONS	ADVERSE EFFECTS	CONTRAINDICATIONS
Mechanism: *Oral forms of iron to replace iron in hemoglobin, myoglobin, and other enzymes; prevents microcytic anemia*			
Ferrous fumarate Ferrous gluconate Ferrous sulfate Polysaccharide-iron complex	Prevention and treatment of iron-deficiency anemias	Constipation GI irritation Epigastric pain Dark stools Nausea and vomiting Stomach cramping	Hypersensitivity Hemochromatosis Hemolytic anemia
Mechanism: *Parenteral forms of iron to replace iron in hemoglobin, myoglobin, and other enzymes; prevents microcytic anemia*			
Ferric gluconate Iron dextran complex Iron sucrose	Treatment iron-deficiency anemias when oral administration is infeasible or ineffective	Hypotension Anaphylactoid reactions Metallic taste Flushing	Hypersensitivity Hemochromatosis Hemolytic anemia
Mechanism: *Required for hematopoiesis; prevents macrocytic anemia*			
Folic acid	Treatment of megaloblastic or macrocytic anemias due to folate deficiency Dietary supplement to prevent neural tube defects	Flushing Pruritus Rash	Hypersensitivity Pernicious anemia
Mechanism: *Folinic acid; a cofactor intermediate beyond the dihydrofolate reductase step in the folate pathway*			
Leucovorin	Antidote for folic acid antagonists Rescue therapy for high-dose methotrexate Given with fluorouracil for colon cancer Treatment of megaloblastic anemias when folic acid can't be used	Increases GI toxicity of fluorouracil Pruritus Rash	Hypersensitivity Pernicious anemia
Mechanism: *A coenzyme for metabolic functions, including odd chain fatty acid metabolism, amino acid synthesis, as well as cell replication and hematopoiesis*			
Cyanocobalamin Hydroxocobalamin	Treatment of pernicious anemia Treatment of vitamin B_{12} deficiency Treatment of cyanide poisoning (hydroxocobalamin)	Erythema Hypertension Headache Nausea	Hypersensitivity
Mechanism: *Promotes erythropoiesis*			
Darbepoetin alfa Epoetin alfa	Anemia of kidney disease Chemotherapy-induced anemia	Hypertension Headache Nausea Fever Arthralgia	Hypersensitivity Uncontrolled hypertension
Mechanism: *Stimulates the production, maturation, and activation of neutrophils*			
Filgrastim Pegfilgrastim	Stimulation of granulocyte production in chemotherapy-induced neutropenia	Fever Headache Nausea Increased alkaline phosphatase Splenomegaly	Hypersensitivity
Mechanism: *Stimulates proliferation, differentiation and functional activity of neutrophils, eosinophils, monocytes, and macrophages*			
Sargramostim	Acute myelogenous leukemia following induction chemotherapy Bone marrow transplant (allogeneic or autologous) failure or engraftment delay Myeloid reconstitution after allogeneic bone marrow transplantation Peripheral stem cell transplantation	Fever Headache Nausea Chills Rash Hyperbilirubinemia Hyperglycemia	Hypersensitivity In patients with excessive leukemic myeloid blasts
Mechanism: *Interleukin (IL)-11 is a growth factor that stimulates multiple stages of megakaryocytopoiesis and thrombopoiesis*			
Oprelvekin	Prevention of severe thrombocytopenia	Tachycardia Edema Fever Headache Nausea Chills Rash	Hypersensitivity

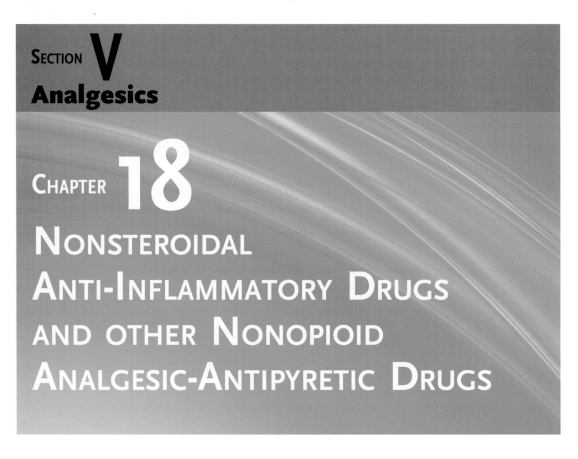

CHAPTER **18**

NONSTEROIDAL ANTI-INFLAMMATORY DRUGS AND OTHER NONOPIOID ANALGESIC-ANTIPYRETIC DRUGS

I. **General Considerations**
   A. **Nonsteroidal anti-inflammatory drugs (NSAIDs)**
   - Inhibit the synthesis of eicosanoids from arachidonic acid (Fig. 18-1; Table 18-1).
   B. **Basic mechanisms**
   1. These drugs primarily inhibit cyclooxygenase (COX), the enzyme responsible for the first step of prostaglandin synthesis.
      a. COX-1 is constituently expressed in many tissues.
      b. COX-2 is induced by cytokines in inflammatory cells and is found in endothelial cells.
      c. COX-3 is a putative isoform found in the brain.
   2. Aspirin is the only irreversible inhibitor of COX.

II. **NSAIDs** (Box 18-1)
   A. **Aspirin and other salicylates**
   1. Aspirin (acetylsalicylic acid), the prototype NSAID, is the standard against which all other NSAIDs are measured.
   2. Mechanism of action
      a. Many effects of aspirin are due to irreversible inhibition of prostaglandin synthesis through acetylation of both COX-1 and COX-2.
      b. Antiplatelet effect (see Chapter 16)
      - Prolonged bleeding time but *no* change in the other coagulation indicators (e.g., prothrombin time [PT], partial thromboplastin time [PTT])
      c. Antithrombotic effect
      - Inhibition of thromboxane A_2 (TXA_2) synthesis (potent platelet aggregator and vasoconstrictor) via irreversible inhibition of platelet COX-1 that lasts for the life span of platelets (see Chapter 16)
   3. Dose-dependent pharmacokinetics
      a. Acetylsalicylic acid ($t_{1/2} = 15$ min) is enzymatically and rapidly metabolized to salicylic acid (a reversible inhibitor of cyclooxygenase).
      b. When conjugation pathways become saturated, small increases in the dose of aspirin can produce relatively large increases in plasma salicylate levels.
      c. A low dose of aspirin (600 mg) gives first-order kinetics, $t_{1/2}$ is 3 to 5 hours (salicylate)
      - Analgesic, antipyretic, platelet inhibitor

COX-1 is constituently expressed.

COX-2 is up-regulated by cytokines in inflammatory cells; also, in endothelial cells.

Aspirin is an irreversible inhibitor of both COX-1 and -2 enzymes.

Aspirin is the only NSAID without a boxed warning of increased cardiovascular events with prolonged use.

The life span of platelets is about 8 days

Aspirin most widely used anti-platelet drug.

Salicylic acid metabolism switches from first to zero-order kinetics at high doses; metabolism becomes dose-dependent.

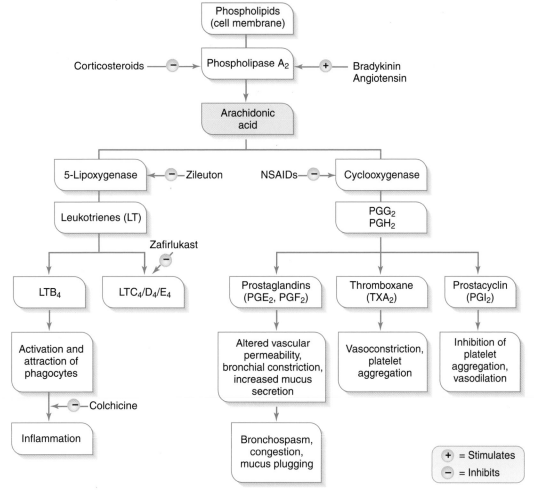

18-1: Schematic representation of the arachidonic acid pathway, which depicts the mediators formed from arachidonic acid, their biologic function, and drugs that stimulate or inhibit their formation. NSAID, nonsteroidal anti-inflammatory drug.

Table 18-1. **Important Actions of Eicosanoid Products**

EFFECTS OF EICOSANOIDS	PGE$_2$	PGF$_{2\alpha}$	PGI$_2$	TXA$_2$	LTB$_4$	LTC$_4$	LTD$_4$
Receptors	EP$_{1-4}$	FP$_{A,B}$	IP	TP$_{\alpha,\beta}$	BLT$_{1,2}$	CysLT$_2$	CysLT$_1$
Vascular tone	↓ or ↑	↓ or ↑	↓↓	↑↑↑	?	↑ or ↓	↑ or ↓
Bronchial tone	↓↓	↑↑	↓	↑↑	?	↑↑↑↑	↑↑↑↑
Uterine tone	↑↑	↑↑↑	↓	↑↑	?	?	?
Platelet aggregation	↓ or ↑	—	↓↓↓	↑↑↑	?	?	?
Leukocyte chemotaxis	?	?	?	?	↑↑↑↑	↑↑	↑↑

↑, G$_q$ pathway = ↑ intracellular Ca^{2+}; ↓, cyclic adenosine monophosphate (cAMP) pathway; LT, leukotriene; PG, prostaglandin; TX, thromboxane.

    d. High dose of aspirin (>4000 mg) gives zero-order kinetics, $t_{1/2}$ greater than 12 hours (salicylate)
      • Anti-inflammatory
    e. Excreted in urine as salicylic acid, salicyluric acid, glucuronic acid conjugates
  4. Uses
    a. Fever, acute rheumatic fever
    b. Headache
    c. Mild pain
    d. Dysmenorrhea
    e. Inflammatory conditions such as osteoarthritis and rheumatoid arthritis (RA)
    f. Prevention of platelet aggregation in:
      (1) Coronary artery disease
      (2) Myocardial infarction
      (3) Atrial fibrillation

Aspirin and other NSAIDs are antipyretic, analgesic, and anti-inflammatory.

COX-1 inhibitors decrease platelet aggregation; COX-2 inhibitors *do not.*

BOX 18-1 NONSTEROIDAL ANTI-INFLAMMATORY DRUGS (NSAIDs) AND OTHER NONOPIOID ANALGESICS	
NSAIDs Aspirin Diclofenac Ibuprofen Indomethacin Ketoprofen Ketorolac (parenteral) Naproxen Oxaprozin Piroxicam Sulindac	**COX-2 Inhibitors (Selective NSAIDs)** Celecoxib Rofecoxib (removed from market) Valdecoxib (removed from market) **Nonopioid and Non-NSAID Analgesic** Acetaminophen

High dose of aspirin produces salicylism (tinnitus, vertigo leading to deafness).

Aspirin overdose causes respiratory alkalosis followed by metabolic acidosis.

Extensive use of NSAIDs can contribute to hypertension.

Aspirin overdose uncouples mitochondrial oxidative phosphorylation leading to hyperthermia.

5. Adverse effects
  a. Gastric irritation, gastrointestinal (GI) bleeding, peptic ulcer disease
    • Occurs to some degree with the use of all NSAIDs
  b. Salicylism (tinnitus, vertigo leading to deafness) with overdose (see Chapter 30); reversible with dosage reduction
  c. Primary respiratory alkalosis often followed by a primary increased anion gap metabolic acidosis
    (1) This is called a mixed blood gas disorder.
      (a) Arterial pH is normal.
      (b) More often occurs in children than in adults
    (2) Respiratory acidosis due to eventual suppression of the medullary respiratory center may also occur as a late finding.
  d. Renal failure
    (1) Possibly due to decrease in prostaglandin E_2 or I_2 production (vasodilators of afferent arterioles)
    (2) Leads to acute ischemic tubular necrosis
  e. Hyperthermia
    (1) Salicylates damage the inner mitochondrial membrane and disrupt oxidative phosphorylation and synthesis of adenosine triphosphate (ATP).
    (2) Energy normally used to synthesize ATP is now converted to heat and increases the core body temperature.
6. Contraindications
  a. Hypersensitivity reactions
    (1) Occurrence in patients (usually women) with aspirin-induced nasal polyps
    (2) Leads to urticaria and bronchoconstriction (aspirin-induced asthma)
    (3) Due to increase in leukotriene production of LTC-D-E4 (potent bronchoconstrictors)
    (4) Treated with zafirlukast
  b. Hemophilia
  c. Risk of Reye's syndrome
    • Encephalopathy and fatty change in the liver
      (1) Aspirin should *not* be given to children with viral infections (e.g., flu, chickenpox)
      (2) Use acetaminophen or ibuprofen as an acceptable substitute.

Patients with aspirin-induced nasal polyps or with sensitivity reactions (e.g., urticaria) to aspirin are at risk of developing bronchoconstriction or anaphylaxis and should not receive aspirin or other NSAIDs.

Drug of choice in children with fever: acetaminophen; do *not* use aspirin (danger of Reye's syndrome)

Ketorolac is often used parenterally for postoperative pain.

B. Other nonselective NSAIDs
  1. Examples
    a. Ibuprofen
    b. Indomethacin
    c. Ketorolac
    d. Naproxen
    e. Piroxicam
    f. Sulindac
  2. Individual differences
    • Mostly in duration of action and potency
      a. Ibuprofen: short half-life (2 hours)
      b. Naproxen: long half-life (14 hours)
      c. Piroxicam: long half-life (45 hours)

Individual NSAIDs differ most in potency and duration of action.

3. The U.S. Food and Drug Administration (FDA) issued a warning that long-term use of a nonselective NSAID, such as naproxen and other NSAIDs, may be associated with an increased cardiovascular (CV) risk compared with placebo; likely due to effects on kidney, decreasing renal blood flow.

4. Mechanism of action
   a. These NSAIDs reversibly bind to both COX-1 and COX-2, exhibiting antipyretic, analgesic, and anti-inflammatory effects that are similar to aspirin.
   b. Antipyretic effects involve blocking the production of prostaglandins in the central nervous system to reset the hypothalamic temperature control, facilitating heat dissipation by vasodilation.

5. Uses
   a. Mild to moderate pain, bone and joint trauma
   b. Inflammatory syndromes (e.g., RA, gout)
   c. Fever
   d. Closure of patent ductus arteriosus (indomethacin)

6. Adverse effects
   a. Gastric upset and GI bleeding, due in part to inhibited synthesis of prostaglandins involved in production and maintenance of the mucus-bicarbonate barrier against acid.
   b. Possibly decreased renal function, especially in patients with underlying renal disease, leading to renal failure (e.g., acute tubular necrosis)
   c. Risk of premature closure of patent ductus arteriosus in the fetus
      • Use after 20 weeks of pregnancy is *not* recommended
   d. Hypocalcemia
      • Decreased production of prostaglandins that have osteoclast-activating activity

C. **Cyclooxygenase 2 (COX-2) inhibitors**
   1. Examples
      a. Celecoxib
      b. Rofecoxib (withdrawn from market)
      c. Valdecoxib (withdrawn from market)
   2. The FDA issued a warning in late 2004 that the COX-2 inhibitors may be associated with an increased risk of serious cardiovascular events (heart attack and stroke), especially when used chronically or in very high risk settings (e.g., after open heart surgery).
   3. Mechanism of action
      • These agents are selective inhibitors of COX-2; whereas, most other NSAIDs are nonselective COX-1 and COX-2 inhibitors
   4. Uses
      a. Rheumatoid arthritis (RA)
      b. Osteoarthritis (OA)
      c. Acute pain
      d. Dysmenorrhea
   5. Adverse effects
      a. GI bleeding
         • Compared with other NSAIDs, COX-2 inhibitors have a lower incidence of gastrointestinal adverse effects
      b. Renal failure
      c. Cardiovascular events
         (1) Cyclooxygenase-2 (COX-2) is the isoform found in endothelial cells required for PGI_2 production
         (2) Its inhibition is the likely cause of increased cardiovascular events associated with COX-2 inhibitors.

III. **Acetaminophen**
   • It has no anti-inflammatory activity, although it has analgesic and antipyretic effects which are similar to those of aspirin
A. **Mechanism of action**
   1. Unknown but some evidence suggests that it inhibits the putative COX-3 isoform in the brain
   2. Produces antipyresis from inhibition of hypothalamic heat-regulating center
B. **Uses**
   1. Osteoarthritis (relieves pain)
   2. Acute pain syndromes
   3. Fever

All NSAIDs, except aspirin, have a boxed warning that they increase cardiovascular events when used at high doses for prolonged periods.

Do not use aspirin in patients with gout; other NSAIDs are used.

Do *not* use aspirin and other NSAIDs after 20 weeks of pregnancy.

Indomethacin given intravenously for closure of patent ductus arteriosus; prostaglandins keep it open

The selective COX-2 inhibitors increase the TXA_2/PGI_2 (thomboxane A-2/prostacyclin) ratio to an unfavorable balance.

There is a lower incidence of life-threatening bleeds with the selective COX-2 inhibitors.

Acetaminophen is the drug of choice for analgesic treatment of the elderly

C. Adverse effects
  1. Hepatic necrosis is the most serious result of acute overdose.
     a. Most common cause of drug-induced fulminant liver failure
     b. A small fraction of the drug is oxidized by CYP2E1 to N-acetyl-*p*-benzoquinone imine (NAPQI) in the liver, which damages the hepatocytes.
     c. Glutathione (GSH), a reactive sulfhydryl compound, is used up in neutralizing NAPQI.
  2. Acetylcysteine is used to prevent hepatotoxicity after acute overdose (see Table 30-2).
     • It increases the synthesis of GSH to help neutralize the toxic intermediate NAPQI.
  3. Chronic alcohol consumption potentiates the liver toxicity of acetaminophen.
  4. Acetaminophen *neither* produces gastric irritation *nor* affects platelet function.
IV. Therapeutic summary of selected nonsteroidal anti-inflammatory and related drugs (Table 18-2)
V. Drugs Used to Treat Migraine Headache (Box 18-2)
  A. Migraine has two phases
    1. First phase is vasoconstriction of intracranial arteries, associated with the prodrome of the attack (aura).
    2. Second phase is vasodilation of the extracranial arteries during which headache occurs.
  B. Treatment of migraine
    1. Drugs for symptomatic treatment
       a. Sumatriptan is the prototype drug; all others end in -triptan
          (1) Mechanism of action
              (a) Highly selective agonist of 5-HT$_{1D}$ receptors
              (b) The drug is *not* an analgesic; direct vasoconstriction is responsible for the decrease of pain.
          (2) Adverse effects
              (a) Coronary artery vasospasm, arrhythmias, cardiac arrest
              (b) Cerebral vasospasm
              (c) Peripheral vascular ischemia and bowel ischemia

Chronic alcohol increases CYP2E1, thereby, increasing NAPQI formation from acetaminophen and hepatotoxicity.

Acetaminophen: most common cause of drug-induced fulminant liver failure; Rx with acetylcysteine

Note the common ending -triptan for 5-hydroxytryptamine (5-HT$_{1D}$) agonists.

All the other "triptans" are similar to sumatriptan, with slightly different pharmacokinetics and adverse effect profile.

Table 18-2. Therapeutic Summary of Selected Nonsteroidal Anti-inflammatory and Related Drugs

DRUGS	CLINICAL APPLICATIONS	ADVERSE EFFECTS	CONTRAINDICATIONS
Mechanism: *Irreversible cyclooxygenase (COX) inhibitor; anti-inflammatory, analgesic; antipyretic; platelet inhibitor*			
Aspirin	Fever, acute rheumatic fever, headache, mild pain, dysmenorrhea Inflammatory conditions such as osteoarthritis and RA Prevention of platelet aggregation in coronary artery disease, myocardial infarction, atrial fibrillation	GI effects Bleeding Tinnitus Primary respiratory alkalosis followed by primary metabolic acidosis in overdose	Hypersensitivity Bleeding disorders In children (<16 years of age) for viral infections (danger Reye's syndrome) Pregnancy (especially 3rd trimester)
Mechanism: *Reversible cyclooxygenase inhibitor; anti-inflammatory, analgesic; antipyretic*			
Diclofenac Ibuprofen Indomethacin Ketoprofen Ketorolac (parenteral) Naproxen Oxaprozin Piroxicam Sulindac	Fever, acute rheumatic fever, headache, mild pain, dysmenorrhea Inflammatory conditions such as osteoarthritis and RA Closure of patent ductus arteriosus (indomethacin)	GI effects Bleeding Tinnitus Fluid retention Hypocalcemia	Hypersensitivity Pregnancy (especially 3rd trimester)
Mechanism: *Selective COX-2 inhibitor: anti-inflammatory, analgesic; antipyretic*			
Celecoxib	Rheumatic arthritis Osteoarthritis Acute pain Dysmenorrhea	Hypertension Diarrhea GI distress	Hypersensitivity Sulfonamide allergies Pregnancy (especially 3rd trimester)
Mechanism: *Inhibits the synthesis of prostaglandins in the central nervous system relieving pain; produces antipyresis from inhibition of hypothalamic heat-regulating center*			
Acetaminophen (only analgesic & antipyretic)	Treatment of mild-to-moderate pain and fever	Hepatotoxicity	Hypersensitivity

GI, gastrointestinal; RA, rheumatoid arthritis.

BOX 18-2 DRUGS USED TO TREAT MIGRAINE HEADACHE

Treatment of an Acute Attack
Dihydroergotamine
Eletriptan
Ergotamine
Frovatriptan
Naratriptan
Rizatriptan
Sumatriptan
Zolmitriptan

Analgesics Used to Treat the Pain
Acetaminophen
Butorphanol (intranasally)

Codeine
Ibuprofen
Ketorolac
Naproxen

Drugs Used for Migraine Prophylaxis
Amitriptyline
Propranolol
Topiramate
Valproic acid
Verapamil

(d) Raynaud's phenomenon
  • Digital vessel constriction produces pain and color changes in the digits.
  (3) Contraindications
    (a) Breast feeding
    (b) Cardiac disease
    (c) Cerebrovascular disease
    (d) Coronary artery disease (CAD)
    (e) Pregnancy
    (f) Renal impairment
    (g) Tobacco smoking

"Triptans" contraindicated in patients with CAD.

b. Ergotamine and dihydroergotamine
  (1) Bind to 5-HT$_{1D}$ receptors, but *not* as specific as the -triptans
    • Also agonists on alpha receptors
  (2) Administered orally or intranasally, sublingual (ergotamine), or by parenteral routes
  (3) Adverse effects are due to vasoconstriction.
  (4) Contraindications
    (a) Peripheral vascular disease
    (b) Ischemic heart disease
    (c) Peptic ulcers
    (d) Pregnancy

Response to dihydroergotamine is diagnostic for migraine headache.

c. Analgesics used to treat the pain (see Box 18-2)
d. Drugs for migraine prophylaxis (see Box 18-2)
  (1) Decrease the occurrence of acute attacks
  (2) *No* uniform medication for prophylaxis
  (3) Agents used
    (a) Beta blockers (see Chapter 5)
    (b) Calcium channel blockers (see Chapter 12)
    (c) Antidepressants (see Chapter 10)
    (d) Anticonvulsants (see Chapter 9)

Some anticonvulsants, beta blockers, calcium channel blockers, and antidepressants have proven beneficial for migraine prophylaxis.

C. **Therapeutic summary of selected drugs used to treat migraine** (Table 18-3)

Table 18-3. **Therapeutic Summary of Selected Drugs Used to Treat Migraine**

DRUGS	CLINICAL APPLICATIONS	ADVERSE EFFECTS	CONTRAINDICATIONS
Mechanism: *Selective agonist for serotonin (5-HT$_{1D}$ receptor) in cranial arteries to cause vasoconstriction*			
Eletriptan	Acute treatment of migraine with	Coronary artery vasospasm	Hypersensitivity
Frovatriptan	or without aura	Arrhythmias	Breastfeeding
Naratriptan	Acute treatment of cluster	Cardiac arrest	Cardiac disease
Rizatriptan	headache	Cerebral vasospasm	Cerebrovascular disease
Sumatriptan		Peripheral vascular ischemia	Coronary artery disease
Zolmitriptan		Bowel ischemia	Pregnancy
			Renal impairment
			Tobacco smoking

(Continued)

Table 18-3. **Therapeutic Summary of Selected Drugs Used to Treat Migraine—Cont'd**

DRUGS	CLINICAL APPLICATIONS	ADVERSE EFFECTS	CONTRAINDICATIONS
Mechanism: *Bind to 5-HT₁D receptors, but not as specific as the–triptans*			
Dihydroergotamine Ergotamine	Acute treatment of migraine with or without aura Acute treatment of cluster headache	Vasoconstriction Pleural and retroperitoneal fibrosis	Hypersensitivity Cardiac disease Cerebrovascular disease Coronary artery disease Pregnancy Renal impairment Hepatic disease
Mechanism: *Analgesics*			
Acetaminophen Butorphanol (intranasally) Codeine Ibuprofen Ketorolac Naproxen	Acute treatment of migraine with or without aura Acute treatment of cluster headache	Discussed above and in Chapter 19	Discussed above and in Chapter 19
Mechanism: *Migraine prophylaxis through complex central actions*			
Amitriptyline Propranolol Topiramate Valproic acid Verapamil	Migraine prophylaxis	Beta blockers (see Chapter 5) Calcium channel blockers (see Chapter 12) Antidepressants (see Chapter 10) Anticonvulsants (see Chapter 9)	Hypersensitivity See other chapters

CHAPTER 19
OPIOID ANALGESICS AND ANTAGONISTS

I. Opioid Agonists (Box 19-1)
- Classified into three categories; strong, moderate, and weak
A. General features
1. Mechanism of action
   a. The effects of endogenous opioid peptides (endorphins and enkephalins) and exogenous opioids result from activation of specific opioid receptors (Table 19-1).
   b. Opioid analgesics activate the intrinsic analgesic system (endogenous pain control system; Fig. 19-1).
      - Reviewed in Rapid Review Neuroscience
         (1) Electrical stimulation of the midbrain periaqueductal gray (PAG) produces analgesia without affecting fine touch.
         (2) PAG activates serotonergic neurons in medullary raphe nuclei.
         (3) Raphe nuclei project to enkephalin interneurons in spinal cord posterior horn.
         (4) Enkephalin interneurons inhibit presynaptic nociceptor terminals and posterior horn pain transmission neurons.
         (5) Morphine suppresses input from pain fibers; this can be reversed by the opioid antagonist naloxone.
   c. Major subtypes of opioid receptors have varying effects (Table 19-2).
      (1) Subtypes include:
         (a) Delta (δ)
         (b) Kappa (κ)
         (c) Mu (μ)
      (2) All are Gi-protein coupled.
      (3) Close Ca^{2+} channels, reducing evoked transmitter release (presynaptic)
      (4) Open K^+ channels, hyperpolarizing membranes (postsynaptic)
2. Pharmacologic actions of opioid agonists (Box 19-2)
3. Uses
   a. Relief of severe pain
   b. Sedation and relief from anxiety (e.g., preoperatively)
   c. Cough suppression
   d. Diarrhea suppression
   e. Analgesic supplement in maintenance of balanced general anesthesia
4. Adverse effects (primarily extensions of pharmacologic actions)
   a. Respiratory depression and coma
   b. Sedation and central nervous system (CNS) depression
   c. Nausea and vomiting (stimulation of chemosensitive trigger zone, [CTZ])
   d. Constipation
   e. Acute postural hypotension (histamine release)
   f. Miosis ("pinpoint pupil")
   g. Elevated intracranial pressure
      - Increased CO_2 leads to vasodilation, which increases cerebral blood flow and leads to increased intracranial pressure.

Opioid receptors: delta; kappa; mu.

Opioid presynaptic receptors close Ca^{2+} channels; decreased transmitter release.

Opioid postsynaptic receptors open K^+ channels; hyperpolarizing signal leads to decreased electrical activity.

Respiratory and CNS depression: most important adverse effects of opioid analgesics

Morphine is noted for causing histamine release in some patients; symptoms can be reduced with diphenhydramine.

Triad of respiratory depression, coma, and "pinpoint pupil" is classic sign of opioid overdose.

BOX 19-1 OPIOID AGONISTS

Strong Opioid Agonists
Fentanyl (parenteral, transdermal, transmucosal)
Hydromorphone (parenteral, oral)
Levorphanol (parenteral, oral)
Meperidine (parenteral, oral)
Methadone (parenteral, oral)
Morphine (parenteral, oral, rectal)
Oxymorphone (parenteral, oral)

Moderate Opioid Agonists
Codeine (oral)
Hydrocodone (oral)
Oxycodone (oral)

Weak Opioid Agonists
Dextromethorphan (oral)
Diphenoxylate (oral with atropine)
Loperamide (oral)
Propoxyphene (oral)
Tramadol (oral)

Opioid Agonists as Adjuncts to Anesthesia
(See Chapter 8)
Alfentanil (parenteral)
Fentanyl (parenteral)
Sufentanil (parenteral)

TABLE 19-1. Effects of Representative Opioids on Opioid Receptor Subtypes

OPIOID	RECEPTOR SUBTYPE		
	MU (μ)	DELTA (δ)	KAPPA (κ)
Buprenorphine	Partial agonist		Antagonist
Butorphanol	Partial agonist		Agonist
Fentanyl	Agonist		Weak agonist
Meperidine	Agonist		Strong agonist
Morphine	Agonist	Weak agonist	Weak agonist
Nalbuphine	Antagonist		Agonist
Nalmefene	Antagonist	Antagonist	Antagonist
Naloxone	Antagonist	Antagonist	Antagonist
Naltrexone	Antagonist	Antagonist	Antagonist
Pentazocine	Partial agonist		Agonist

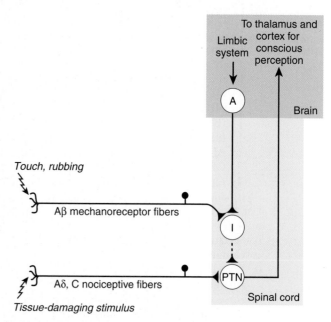

19-1: Endogenous analgesia systems. Nociceptors (Aδ and C fibers) excite pain transmission neurons (PTN). Large, myelinated mechanoreceptors (Aβ fibers) excite inhibitory (e.g., enkephalinergic) interneurons (I) that inhibit pain transmission at the first synapse. Pain transmission neurons (anterolateral system) project to thalamus with collaterals to brain stem. Limbic cortex contributes to activation of periaqueductal gray intrinsic analgesia circuitry. Periaqueductal gray (A) projects to medullary raphe, which project to posterior horn to inhibit pain transmission. *(From Weyhenmeyer JA and Gallman EA: Rapid Review Neuroscience. Philadelphia, Mosby, 2007, Figure 7-10.)*

    h. Abuse, physical and psychological dependence
    i. Abstinence syndrome on withdrawal of the drug
        • Symptoms and treatment of opioid overdose (see Chapter 30)
  B. Selective specific opioid agonists
    1. Morphine
        • The prototype opioid agonist; the standard against which all other analgesics are measured

TABLE 19-2. **Opioid Receptors and their Associated Effects**

RECEPTOR	EFFECTS OF ACTIVATION
Mu (μ) receptor	Analgesia, euphoria, respiratory depression, miosis, decreased gastrointestinal motility, and physical dependence
Kappa (κ) receptor	Analgesia, miosis, respiratory depression, dysphoria, and some psychomimetic effects
Delta (δ) receptor	Analgesia (spinal and supraspinal)

BOX 19-2   PHARMACOLOGIC ACTIONS OF OPIOID AGONISTS

Central Nervous System Effects
Analgesia
Euphoria or dysphoria
Inhibition of cough reflex
Miosis (pinpoint pupils)
Physical dependence
Respiratory depression (inhibit respiratory center in medulla)
Sedation

Cardiovascular Effects
Decreased myocardial oxygen demand
Vasodilation and orthostatic hypotension (histamine release)

Gastrointestinal and Biliary Effects
Decreased gastric motility and constipation (increased muscle tone leads to diminished propulsive peristalsis in colon)
Biliary colic from increased sphincter tone and pressure
Nausea and vomiting (from direct stimulation of chemoreceptor trigger zone)

Genitourinary Effects
Increased bladder sphincter tone
Increased urine retention

---

   a. Administration
      (1) Intravenous, intramuscular, or rectal (the drug is less effective orally
      (2) Oral-extended release products are also used
   b. Primary use
      • Relief of severe pain associated with trauma, myocardial infarction (MI), or cancer
   c. Other use
      • Acute pulmonary edema to reduce perception of shortness of breath, anxiety, and cardiac preload and afterload
2. Codeine, oxycodone, hydrocodone
   a. Relative to morphine
      • Less potent and less likely to cause physical dependence
   b. Codeine and codeine derivatives do *not* bind to μ receptors.
      (1) Requires metabolism by CYP2D6 to the corresponding morphine derivatives
      (2) Genetic polymorphism of CYP2D6 gives variable responses for this class
   c. Uses
      (1) Antitussive agent (codeine)
      (2) Analgesic (mild to moderate pain)
         • Commonly given in combination with aspirin or acetaminophen
3. Meperidine
   a. Uses
      (1) Statement from The Agency for Health Care Policy and Research Clinical Practice
         (a) Meperidine is recommended for use *only* in very brief courses in patients who are healthy or have problems with other opiate agonists.
         (b) It is considered a second-line agent for the treatment of acute pain.
      (2) Obstetric analgesia (may prolong labor)
      (3) Acute pain syndromes, such as MI, neuralgia, painful procedures (short-term treatment)

Morphine: high first-pass effect

Codeine is the most constipating opioid.

Fluoxetine and paroxetine are 2 selective serotonin reuptake inhibitors (SSRIs) that inhibit CYP2D6 and prevent the bioactivation of codeine, hydrocodone, and oxycodone.

Use meperidine, rather than morphine, for pancreatitis; it produces less spasm of the sphincter of Oddi.

Normeperidine, a metabolite of meperidine, may cause seizures in patients with compromised renal function

Meperidine is contraindicated to take with monoamine oxidase inhibitors (tranylcypromine, phenelzine); produce serotonin syndrome;

Fentanyl is available as transdermal patches, lozenges, and buccal tablets.

Tramadol is used for neuropathic pain.

Loperamide and diphenoxylate are used to treat diarrhea.

Atropine is added to diphenoxylate to deter abuse.

Dextromethorphan and codeine are used to suppress cough.

Propoxyphene is often overused in the geriatric population.

Partial agonists of the μ receptor may precipitate withdrawal reaction in opioid addicts.

        (4) Used to interrupt post administration shivering and shaking chills caused by amphotericin B
   b. Specific adverse effect
      • Anxiety and seizures due to accumulation of a metabolite (normeperidine)
  4. Methadone
   a. Relative to morphine
      • Longer duration of action and milder withdrawal symptoms
   b. Orally effective
   c. Uses
      (1) Maintenance therapy for heroin addicts
      (2) Control of withdrawal symptoms from opioids
      (3) Neuropathic pain
      (4) Oral agent for severe pain
  5. Fentanyl and its derivatives
   a. Fentanyl is available as solution for injection, long-acting transdermal patch for continuous pain relief.
   b. *Also* available as buccal tablets and lozenge for treatment of breakthrough cancer pain
   c. Relative to morphine, fentanyl produces less nausea
   d. Uses
      (1) Analgesia
      (2) Anesthesia, in some cases (cardiovascular surgery)
      (3) Other drugs for anesthesia
         (a) Alfentanil
         (b) Sufentanil
  6. Tramadol
   a. Mechanism of action
      (1) Tramadol is a μ receptor partial agonist
      (2) Also, inhibits neuronal reuptake of norepinephrine and serotonin, similar to antidepressants; may help for pain-induced anxiety
   b. Use
      • Acute and chronic pain syndromes
   c. Adverse effect
      • Decreased seizure threshold
  7. Loperamide and diphenoxylate
   a. Drugs with minimal analgesic activity; used in the treatment of diarrhea
   b. Diphenoxylate formulation contains a subtherapeutic amount of atropine to discourage abuse.
   c. Loperamide does not pass the blood brain barrier
  8. Dextromethorphan
   a. Drug with minimal analgesic activity
   b. Used as an antitussive agent
   c. The U.S. Food and Drug Administration (FDA) has issued a Public Health Advisory reminding that over-the-counter (OTC) cough and cold medications should *not* be used to treat infants and children younger than 2 years of age.
  9. Propoxyphene
   a. Weak opioid agonist at the μ receptor
   b. Often combined with acetaminophen or aspirin

II. Mixed Opioid Agonists-Antagonists (Box 19-3)
  A. General considerations
   1. React with a particular receptor subtype (e.g., strong κ but weak μ agonist)
   2. Effective analgesics
   3. Respiratory depressant effects do *not* rise proportionately with increasing doses.
   4. Associated with a much lower risk of drug dependence than morphine

---

BOX 19-3 MIXED OPIOID AGONISTS-ANTAGONISTS

Buprenorphine (parenteral, oral)
Butorphanol (parenteral, intranasal)
Nalbuphine (parenteral)
Pentazocine (parenteral, oral)

B. **Buprenorphine** (partial agonist on the μ receptor)
   1. Used for relief of moderate or severe pain
   2. Maintenance for opioid-dependent patients
C. **Butorphanol** (κ agonist)
   1. Used pain relief (parenterally)
   2. Used for migraine headaches (nasal spray)
D. **Nalbuphine** (κ agonist, μ antagonist)
   1. Used for relief of moderate to severe pain associated with acute and chronic disorders such as cancer, renal or biliary colic, and migraine or vascular headaches, as well as surgery
   2. Used as obstetric analgesia during labor and delivery
E. **Pentazocine** (κ agonist)
   • Oldest mixed opioid agonist-antagonist
   1. Used for relief of moderate to severe pain
   2. CNS effects such as disorientation and hallucinations limit use.
III. **Opioid Antagonists** (Box 19-4)
  A. **Mechanism of action**
   • Competition with opioid agonists for μ receptors to rapidly reverse the effects of morphine and other opioid agonists
  B. **Uses**
   1. Treatment of opioid overdose
    a. Naloxone: short acting (1 to 2 hours)
    b. Naltrexone: long acting (up to 24 hours), oral administration
    c. Nalmefene: long acting (up to 48 hours)
   2. Treatment of ethanol and opioid dependence; naltrexone given orally
  C. **Problems**
   • Precipitation of a withdrawal syndrome when given to chronic users of opioid drugs
IV. **Therapeutic summary of selected opioid drugs** (Table 19-3)

> Butorphanol available as a nasal spray.

> Naloxone given parenterally to treat opioid overdose; must give repeated doses because of short half-life.

> Oral naltrexone for treatment of substance abuse, dependence.

BOX 19-4   OPIOID ANTAGONISTS

Nalmefene (parenteral)
Naloxone (parenteral)
Naltrexone (oral)

TABLE 19-3. **Therapeutic Summary of Selected Opioid Drugs**

DRUGS	CLINICAL APPLICATIONS	ADVERSE EFFECTS	CONTRAINDICATIONS
Mechanism: *Strong agonists at opioid receptors*			
Fentanyl Hydromorphone Levorphanol Meperidine Methadone Morphine Oxymorphone	Relief of moderate to severe acute and chronic pain Preanesthetic medication Relief of pain of myocardial infarction (morphine) Relief of dyspnea of acute left ventricular failure and pulmonary edema (morphine) Detoxification and maintenance treatment of opioid addiction (methadone)	CNS depression Respiratory depression Miosis Constipation Pruritus Physical and psychological dependence Abstinence syndrome on withdrawal of the drug Seizures (meperidine)	Hypersensitivity Head injuries Obstructive airway disease
Mechanism: *Moderate agonists at opioid receptors*			
Codeine Hydrocodone Oxycodone	Treatment of mild-to-moderate pain; usually given with acetaminophen or aspirin Antitussive (codeine)	Constipation CNS depression Respiratory depression Miosis Lower incidence than with morphine	Hypersensitivity
Mechanism: *Weak agonists at opioid receptors*			
Dextromethorphan Diphenoxylate Loperamide Propoxyphene Tramadol	Cough (dextromethorphan) Diarrhea (diphenoxylate, loperamide) Mild pain (propoxyphene) Chronic pain (tramadol)	Lower incidence than with morphine	Hypersensitivity

(Continued)

TABLE 19-3. **Therapeutic Summary of Selected Opioid Drugs—Cont'd**

DRUGS	CLINICAL APPLICATIONS	ADVERSE EFFECTS	CONTRAINDICATIONS
Mechanism: *Partial agonists at opioid receptors*			

Buprenorphine
Butorphanol
Nalbuphine
Pentazocine
	Management of moderate to severe pain
	Treatment of opioid dependence
	  (buprenorphine)
	Obstetrical analgesia (buprenorphine,
	  butorphanol)
	Migraine headache pain (butorphanol)
		Lower incidence than with
		  morphine
			Hypersensitivity
			Head injuries

Mechanism: *Opioid antagonists*			

Nalmefene
Naloxone
Naltrexone
	Opioid overdose (naloxone, nalmefene)
	Treatment of ethanol and opioid dependence
	  (naltrexone)
		May induce withdrawal in
		  dependent patient
			Hypersensitivity

CNS, central nervous system.

Drugs That Affect the Respiratory and Gastrointestinal Systems and are Used to Treat Rheumatic Disorders and Gout

CHAPTER **20**

Drugs Used in the Treatment of Asthma, Chronic Obstructive Pulmonary Disease and Allergies

I. General Considerations

A. Asthma

1. An obstructive airway disorder resulting from:
   a. Smooth muscle hypertrophy
   b. Bronchospasm
   c. Inflammation
   d. Increased mucus secretion
   e. Mucosal edema
2. Both nonimmunogenic (Box 20-1) and immunogenic factors (Fig. 20-1) play a role in the pathogenesis of asthma.
3. Drug therapy, which includes anti-inflammatory agents and bronchodilators, affects these factors.
4. Clinical symptoms include:
   a. Episodic bouts of coughing associated with dyspnea
   b. Wheezing
   c. Chest tightness
5. A variety of drugs are used in the pharmacotherapy of asthma (Box 20-2; Table 20-1).

B. Chronic obstructive pulmonary disease (COPD)

1. This progressive obstructive airway disorder, which usually results from smoking, is marked by airway reactivity.
2. COPD involves chronic bronchitis, emphysema, and bronchiectasis.
3. Clinical symptoms of COPD:
   a. Chronic bronchitis and bronchiectasis are associated with chronic cough with increased sputum production and dyspnea.
   b. Emphysema is associated with dyspnea.

II. Anti-inflammatory Agents Used to Treat Asthma (see Box 20-2; Fig. 20-1)

A. Corticosteroids

1. Mechanism of action
   a. Corticosteroids generally inhibit the inflammatory response, thereby preventing bronchoconstriction and producing smooth muscle relaxation.

Asthma involves both bronchoconstriction and underlying inflammation.

Asthma therapy: β_2 agonists are referred to as *Relievers*, anti-inflammatory agents are referred to as *Controllers*.

Smoking is a major cause of COPD.

BOX 20-1   FACTORS THAT MAY CAUSE ASTHMA

β-Adrenergic receptor antagonists
Aspirin
Dyes in food and medications
Emotional stress
Environmental pollutants
Exercise
Immunogenic factors
Metal salts
Nitrogen dioxide
Occupational factors
Ozone
Pharmacologic stimuli
Viral infections
Wood, animal, and insect dust

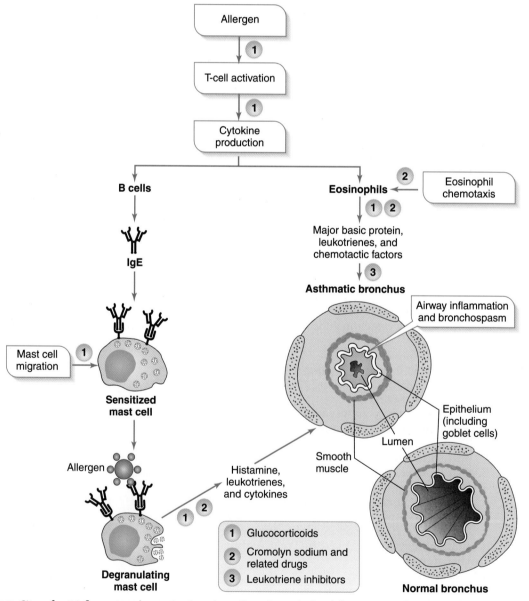

20-1: Sites of anti-inflammatory drug action in asthma. Cromolyn and related drugs prevent the release of mediators from mast cells and eosinophils. IgE, immunoglobin E.

BOX 20-2 Anti-Inflammatory Agents	
Inhaled Corticosteroids Beclomethasone Budesonide Ciclesonide Flunisolide Fluticasone Mometasone Triamcinolone **Systemic Corticosteroids** Methylprednisolone Prednisone Triamcinolone	**Mast Cell Stabilizers** Cromolyn Ketotifen (eye) Lodoxamide (eye) Nedocromil Pemirolast (eye) **Leukotriene Inhibitors** Montelukast Zafirlukast Zileuton **Monoclonal Antibody** Omalizumab

TABLE 20-1. **Asthma Pharmacotherapy**

DRUG TYPE	EXAMPLE	USE
Daily Medications for Long-Term Control		
Inhaled corticosteroids	Beclomethasone	First-line treatment
Systemic corticosteroids	Triamcinolone	Used to gain prompt control when initiating long-term inhaled corticosteroids
Mast cell stabilizers	Cromolyn	May be initial choice in children Also used as prevention before exercise or allergen exposure
Long-acting β_2-receptor agonist	Salmeterol	Given concomitantly with anti-inflammatory agents Not used for acute symptoms
Methylxanthines	Theophylline	Adjunct to inhaled corticosteroids
Leukotriene inhibitors	Zafirlukast	Prophylaxis and long-term management (alone or in combination)
"Rescue" Medications Useful in Acute Episode		
Short-acting β_2-receptor agonists	Albuterol Pirbuterol Should be prescribed for all patients	First choice for acute symptoms Prevention of exercise-induced bronchospasm
Anticholinergic	Ipratropium	Additive benefit to inhaled β_2-receptor agonists in severe exacerbations Alternative for patients intolerant to β_2-receptor agonists

b. Inhibition of the release of arachidonic acid by increasing the synthesis of lipocortin, which inhibits phospholipase A_2 activity

c. Decreased synthesis of cyclooxygenase-2 (COX-2), an inducible form of COX in inflammatory cells

d. Inhibition of the production of cytokines involved in the inflammatory cascade (interferon-γ, interleukin 1, interleukin 2)

e. Effects the concentration, distribution, and function of peripheral leukocytes:
  (1) Increased concentration in circulating
    • Neutrophils
  (2) Decreased concentration in circulating
    (a) Granulocytes
    (b) Lymphocytes
    (c) Monocytes

2. Uses
  a. Mild or moderate asthma or COPD
    (1) Inhaled steroids are first-line maintenance therapy
    (2) Agents include:
      (a) Beclomethasone
      (b) Budesonide
      (c) Flunisolide
      (d) Fluticasone
      (e) Mometasone
      (f) Triamcinolone

Glucocorticoids have multiple actions that relieve inflammation.

Inhaled corticosteroids: fewer adverse effects than systemic corticosteroids

(3) Prodrug
Ciclesonide
   (a) An inhaled prodrug that is activated by esterases in bronchial epithelial cells
   (b) Tight binding to serum proteins limits its access to glucocorticoid receptors in skin, eye, and bone.
b. Severe airway obstruction despite optimal bronchodilator therapy
   • Systemic (oral or intravenous) steroids often required
c. Asthma or COPD
   • Often treated with a combination of inhaled steroids with selective β_2-adrenergic receptor agonists such as salmeterol
d. Emergency treatment
   (1) Oral (prednisone) or parenteral steroids (methylprednisolone) are used for severe asthma or COPD if bronchodilators do not resolve the airway obstruction.
   (2) See Chapter 22 for the discussion of the use of these agents in rheumatic disorders.
3. Adverse effects
   a. Inhaled steroids
      (1) Oropharyngeal candidiasis
      (2) Hoarseness from affects on vocal cords
   b. Systemic effects
      • Rare from inhaled preparations
      (1) Iatrogenic Cushing's syndrome, diabetes mellitus, hypertension, peptic ulcer disease, hypomania, psychosis, adrenal insufficiency on abrupt cessation of therapy (see Chapter 22)
      (2) To prevent adrenal insufficiency, patients who have been receiving oral corticosteroid treatment for longer than 1 week should be given diminishing doses.

B. Mast cell stabilizers
1. Examples
   a. Cromolyn
   b. Nedocromil
2. Pharmacokinetics
   • Administration in the form of an aerosol before exposure to agents that trigger asthma
3. Mechanism of action (Fig. 20-2)
   a. Stabilize the plasma membranes of mast cells and eosinophils, preventing release of:
      (1) Histamine
      (2) Leukotrienes
      (3) Other mediators of airway inflammation
   b. Decrease activation of airway nerves (nedocromil)
4. Uses
   a. Prevention of asthmatic episodes, such as before exercise or in cold weather (cromolyn, nedocromil)
   b. Less effective in reducing bronchial reactivity in acute settings
   c. Prevention of allergic rhinitis and seasonal conjunctivitis (cromolyn; *not* first-line agents)
   d. Ophthalmic use
      (1) Treatment of itching associated with allergic conjunctivitis (cromolyn, ketotifen, pemirolast)
      (2) Treatment of vernal keratoconjunctivitis, vernal conjunctivitis, and vernal keratitis (lodoxamide)
5. Adverse effects
   a. Nausea and vomiting
   b. Dysgeusia (bad taste in mouth)
   c. Cough

C. Leukotriene inhibitors
1. Leukotriene synthesis inhibitor
   a. Example
      • Zileuton
   b. Mechanism of action
      • Selective inhibitor of 5-lipoxygenase, which catalyzes leukotriene formation (Fig. 20-3; see also Fig. 20-1)
   c. Use
      • Given orally for prophylaxis and chronic treatment of asthma in children 12 years of age and older and adults

---

Use a spacer and rinse mouth after using inhaled steroids to prevent oropharyngeal candidiasis.

Taper the dose of oral corticosteroids in patients who have been taking the drug for longer than 1 week.

Mast cell stabilizers are used to prevent asthmatic episodes and relieve allergic nasal and eye responses.

Leukotriene inhibitors are used prophylactically.

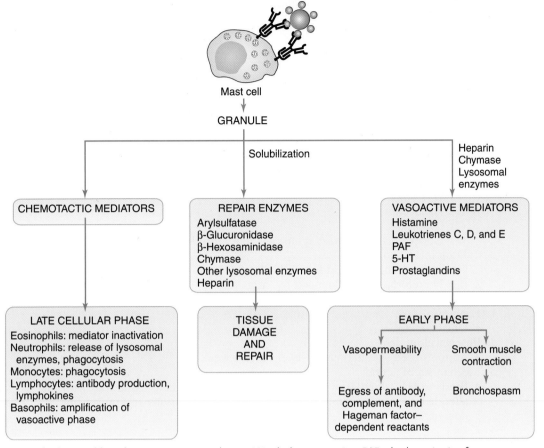

Mast cell

GRANULE

Solubilization

Heparin
Chymase
Lysosomal
enzymes

| CHEMOTACTIC MEDIATORS | REPAIR ENZYMES | VASOACTIVE MEDIATORS |

REPAIR ENZYMES
Arylsulfatase
β-Glucuronidase
β-Hexosaminidase
Chymase
Other lysosomal enzymes
Heparin

VASOACTIVE MEDIATORS
Histamine
Leukotrienes C, D, and E
PAF
5-HT
Prostaglandins

LATE CELLULAR PHASE
Eosinophils: mediator inactivation
Neutrophils: release of lysosomal
  enzymes, phagocytosis
Monocytes: phagocytosis
Lymphocytes: antibody production,
  lymphokines
Basophils: amplification of
  vasoactive phase

**TISSUE
DAMAGE
AND
REPAIR**

EARLY PHASE
Vasopermeability   Smooth muscle
                        contraction

Egress of antibody,   Bronchospasm
complement, and
Hageman factor–
dependent reactants

20-2: Early-phase and late-phase responses in asthma. 5-HT, 5-hydroxytryptamine; PAF, platelet activating factor.

    d. Adverse effects
        • Hepatotoxicity
2. Leukotriene receptor antagonists
    a. Examples
        (1) Zafirlukast
        (2) Montelukast
    b. Pharmacokinetics
        • Oral administration
    c. Mechanism of action (see Figure 20-1 and Figure 20-3)

Zileuton is hepatotoxic.

*Note the common ending:
-lukast*

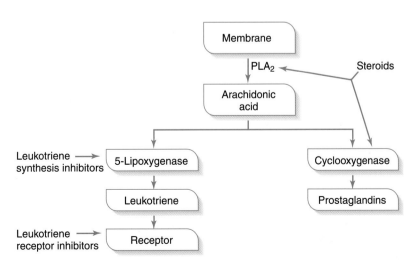

Membrane

PLA$_2$ Steroids

Arachidonic
acid

Leukotriene → 5-Lipoxygenase   Cyclooxygenase
synthesis inhibitors

Leukotriene   Prostaglandins

Leukotriene → Receptor
receptor inhibitors

20-3: Role of prostaglandins and leukotrienes in asthma. Zileuton is a leukotriene synthesis inhibitor. Zafirlukast is a leukotriene receptor inhibitor. PLA$_2$, phospholipase A$_2$.

(1) Selective inhibition of binding of leukotrienes to their receptors
(2) Reducing the airway inflammation that leads to:
  (a) Edema
  (b) Bronchoconstriction
  (c) Mucus secretion
d. Uses
(1) Prophylaxis and chronic treatment of asthma
(2) Relief of symptoms of seasonal allergic rhinitis and perennial allergic rhinitis (montelukast)
(3) Prevention of exercise-induced bronchospasm
(4) *Not* effective in acute bronchospasm
(5) Useful for aspirin-induced asthma
(6) Useful for children who comply poorly with inhaled therapies
e. Adverse effects
(1) Headache
(2) Gastritis
(3) Upper respiratory tract symptoms (e.g., flu-like symptoms)
f. Drug interactions
(1) Both are metabolized by CYP2C9.
(2) Therefore, dose influenced by drugs that induce or inhibit this enzyme

D. Monoclonal antibody
1. Example
   - Omalizumab
2. Pharmacokinetics
   - Administered subcutaneously every 2 to 4 weeks
3. Mechanism of action
   - Binds to IgE's high affinity Fc receptor (FcεRI), on cells associated with the allergic response, lowering free serum IgE concentrations and preventing degranulation
4. Uses
   - Treatment of moderate to severe allergic asthma triggered by responses to allergens such as:
     a. Pollen
     b. Mold
     c. Dust mites
     d. Pet dander

E. Therapeutic summary of selected anti-inflammatory agents used to treat asthma: (Table 20-2)

III. Bronchodilators (Box 20-3)

A. β₂-Adrenergic receptor agonists
1. General considerations (see Chapter 5)
2. Examples
   a. Albuterol
   b. Levalbuterol
   c. Salmeterol
   d. Terbutaline
3. Pharmacokinetics
   a. Administration
   (1) Via a metered-dose inhaler or nebulizer
   (2) Provides the greatest local effect on airway smooth muscle with the fewest systemic adverse effects
   (3) Terbutaline
       - Also, available for oral and subcutaneous injection
   b. Duration of action
   (1) Rapid-acting agents attain their maximal effect in 30 minutes
   (2) Action persists for 3 to 4 hours
   (3) Long-acting maintenance agents (inhaled powder)
     (a) Salmeterol
     (b) Salmeterol/fluticasone
     (c) Formoterol
     (d) Arformoterol

Leukotriene antagonists are used to treat aspirin-induced asthma.

Orally administered leukotriene antagonists are good to treat children who have difficulty using inhalers.

Omalizumab targets IgE in asthma.

β₂-Receptor agonists: the only bronchodilators used to counteract acute asthma attacks

TABLE 20-2. **Therapeutic Summary of Selected Anti-inflammatory Agents Used to Treat Asthma**

DRUGS	CLINICAL APPLICATIONS	ADVERSE EFFECTS	CONTRAINDICATIONS
Mechanism: *Inhaled steroids; anti-inflammatory*			
Beclomethasone Budesonide Ciclesonide (prodrug) Flunisolide Fluticasone Mometasone Triamcinolone	Controller agents to treat and prevent asthma and COPD	Oropharyngeal candidiasis Throat irritation Steroid adverse effects much less with inhaled preparations Upper respiratory tract infection	Hypersensitivity Acute treatment of bronchospasm Status asthmaticus
Mechanism: *Systemic steroids; anti-inflammatory*			
Methylprednisolone Prednisone Triamcinolone	Short term use for severe asthma or COPD	Iatrogenic Cushing's syndrome with long use: diabetes mellitus, hypertension, peptic ulcer disease, hypomania, psychosis, adrenal insufficiency on abrupt cessation of therapy	Hypersensitivity Serious infections
Mechanism: *Mast cell stabilizers; anti-inflammatory*			
Cromolyn Nedocromil	Adjunct in the prophylaxis of allergic disorders, including asthma Prevention of exercise-induced bronchospasm	Nausea and vomiting Dysgeusia (bad taste in mouth) Cough	Hypersensitivity Acute treatment of bronchospasm Status asthmaticus
Mechanism: *Selective inhibitor of 5-lipoxygenase; anti-inflammatory*			
Zileuton	Prophylaxis and chronic treatment of asthma in children $\geq$12 years of age and adults	Hepatotoxicity	Hypersensitivity Liver disease
Mechanism: *Receptor antagonist of leukotriene D_4 and E_4 (LTD$_4$ and LTE$_4$); anti-inflammatory*			
Zafirlukast Montelukast	Prophylaxis and chronic treatment of asthma Aspirin-induced asthma	Headache Gastritis Upper respiratory tract symptoms (e.g., flu-like symptoms)	Hypersensitivity
Mechanism: *Monoclonal antibody that inhibits IgE binding to the high-affinity IgE receptor on mast cells and basophils; anti-inflammatory*			
Omalizumab	Treatment of moderate-to-severe, not adequately controlled with inhaled corticosteroids	Headache Upper respiratory tract infection	Acute treatment of bronchospasm Status asthmaticus

COPD, chronic obstructive pulmonary disease.

BOX 20-3   BRONCHODILATORS

Methylxanthines
Aminophylline
Dyphylline
Theophylline

β₂-Adrenergic Receptor Agonists
Arformoterol
Albuterol
Fenoterol
Formoterol

Levalbuterol
Metaproterenol
Pirbuterol
Salmeterol
Terbutaline

Anticholinergic Drugs
Ipratropium
Tiotropium

---

4. Mechanism of action
   a. These potent bronchodilators stimulate β_2 receptors
   b. Leading to the activation of adenylyl cyclase
   c. Increasing cyclic adenosine monophosphate (cAMP) levels (Fig. 20-4)
   d. Relaxing constricted bronchial smooth muscle (see Fig. 20-1)
5. Uses
   a. Treatment of acute asthma attacks
   b. Prevention or treatment of bronchospasm caused by asthma or COPD
   c. Asthma prophylaxis (oral albuterol, metaproterenol)

Albuterol is a "rescue" medication.

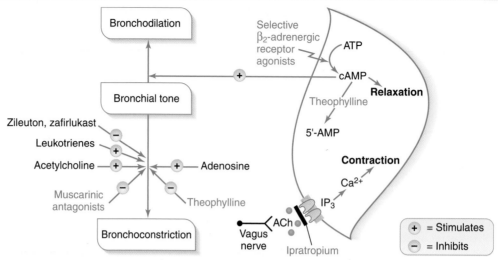

20-4: Mechanism of action of bronchodilators. ACh, acetylcholine; 5'-AMP, 5'-adenosine monophosphate; ATP, adenosine triphosphate; cAMP, cyclic adenosine monophosphate; IP$_3$, inositol triphosphate.

> d. Emergency treatment of severe bronchospasm (subcutaneous terbutaline)
> e. Delay of premature labor (see Chapter 26)
> - Terbutaline
6. Adverse effects
> a. Tremor with inhaled agents
> b. Systemic adverse effects occur with overdose
> c. Many of these systemic effects are related to activation of the sympathetic nervous system, such as:
> > (1) Anxiety
> > (2) Excitability
> > (3) Hyperglycemia
> > (4) Hypokalemia
> > (5) Palpitations
> > (6) Tachycardia
> > (7) Tremor

B. Specific considerations of some β$_2$-adrenergic receptor agonists
1. Salmeterol, arformoterol, and formoterol: longer acting drugs (12 hours)
> a. Should *not* be used to treat acute asthma attacks
> b. Boxed warning in the United States
> > - Long-acting β$_2$-agonists may increase the risk of asthma-related deaths; especially among African Americans
2. Levalbuterol
> a. R-isomer and active form of racemic albuterol
> b. Inhalant which is claimed to have fewer central nervous system (CNS) and cardiac adverse effects

C. Epinephrine
- Used in emergency settings as subcutaneous injection or microaerosol for rapid bronchodilation in severe airway obstruction (see Chapter 5)

D. Methylxanthines
1. Examples
> a. Theophylline
> b. Aminophylline
> c. Dyphylline
2. Pharmacokinetics
> a. Decreasing hepatic function or drugs that inhibit the cytochrome P450 system (e.g., beta blockers, erythromycin, fluoroquinolones) increase the half-life ($t_{1/2}$) of theophylline
> b. Drugs that induce the cytochrome P450 system (e.g., barbiturates, phenytoin, rifampin) hasten the elimination of theophylline
> c. Because of narrow therapeutic index, plasma levels are often determined.
> > (1) Therapeutic range: 5 to 20 mg/L

Tremor is the most frequent adverse effect with inhaled β$_2$ agonists.

Long-acting β$_2$-receptor agonists have been associated with sudden death from an asthmatic attack; especially in African Americans.

Long-acting β$_2$-receptor agonists should be combined with inhaled steroids to prevent receptor downregulation

(2) Mild toxicities (nausea vomiting anxiety, and headache): >15 mg/L
(3) Frequent toxicities: >20 mg/L
(4) Severe toxicities (seizures and arrhythmias): >40 mg/L
3. Mechanism of action (see Fig. 20-4)
   a. Antagonize adenosine receptors
   b. Inhibit phosphodiesterase, an enzyme that catalyzes degradation of cAMP; probably causes bronchodilation
   c. Improve contractility of skeletal muscle (strengthen diaphragm contraction, beneficial in COPD)
   d. Other effects include
      (1) CNS stimulation
      (2) Cardiovascular actions
      (3) Diuresis (slight)
4. Uses
   a. Adjunctive treatment of acute asthma
   b. Prevention of bronchospasm associated with asthma or COPD
5. Adverse effects
   a. Anxiety
   b. Diuresis
   c. Gastrointestinal (GI) irritation
   d. Headache
   e. Palpitations
   f. Premature ventricular contractions
   g. Seizures
6. Use with precaution in patients with:
   a. Heart disease
   b. Liver disorders
   c. Seizure disorders
   d. Peptic ulcer disease
E. **Anticholinergic agents** (muscarinic receptor antagonist; see Chapter 4)
   1. Examples
      a. Ipratropium
      b. Tiotropium
   2. Pharmacokinetics
      • Administration via aerosol for local effects at muscarinic receptors in the airway
   3. Mechanism of action
      • Blockade of the effects of vagus nerve stimulation
   4. Uses
      a. Prevention of bronchoconstriction in COPD (often given in combination with β_2-adrenergic receptor agonists)
      b. Treatment of asthma (less effective than β_2-adrenergic receptor agonists)
      c. Tiotropium can be given once a day for the maintenance treatment of COPD.
   5. Adverse effects
      a. Airway irritation
      b. Anticholinergic effects
         (1) GI upset
         (2) Xerostomia
         (3) Urinary retention
         (4) Increased ocular pressure
   F. **Therapeutic summary of selected bronchodilator drugs:** (Table 20-3)
IV. **Antihistamines Used in the Treatment of Allergies** (Box 20-4)
   A. **H_1 antagonists**
      1. Pharmacokinetics
         a. These antihistamines are available orally and topically and have short effective half-lives of 4 to 6 hours.
         b. First-generation antihistamines cross the blood-brain barrier and produce sedation.
         c. The second-generation antihistamines have lesser propensity to cross the blood-brain barrier and cause sedation.
      2. Pharmacodynamics
         a. Competitive blockers of H_1 receptors to reduce edema and itching
         b. *No* profound effect on gastric acid secretions in contrast to H_2 blockers
         c. First generation *also* block muscarinic receptors

The $t_{1/2}$ of theophylline is decreased in adults who smoke and in children.

Theophylline has a narrow therapeutic index; levels need to be monitored closely when therapy is initiated.

Theophylline has a narrow therapeutic index; often have to monitor blood levels.

Anticholinergics are better for COPD than for asthma.

Remember these anticholinergic effects because they occur with many classes of drugs: antihistamines; phenothiazines; tricyclic

Second-generation antihistamines are often referred to as nonsedating antihistamines.

TABLE 20-3. **Therapeutic Summary of Selected Bronchodilator Drugs**

DRUGS	CLINICAL APPLICATIONS	ADVERSE EFFECTS	CONTRAINDICATIONS
Mechanism: *Selective β_2 agonists; bronchodilator*			

Arformoterol
Albuterol
Fenoterol
Formoterol
Levalbuterol
Metaproterenol
Pirbuterol
Salmeterol
Terbutaline
	Bronchodilator in reversible airway
	  obstruction and bronchial asthma
	Tocolytic agent (terbutaline)
		Tremor (inhaled agents)
		Tachycardia
			Hypersensitivity
			Cardiac arrhythmias
			Risk of asthma-
			  related deaths
			  (salmeterol,
			  formoterol)

Mechanism: *Anticholinergic; bronchodilator*			

Ipratropium
Tiotropium
	Bronchospasm associated with COPD,
	  bronchitis, and emphysema
		Airway irritation
		Anticholinergic effects; GI upset,
		  xerostomia, urinary retention,
		  increased ocular pressure
			Hypersensitivity

Mechanism: *Inhibits phosphodiesterase to increase cAMP; bronchodilator*			

Aminophylline
Dyphylline
Theophylline
	Treatment of symptoms and reversible
	  airway obstruction due to chronic
	  asthma, chronic bronchitis, or COPD
		Anxiety
		Arrhythmias
		Seizures
			Hypersensitivity

cAMP, cyclic adenosine monophosphate; COPD, chronic obstructive pulmonary disease; GI, gastrointestinal.

BOX 20-4 ANTIHISTAMINES USED IN THE TREATMENT OF ALLERGIES

First-Generation Antihistamines
Carbinoxamine
Brompheniramine
Chlorpheniramine
Cyproheptadine (also blocks serotonin receptors)
Cyclizine
Dimenhydrinate
Diphenhydramine
Hydroxyzine

Meclizine
Promethazine

Second-Generation Antihistamines
Azelastine
Cetirizine
Desloratadine
Fexofenadine
Loratadine

Cyproheptadine is also useful in treating serotonin syndrome.

    d. First generation *also* block α-adrenergic receptors
    e. Cyproheptadine *also* blocks serotonin receptors
  3. Adverse effects
    a. CNS
      (1) First generation drugs are very sedating.
      (2) Cycle between coma and seizures when taken in large overdose; especially in children
    b. GI
      (1) Nausea
      (2) Vomiting
      (3) Constipation
      (4) Diarrhea
    c. Atropine-like effects (first generation)
  4. Uses
    a. Treatment of allergic reactions
    b. Motion sickness
      (1) Dimenhydrinate
      (2) Diphenhydramine
      (3) Meclizine (lower sedation)
      (4) Cyclizine (lower sedation)
      (5) Scopolamine (an anticholinergic is *also* used)
    c. Over-the-counter sleeping medications (diphenhydramine)
    d. Treatment of nausea and vomiting (promethazine)
    e. Azelastine is available as a nasal spray for the treatment of the symptoms of seasonal
      allergic rhinitis such as rhinorrhea, sneezing, and nasal pruritus
    f. Serotonin syndrome (cyproheptadine)

First generation: diphenhydramine; dimenhydrinate; chlorpheniramine; tripelennamine; second generation: azelastine; fexofenadine; loratadine; cetirizine, desloratadine

5. Precautions
   a. Machine operation should be curtailed as drowsiness is common (first generation).
   b. Sedative effect is cumulative with other CNS sedative drugs (first generation).
   c. The U.S. Food and Drug Administration (FDA) has issued a Public Health Advisory reminding that over-the-counter (OTC) cough and cold medications (many contain antihistamines) should *not* be used to treat infants and children younger than 2 years of age.
   d. Ethanol and first generation antihistamines synergistically reduce reaction time when driving.

B. **Therapeutic summary of selected antihistamines used in the treatment of allergies:** (Table 20-4)

Don't drive or operate machinery when taking first generation antihistamines.

TABLE 20-4. **Therapeutic Summary of Selected Antihistamines Used in the Treatment of Allergies**

DRUGS	CLINICAL APPLICATIONS	ADVERSE EFFECTS	CONTRAINDICATIONS
Mechanism: *First generation blockers of histamine H_1-receptors; sedating*			
Carbinoxamine Brompheniramine Chlorpheniramine Cyproheptadine (also blocks serotonin receptors) Dimenhydrinate Diphenhydramine Hydroxyzine Meclizine Promethazine	Treatment of allergic reactions Motion sickness (dimenhydrinate, meclizine) Over-the-counter sleeping medications (diphenhydramine) Treatment of nausea and vomiting (promethazine) Azelastine is a nasal spray for the treatment of the symptoms of seasonal allergic rhinitis Serotonin syndrome (cyproheptadine)	Sedation Anticholinergic effects; gastrointestinal upset, xerostomia, urinary retention, increased ocular pressure	Hypersensitivity Acute asthma Neonates or premature infants Breast-feeding
Mechanism: *Second generation blockers of histamine H_1-receptors; non-sedating*			
Azelastine Cetirizine Desloratadine Fexofenadine Loratadine	Treatment of seasonal allergic rhinitis Treatment of chronic idiopathic urticaria	Headache Fatigue Dyspepsia	Hypersensitivity

CHAPTER **21**

DRUGS USED IN THE TREATMENT OF GASTROINTESTINAL DISORDERS

I. Peptic Disorders

    A. Pathology; diseases include

        1. Ulcers of the stomach, esophagus, and duodenum

        2. Zollinger-Ellison syndrome

        3. Gastroesophageal reflux disease (GERD)

        4. Gastritis

        5. Esophagitis

    B. Physiology; (Fig. 21-1) physiologic stimulants of gastric acid secretion include:

        1. Gastrin

        2. Acetylcholine

        3. Histamine

        4. Prostaglandins

II. Drugs That Decrease Gastric Acidity (Box 21-1)

    A. Histamine H$_2$-receptor antagonists

        1. Cimetidine

            a. Mechanism of action

               (1) Blocks histamine action at the H$_2$-receptor site on parietal cells, thus inhibiting gastric acid secretion (see Fig. 21-1)

               (2) Decreases production of pepsin

               (3) Inhibits postprandial and basal gastric acid secretion

            b. Uses

               (1) Healing of duodenal and gastric ulcers and prevention of their recurrence

                 • Intractable peptic ulcers may require higher doses or combination therapy.

               (2) Control of secretory conditions such as Zollinger-Ellison syndrome and GERD

                 • Especially effective against nocturnal secretion (i.e., 90% reduced)

            c. Adverse effects

               • Antiandrogenic effects (gynecomastia and male sexual dysfunction)

            d. Drug interactions

               • Inhibition of liver microsomal metabolism of many drugs that utilize the cytochrome P450 system (e.g., beta blockers, benzodiazepines, calcium channel blockers, opioid agonists, tricyclic antidepressants)

        2. Other H$_2$-receptor antagonists

            a. Examples

               (1) Ranitidine

               (2) Famotidine

               (3) Nizatidine

            b. Therapeutic effects are similar to cimetidine

            c. Drug interactions and antiandrogenic effects occur much less frequently than with cimetidine

            d. All three are more potent than cimetidine

               (1) Control of secretory conditions such as Zollinger-Ellison syndrome and GERD; especially effective against nocturnal secretion (i.e., 90% reduced)

Helicobacter pylori often responsible for causing ulcers.

Cimetidine can cause gynecomastia in men.

Cimetidine extends the half-life ($t_{1/2}$) of many drugs that are metabolized in the liver.

Note common ending -tidine for all H$_2$-receptor antagonists

H$_2$-receptor blockade: more than 90% reduction in basal, food-stimulated, and nocturnal gastric acid secretions.

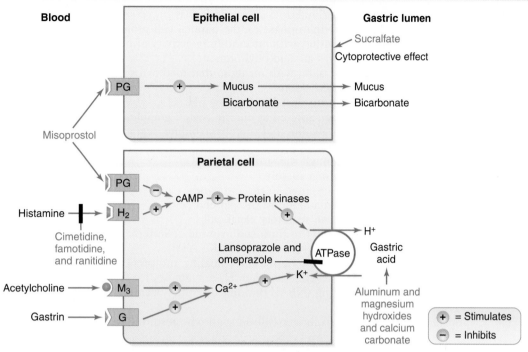

21-1: Gastric acid secretion and sites of drug action. ATPase, adenosine triphosphatase; cAMP, cyclic adenosine monophosphate; G, gastrin receptor; H₂, histamine H₂-receptor; M₃, muscarinic M₃ receptor; PG, prostaglandin receptor.

BOX 21-1 DRUGS THAT DECREASE GASTRIC ACIDITY	
H₂-Receptor Antagonists Cimetidine Famotidine Nizatidine Ranitidine **Proton Pump Inhibitors** Esomeprazole Lansoprazole Omeprazole	Pantoprazole Rabeprazole **Antacids** Aluminum hydroxide Calcium carbonate Magnesium hydroxide Sodium bicarbonate

  (2) Use
    • Treatment of duodenal ulcers associated with *Helicobacter pylori* (given with
      a bismuth compound and an antibiotic)
  (3) Adverse effect
    • Thrombocytopenia
  (4) Famotidine
    • Most potent H₂-receptor antagonist
B. Proton pump inhibitors (PPIs) (see Box 21-1)
  1. Examples
    a. Esomeprazole
    b. Lansoprazole
    c. Omeprazole
    d. Pantoprazole
    e. Rabeprazole
  2. Mechanism of action (see Fig. 21-1)
    a. Intragastric pH is higher and remains elevated longer than with H₂-receptor
      antagonist therapy.

Note common ending
-prazole to all PPIs; *but*
aripiprazole is a partial D₂
agonist

b. These drugs are benzimidazole compounds that irreversibly inhibit H^+/K^+ ATPase (adenosine triphosphatase), the parietal cell proton pump.

c. These drugs are prodrugs without inhibitory activity at neutral pH.

   (1) Activation requires an acid environment

   (2) They should be taken with meals so that food can stimulate acid secretion required for bioactivation.

d. Because these drugs are unstable at a low pH

   (1) Dosage forms are supplied as enteric coated granules.

   (2) Dissolve only at alkaline pH thereby avoiding degradation by acid in the esophagus and stomach

   (3) After passing through the stomach

   (4) The enteric coatings dissolve

   (5) The prodrug is absorbed in the intestines.

   (6) Carried by the circulation to the parietal cells

   (7) Accumulates in the secretory canaliculi

   (8) Activated at acid pH to form sulfonamide or sulfenic acid

   (9) It binds to sulfhydryl groups on H^+/K^+ ATPase.

e. These drugs will promote peptic ulcer healing and prevent ulcer recurrence

f. These drugs are more effective than H_2 antagonists for GERD or nonsteroidal anti-inflammatory drug (NSAID)-induced peptic ulcers.

  3. Uses

    a. Drugs of choice for Zollinger-Ellison syndrome resulting from gastrin-secreting tumors

    b. Most effective agents for GERD

    c. Duodenal ulcer, esophagitis, and gastric ulcer

      (1) When used to treat peptic ulcer disease, these drugs promote healing, but relapse may occur.

      (2) Proton pump inhibitors must be given in combination with agents that eliminate *H. pylori*.

C. Antacids: weak bases

  1. Examples

    a. Sodium bicarbonate

    b. Aluminum hydroxide

    c. Magnesium hydroxide

    d. Calcium carbonate

  2. Mechanism of action

    • Neutralize gastric hydrochloric acid and generally raise stomach pH from 1 to 3.0 to 3.5

  3. Uses

    • Symptomatic relief of acid indigestion, heartburn, GERD

  4. Adverse effects

    a. Diarrhea for magnesium

    b. Constipation for aluminum and calcium

    c. Cation absorption producing systemic alkalosis in patients with impaired renal function

    d. Sodium bicarbonate causes reflex hyperacidity; contraindicated in peptic ulcer disease.

III. Cytoprotective Agents (Box 21-2)

  • These drugs act by binding to ulcers; providing a protective coating against digestion by acid and pepsin

A. Sucralfate (aluminum sucrose sulfate)

  1. Pharmacokinetics

    a. Poorly soluble molecule that polymerizes in acid environment

    b. *No* significant absorption and *no* systemic effect

PPIs are administered as enteric coated formulations to prevent dissolution and bioactivation in the acidic stomach prior to absorption.

PPIs are prodrugs that are bioactivated in the acidic environment of the parietal cell to an intermediate that irreversibly binds to the proton pump.

Proton pump inhibitors are more effective than H_2-receptor blockers for treatment of peptic ulcer disease and GERD.

Antacids affect the absorption of many drugs, such as fluoroquinolones and tetracyclines.

Magnesium salts produce diarrhea while aluminum and calcium salts produce constipation.

BOX 21-2 CYTOPROTECTIVE DRUGS

Sucralfate
Prostaglandin analogues (e.g., misoprostol)
Colloidal bismuth compounds (e.g., bismuth subsalicylate)

2. Mechanism of action
   a. Selectively binds to necrotic ulcer tissue
   b. Acts as barrier to acid, pepsin, and bile
   c. Allows duodenal ulcers time to heal
   d. Stimulates synthesis of prostaglandins, which have cytoprotective effects on the gastrointestinal tract
3. Uses
   a. Treatment of active peptic ulcer disease
   b. Suppression of recurrence

B. Misoprostol
- Synthetic, oral prostaglandin E_1 analogue
1. Mechanism of action
   a. Inhibits secretion of gastrin
   b. Promotes secretion of mucus and bicarbonate
2. Uses
   a. Prevention of NSAID and steroid-induced gastric ulcers
   b. Medical termination of pregnancy of 49 days or less (in combination with mifepristone)
   c. Unlabeled uses
      (1) Cervical ripening and labor induction
      (2) NSAID-induced nephropathy
      (3) Fat malabsorption in cystic fibrosis
3. Adverse effects
   a. Abdominal cramps
   b. Diarrhea
   c. Vaginal bleeding
   d. Contraindication
     - Pregnancy (can induce labor and uterine rupture)

C. Colloidal bismuth compounds
1. Example
   - Bismuth subsalicylate
2. Mechanism of action
   a. Selectively binds to ulcer coating
   b. Protects the ulcer from gastric acid
3. Uses
   a. Control of nonspecific diarrhea
   b. Prophylaxis of traveler's diarrhea, dyspepsia, and heartburn
   c. Control of *H. pylori* (in combination therapy)
4. Adverse effects
   - Darken the tongue and stools because the bismuth sulfide formed is a black solid

IV. Drugs Used in the Treatment of *H. pylori* Infection (see Chapter 27)
- *H. pylori* organisms can be identified in antral samples from most patients with duodenal and gastric ulcers.

A. Eradication
- Requires multiple drug therapy to enhance the rate of ulcer healing

B. Therapeutic regimens
1. Usually includes a proton pump inhibitor (e.g., rabeprazole) in combination with two or more of the following drugs:
   a. Amoxicillin
   b. Bismuth
   c. Clarithromycin
   d. Metronidazole
   e. Tetracycline
   f. Tinidazole
2. Pharmacology of antimicrobials (see Chapters 27 and 28).

V. Therapeutic summary of selected drugs used to treat diseases of hyperacidity: (Table 21-1)

V1. Antidiarrheal Drugs (Box 21-3)

A. Inhibitors of acetylcholine (ACh) release
1. Examples
   a. Diphenoxylate
   b. Loperamide

Margin notes:

Sucralfate requires acid pH for activation and should *not* be administered with antacids, H_2-receptor antagonists, or PPIs.

Don't use misoprostol during pregnancy; it can cause the fetus to abort.

Misoprostol causes severe gastrointestinal (GI) effects.

Bismuth effective for both diarrhea and ulcers.

Bismuth darkens tongue and stools, may produce hypersensitivity reactions in salicylate-sensitive patients

Triple drug therapy with metronidazole; a bismuth compound; and an antibiotic such as tetracycline, amoxicillin, or clarithromycin is recommended in some patients, to overcome drug resistance.

Loperamide produces less sedation and less abuse potential than diphenoxylate; atropine is added to diphenoxylate to act as a deterrent of abuse.

TABLE 21-1. **Therapeutic Summary of Selected Drugs Used to Treat Diseases of Hyperacidity**

DRUGS	CLINICAL APPLICATIONS	ADVERSE EFFECTS	CONTRAINDICATIONS
Mechanism: *Histamine H₂ antagonists*			
Cimetidine Famotidine Nizatidine Ranitidine	Short-term treatment of active duodenal ulcers and benign gastric ulcers Long-term prophylaxis of duodenal ulcer Gastric hypersecretory states Gastroesophageal reflux OTC use for prevention or relief of heartburn, acid indigestion, or sour stomach	Antiandrogenic effects; gynecomastia and male sexual dysfunction (cimetidine)	Hypersensitivity Many drug-drug interactions (cimetidine)
Mechanism: *Proton pump inhibitors (PPIs)*			
Esomeprazole Lansoprazole Omeprazole Pantoprazole Rabeprazole	Short-term treatment of active duodenal ulcers and benign gastric ulcers Long-term prophylaxis of duodenal ulcer Gastric hypersecretory states Gastroesophageal reflux OTC use for prevention or relief of heartburn, acid indigestion, or sour stomach Multidrug regimen for *Helicobacter pylori* Healing NSAID-induced ulcers Prevention of NSAID-induced ulcers OTC for short-term treatment of frequent, uncomplicated heartburn occurring ≥2 days/week	Headache GI distress	Hypersensitivity
Mechanism: *Nonsystemic antacids; neutralize stomach acid*			
Aluminum hydroxide Calcium carbonate Magnesium hydroxide	Treatment of hyperacidity	Diarrhea for magnesium Constipation for aluminum and calcium	Hypersensitivity
Mechanism: *Systemic antacid; neutralize stomach acid*			
Sodium bicarbonate	Treatment of hyperacidity	Edema Belching Milk-alkali syndrome Metabolic alkalosis	Alkalosis Hypernatremia Severe pulmonary edema Hypocalcemia Abdominal pain of unknown origin
Mechanism: *Gastric cytoprotective agents*			
Sucralfate Misoprostol Bismuth subsalicylate	Duodenal ulcers NSAID-induced gastric ulcers (misoprostol) Diarrhea (bismuth)	GI distress Vaginal bleeding (misoprostol)	Hypersensitivity Pregnancy (misoprostol, bismuth) Salicylate hypersensitivity (bismuth)
Mechanism: *Antimicrobial for H. pylori*			
Amoxicillin Bismuth Clarithromycin Metronidazole Tetracycline Tinidazole	Antimicrobial for *H. pylori*	See Chapter 27	Hypersensitivity

GI, gastrointestinal; NSAID, nonsteroidal anti-inflammatory drug; OTC, over-the-counter.

BOX 21-3 ANTIDIARRHEAL DRUGS

Opioids
Diphenoxylate with atropine
Loperamide

Locally Acting Drugs
Bismuth subsalicylate
Kaolin-pectin
Polycarbophil

2. These drugs are also known as opioid antidiarrheals (see Chapter 19).
3. Mechanism of action
   a. These drugs inhibit ACh release through presynaptic opioid receptors in the enteric nervous system; this:
      (1) Disrupts peristalsis
      (2) Decreases intestinal motility
      (3) Increases intestinal transit time
   b. Loperamide does *not* cross the blood-brain barrier.
4. Uses
   a. Control and relief of acute, nonspecific diarrhea
   b. Treatment of chronic diarrhea associated with inflammatory bowel disease
5. Contraindication
   • Ulcerative colitis (can induce toxic megacolon)

B. Locally acting agents
1. Mechanism of action
   a. Inhibit intestinal secretions
   b. Adsorb water and other substances
2. Uses
   a. Bismuth
      • Management of infectious diarrhea, especially traveler's diarrhea
   b. Adsorbents (kaolin-pectin)
      • Can also bind potentially toxic substances

C. Therapeutic summary of selected antidiarrheal drugs: (Table 21-2)

VII. Prokinetic Drugs (Box 21-4):

A. Examples
1. Metoclopramide
2. Cisapride

B. Metoclopramide
1. Mechanism of action
   a. Enhances gastric motility without stimulating gastric secretions
   b. Augments cholinergic release of ACh from postganglionic nerve endings, sensitizing muscarinic receptors on smooth muscle cells
   c. Blocks dopamine D_2 and 5-hydroxytryptamine ($5\text{-}HT_3$) receptors (antiemetic action)
2. Uses and clinical effects
   a. GERD
      • Reduced reflux and increased gastric emptying due to the decrease of the resting tone of the lower esophageal sphincter
   b. Nausea and vomiting
      • Antiemetic effect produced by blockade of dopamine D_2 receptors in the chemoreceptor trigger zone (CTZ)
   c. Gastroparesis
      • Promotion of motility
3. Adverse effects
   • Extrapyramidal or dystonic reactions

Margin notes:

Opioid antidiarrheals are contraindicated in ulcerative colitis.

Kaolin-pectin absorbs toxins that induce diarrhea.

Metoclopramide has both antiemetic and prokinetic actions.

Metoclopramide noted for producing acute dystonia.

TABLE 21-2. Therapeutic Summary of Selected Antidiarrheal Drugs

DRUGS	CLINICAL APPLICATIONS	ADVERSE EFFECTS	CONTRAINDICATIONS
Mechanism: Antidiarrheal opioids; inhibit ACh release through presynaptic opioid receptors in the enteric nervous system			
Diphenoxylate with atropine Loperamide	Diarrhea	Constipation Abdominal cramping Nausea	Hypersensitivity Avoid use as primary therapy in acute dysentery, acute ulcerative colitis, bacterial enterocolitis, pseudomembranous colitis
Mechanism: Local actions; bind toxins			
Bismuth subsalicylate Kaolin-pectin Polycarbophil	Diarrhea	Constipation Abdominal cramping Nausea Black tongue (bismuth)	Hypersensitivity Pregnancy (bismuth) Severe GI bleed

ACh, acetylcholine; GI, gastrointestinal.

BOX 21-4 PROKINETIC AND ANTIEMETIC DRUGS	
Prokinetic drugs Cisapride Metoclopramide **Anticholinergic Drugs** Scopolamine **Antihistamines** Dimenhydrinate Diphenhydramine Cyclizine Meclizine Hydroxyzine **Dopamine D$_2$-Receptor Antagonists** Droperidol Metoclopramide Perphenazine Prochlorperazine Promethazine Trimethobenzamide	**Serotonin 5-HT$_3$ Receptor Antagonists** Alosetron Dolasetron Granisetron Ondansetron Palonosetron **Cannabinoid receptor (CB1) agonists** Dronabinol Nabilone **Neurokinin 1 (NK1) Receptor Antagonists** Aprepitant Fosaprepitant

C. **Cisapride**
- Available in United States only via limited-access protocol (1-800-JANSSEN).
1. Mechanism of action
   a. Enhances the release of acetylcholine at the myenteric plexus
   b. 5-HT$_4$ agonist properties
      (1) Increases gastrointestinal motility and cardiac rate
      (2) Increases lower esophageal sphincter contraction and lowers esophageal peristalsis
   c. Accelerates gastric emptying of both liquids and solids
2. Uses
   a. Nocturnal symptoms of gastroesophageal reflux disease (GERD)
   b. Effective for gastroparesis
   c. Effective for refractory constipation
   d. Effective for non-ulcer dyspepsia
3. Adverse effects
   a. Boxed warning
      - Serious cardiac arrhythmias including ventricular tachycardia, ventricular fibrillation, torsade de pointes, and QT prolongation have been reported in patients taking this drug.
   b. Diarrhea, GI cramping, dyspepsia, flatulence, nausea, xerostomia
   c. Increased liver function tests (LFTs)
   d. Hematologic
      (1) Thrombocytopenia
      (2) Pancytopenia
      (3) Leukopenia
      (4) Granulocytopenia
      (5) Aplastic anemia

VIII. **Antiemetic Drugs** (see Box 21-4)
   A. **Physiology of emesis** (incompletely understood process)
      1. Coordination of stimuli takes place in the vomiting center, located in the reticular formation of the medulla.
      2. Input arises from the CTZ, vestibular apparatus, and afferent nerves.
   B. **Antiemetic drugs**
      1. Serotonin 5-HT$_3$ receptor antagonists
         a. Examples
            (1) Alosetron
            (2) Dolasetron
            (3) Granisetron

Cisapride is a very effective prokinetic agent but it can cause life-threatening cardiovascular effects; so its use is restricted for compassionate use only.

Cisapride can also produce severe hematologic abnormalities.

Blockade of muscarinic, histamine H$_1$, dopamine D$_2$, serotonin 5-HT$_3$, cannabinoid CB1, or neurokinin NK1 receptors all result in decreased emesis.

(4) Ondansetron
(5) Palonosetron
b. Safe and effective antiemetics
c. Uses
(1) The -setrons are used for chemotherapy-induced emesis
(2) Postsurgery nausea and vomiting
(3) Hyperemesis gravidarum (unlabeled use)
(4) Alosetron is used for the treatment of women who exhibit severe diarrhea-predominant irritable bowel syndrome (IBS).
(a) *Only* in those who have failed conventional therapy
(b) *Only* physicians enrolled in Prometheus' Prescribing Program for Lotronex may prescribe this medication.

2. Cannabinoid derivatives
a. Examples
(1) Dronabinol
(2) Nabilone
b. Mechanism of action
• Antiemetic activity may be due to effect on cannabinoid receptors (CB1) within the CNS.
c. Use
• Nausea and vomiting in patients with acquired immunodeficiency syndrome (AIDS) or cancer
d. Adverse effects
(1) Dizziness
(2) Drowsiness
(3) Vertigo
(4) Euphoria

3. Dopamine D_2 receptor antagonists
a. Examples
(1) Droperidol
(2) Metoclopramide
(3) Phenothiazines (perphenazine, prochlorperazine, promethazine)
(4) Trimethobenzamide
b. Pharmacology of phenothiazines discussed in Chapter 10
c. Metoclopramide is discussed above
• Trimethobenzamide has similar actions as an antiemetic
d. Phenothiazines have multiple uses:
(1) Antiemetic
(2) Symptomatic treatment of various allergic conditions
(3) Motion sickness
(4) Sedative
(5) Postoperative pain (adjunctive therapy)
(6) Anesthetic (adjunctive therapy)
(7) Anaphylactic reactions (adjunctive therapy

4. Antihistamines
a. Examples
(1) Dimenhydrinate
(2) Diphenhydramine
(3) Cyclizine
(4) Hydroxyzine
(5) Meclizine
b. Use
• Nausea and vomiting associated with motion sickness

5. Anticholinergic
a. Example
• Scopolamine
b. Use
(1) **Transdermal**
• Prevention of nausea/vomiting associated with motion sickness and recovery from anesthesia and surgery
(2) **Injection**
• Preoperative medication to produce amnesia, sedation, tranquilization, antiemetic effects, and decrease salivary and respiratory secretions

Note common ending -setron in 5-HT$_3$ receptor antagonists: ondansetron, granisetron

Setrons are the best antiemetics; especially for chemotherapy-induced emesis.

Setrons are being used to treat morning sickness; expensive option.

Alosetron is used to treat IBS with diarrhea in women.

Marijuana and cannabinoid derivatives are effective antiemetics and stimulate appetite in patients with end-stage cancer or AIDS.

Phenothiazines have multiple uses:

The blockade of both histamine H$_1$ and dopamine D$_2$ receptors by some phenothiazines confer to them sedative antiemetic, and anti-itch properties.

Cyclizine and meclizine are *not* as sedating as dimenhydrinate or diphenhydramine when used to treat motion sickness.

Scopolamine patch behind the ear is effective for motion sickness.

Neurokinin-1 (NK-1) receptor antagonists are the newest class of drugs for treating emesis.

6. Neurokinin 1 (NK-1) receptor antagonist
   a. Examples
      (1) Aprepitant
      (2) Fosaprepitant (prodrug)
   b. Use
      (1) Prevention of acute and delayed nausea and vomiting associated with moderately- and highly-emetogenic chemotherapy (in combination with other antiemetics)
      (2) Prevention of postoperative nausea and vomiting
IX. **Therapeutic summary of selected prokinetic and antiemetic drugs:** (Table 21-3)
X. **Drugs Used to Treat Irritable Bowel Syndrome (IBS)**

IBS mainly occurs in women.

   A. **Tricyclic antidepressants**
      • Low doses of amitriptyline or desipramine are used for treatment of chronic abdominal pain associated with IBS.
   B. **Antispasmodics**
      • Anticholinergics, such as dicyclomine or hyoscyamine, are sometimes used to treat IBS.

TABLE 21-3. **Therapeutic Summary of Selected Prokinetic and Antiemetic drugs**

DRUGS	CLINICAL APPLICATIONS	ADVERSE EFFECTS	CONTRAINDICATIONS
Mechanism: *Prokinetic via multiple actions*			
Cisapride Metoclopramide	Symptomatic treatment of diabetic gastric stasis Gastroesophageal reflux Cisapride restricted for compassionate use	Cardiovascular Acute dystonic reactions Drowsiness Parkinsonian-like symptoms	Hypersensitivity Pheochromocytoma History of seizures Cardiac disease (cisapride)
Mechanism: *Central muscarinic receptor antagonist*			
Scopolamine	Motion sickness Emesis	See Chapter 4	Hypersensitivity
Mechanism: *Central both histamine H₁ receptor and muscarinic antagonists*			
Diphenhydramine Dimenhydrinate Cyclizine Meclizine Hydroxyzine	Motion sickness Emesis Hypnotic Allergies	Dry mouth Sedation Constipation Blurred vision Hypotension Tachycardia	Hypersensitivity Acute asthma Neonates or premature infants Breast-feeding
Mechanism: *Central dopamine D₂ receptor antagonists*			
Droperidol Metoclopramide Perphenazine Prochlorperazine Promethazine Trimethobenzamide	Management of nausea and vomiting Antiemetic in surgical and diagnostic procedures Allergic conditions (promethazine)	Multiple cardiac effects Parkinsonism effects Dystonias Sedation	Hypersensitivity Pheochromocytoma History of seizures
Mechanism: *Central 5-HT₃ receptor antagonists*			
Alosetron Dolasetron Granisetron Ondansetron Palonosetron	Chemotherapy-induced emesis Postsurgery nausea and vomiting Hyperemesis gravidarum Irritable bowel syndrome (alosetron)	Headache Fatigue Constipation ECG changes	Hypersensitivity
Mechanism: *Central cannabinoid receptor (CB1) agonists*			
Dronabinol Nabilone	Nausea and vomiting in patients with acquired immunodeficiency syndrome (AIDS) or cancer Appetite stimulus during the wasting syndrome	Vasodilation/ facial flushing Euphoria Abnormal thinking Paranoia	Hypersensitivity Patients with a history of schizophrenia
Mechanism: *Central neurokinin 1 (NK1) Receptor Antagonists*			
Aprepitant Fosaprepitant	Postoperative nausea and vomiting Prevention of acute and delayed nausea and vomiting associated with emetogenic chemotherapy	Fatigue Constipation Hypotension	Hypersensitivity

ECG, electrocardiogram; 5-HT₃, 5-hydroxytryptamine-3.

TABLE 21-4. **5-Hydroxytrypamine (5-HT) Receptor Subtypes and Important Pharmacology**

RECEPTOR SUBTYPE	DISTRIBUTION	SECOND MESSENGER	AGONISTS	ANTAGONISTS	USES
5-HT$_{1A}$	Raphe nuclei, hippocampus	Multiple, G$_i$ dominates	Buspirone (partial)		Anxiolytic
5-HT$_{1D}$	Brain	G$_i$, ↓ cAMP	Sumatriptan and other triptans, ergots		Migraine
5-HT$_{2A}$	Platelets, smooth and striated muscle, cerebral cortex	G$_q$, ↑ IP$_3$		Clozapine, olanzapine, risperidone	Psychosis
5-HT$_3$	Area postrema, sensory and enteric nerves	Na$^+$-K$^+$ ion channel		Ondansetron, granisetron	Emesis
5-HT$_4$	CNS and myenteric neurons, smooth muscle	G$_s$, ↑cAMP	Metoclopramide, cisapride, tegaserod partial		Prokinetic and irritable bowel syndrome

cAMP, cyclic adenosine monophosphate; CNS, central nervous system; IP$_3$, inositol-triphosphate.

C. **Selective serotonin (5-HT$_4$) partial agonist**
- Tegaserod
1. See Table 21-4 for 5-HT receptor subtypes and their important pharmacology.
2. Tegaserod is only available for emergency treatment of irritable bowel syndrome with constipation (IBS-C) and chronic idiopathic constipation (CIC) in women (younger than 55 years of age) in which *no* alternative therapy exists.
3. Serious cardiovascular events (e.g., myocardial infarction [MI], stroke, unstable angina) may occur with the use of tegaserod.

D. **Serotonin 5-HT$_3$ receptor antagonist**
- Alosetron is used for the treatment of women who exhibit severe diarrhea-predominant IBS and have failed conventional therapy.

E. **Therapeutic summary of selective important drugs used to treat IBS**: (Table 21-5)

XI. **Drugs Used in the Treatment of Inflammatory Bowel Disease (IBD)**

A. **Pathology**
- Crohn's disease and ulcerative colitis are often considered together as inflammatory bowel disease.

B. **Salicylates** (see Chapter 18)
1. 5-Aminosalicylic acid (5-ASA, mesalamine)
- Active anti-inflammatory agent
  a. Mechanism of action
  - Inhibitor of cyclooxygenase (COX) pathway
  b. Uses
    (1) Ulcerative colitis
    (2) Crohn's disease (sometimes)
  c. Adverse effects
    (1) Abdominal pain
    (2) Nausea and vomiting
    (3) Headache
2. Sulfasalazine
- Chemical linkage of sulfapyridine and mesalamine
  a. Mechanism of action
  - Production of beneficial effects due to antibacterial action of sulfapyridine and anti-inflammatory (most important) properties of mesalamine (5-ASA)
  b. Uses
    (1) Ulcerative colitis
    (2) Crohn's disease (maintain remission)
    (3) Rheumatoid arthritis
  c. Adverse effects
    (1) Malaise
    (2) Nausea, abdominal discomfort
    (3) Headache
    (4) Typical sulfonamide adverse effects (e.g., blood dyscrasias, skin reactions, hypersensitivity)

Constipation-dependent IBS (tegaserod); diarrhea-dependent IBS (alosetron).

Local delivery of 5-ASA; useful anti-inflammatory for inflammatory bowel diseases.

Note: many ways of locally delivering 5-ASA in treating inflammatory bowel diseases.

TABLE 21-5. **Therapeutic Summary of Selected Drugs Used to Treat Irritable Bowel Syndrome (IBS)**

DRUGS	CLINICAL APPLICATIONS	ADVERSE EFFECTS	CONTRAINDICATIONS
Mechanism: *Tricyclic antidepressants; therapeutic due to blocking NE and 5-HT reuptake at presynaptic neuron; many adverse effects associated with blocking alpha adrenergic, muscarinic and histaminic receptors*			
Amitriptyline Desipramine	Useful in chronic IBS Endogenous depression Nocturnal enuresis in children (Imipramine) Amitriptyline (Analgesic for certain chronic and neuropathic pain; prophylaxis against migraine headaches) OCD (Clomipramine)	Hypotension Anticholinergic effects Sedation Dangerous in overdose (arrhythmias and seizures)	Hypersensitivity Heart disease With MAO inhibitors can get serotonin syndrome Pregnancy
Mechanism: *Anticholinergics; muscarinic receptor antagonists*			
Dicyclomine Hyoscyamine	Anticholinergics used for IBS	Dry mouth Blurred vision Urinary retention Constipation Tachycardia ↑ intraocular pressure Hyperthermia	Hypersensitivity Narrow angle glaucoma Obstructive uropathy Myasthenia gravis Obstructive GI tract disease
Mechanism: *Selective serotonin (5-HT$_4$) partial agonist*			
Tegaserod	Emergency treatment of IBS with constipation Chronic idiopathic constipation in women (<55 years of age) in which no alternative therapy exists	Serious cardiovascular events (e.g., MI, stroke, unstable angina)	Hypersensitivity Severe renal disease Severe hepatic disease Exclusion criteria under the emergency-IND process: Unstable angina, history of MI or stroke, hypertension, hyperlipidemia, diabetes, age ≥55 years, smoking, obesity, depression, anxiety, or suicidal ideation.
Mechanism: *Selective serotonin 5-HT$_3$ receptor antagonist*			
Alosetron	Treatment of women with severe diarrhea-predominant IBS who have failed to respond to conventional therapy	Headache Fatigue Constipation ECG changes	Hypersensitivity

ECG, electrocardiogram; GI, gastrointestinal; 5-HT, 5-hydroxytryptamine; IBS, irritable bowel syndrome; IND, investigational new drug application; MAO monoamine oxidase; MI, myocardial infarction; NE, norepinephrine; OCD, obsessive compulsive disorder.

    3. Olsalazine
        a. Chemistry
            • Two 5-ASA molecules linked by a diazo bond (RN=NR′), cleaved by bacteria in the colon
        b. Used in the treatment of ulcerative colitis
    C. **Immunosuppressive agents** (see Chapter 17)
        1. Hydrocortisone and other glucocorticoids can induce remission of ulcerative colitis and Crohn's disease
            • Hydrocortisone is available as an enema
        2. Anti-Tumor Necrosis Factor therapy
            a. Infliximab
                • A monoclonal antibody to tumor necrosis factor-α (TNF$_α$) is used to treat moderate to severe Crohn's disease.
            b. Adalimumab
                • Is also used for treatment of moderately- to severely-active Crohn's disease in patients with inadequate response to conventional treatment, or patients who have lost response to or are intolerant of infliximab.
    D. **Therapeutic summary of selected drugs used to treat inflammatory bowel disease (IBD):** (Table 21-6)
XII. **Laxatives** (Table 21-7)
    A. **General considerations**
        1. Laxative abuse occurs frequently.
        2. Contraindications to these drugs include:
            a. Unexplained abdominal pain
            b. Intestinal obstruction

Hydrocortisone can be given as an enema to produce local anti-inflammatory effects in inflammatory bowel diseases.

Anti-TNF$_α$ compounds are very beneficial in severe Crohn's disease.

Cathartics are often abused; especially by the elderly.

TABLE 21-6. **Therapeutic Summary of Selected Drugs Used to Treat Inflammatory Bowel Disease (IBD):**

DRUGS	CLINICAL APPLICATIONS	ADVERSE EFFECTS	CONTRAINDICATIONS
Mechanism: *All locally release 5-aminosalicylic acid; anti-inflammatory*			
Mesalamine Sulfasalazine Olsalazine	Ulcerative colitis Crohn's disease Rheumatoid arthritis (sulfasalazine)	Headache GI distress Photosensitivity Reversible oligospermia	Hypersensitivity Allergies to sulfonamides
Mechanism: *Anti-inflammatory glucocorticoid*			
Hydrocortisone	Adjunctive treatment of ulcerative colitis (often given as enema)	Iatrogenic Cushing's syndrome with long use Diabetes mellitus Hypertension Peptic ulcer disease Hypomania and psychosis Depression Adrenal insufficiency on abrupt cessation of therapy	Hypersensitivity Serious infections
Mechanism: *Monoclonal antibody to tumor necrosis factor-α (TNF$_\alpha$); proinflammatory cytokine*			
Infliximab Adalimumab	Treatment of Crohn's disease Treatment of and maintenance of healing of ulcerative colitis	Headache GI distress Increased risk of infection	Hypersensitivity Congestive heart failure (NYHA Class III/IV)

GI, gastrointestinal; NYHA, New York Heart Association.

TABLE 21-7. **Effects of Common Laxatives**

TYPE	SITE OF ACTION	MECHANISM	USES	ADVERSE EFFECTS
Bulk-Forming				
Psyllium	Small and large intestines	Increase bulk and moisture content in stool, stimulating peristalsis	Prevent straining during defecation	Esophageal or bowel obstruction if taken with insufficient liquid Flatulence
Osmotic				
Lactulose	Colon	Retain ammonia in colon, producing osmotic effect that stimulates bowel evacuation	Prevent and treat portal systemic encephalopathy Treat constipation	Abdominal discomfort Flatulence
Saline cathartics, magnesium citrate	Small intestine	Induce cholecystokinin release from duodenum, producing osmotic effect that produces distention, promoting peristalsis	Evacuate colon before diagnostic examination or surgery Accelerate excretion of parasites or poisons from GI tract	Electrolyte disturbance
Stimulant				
Senna	Colon	Acts directly on intestinal smooth muscle to increase peristalsis	Facilitates defecation in diminished colonic motor response Evacuate colon before diagnostic examination or surgery	Urine discoloration Abdominal cramping Fluid and electrolyte depletion
Stool Softener				
Docusate	Small and large intestine	Lowers surface tension Facilitates penetration of fat and water into stool	Short-term treatment of constipation Evacuate colon before diagnostic examination or surgery Prevent straining during defecation Modify fluid from ileostomy, colostomy	GI cramping

GI, gastrointestinal.

BOX 21-5 LAXATIVES	

Bulk-Forming Laxatives
Methylcellulose
Psyllium
 	
Osmotic Laxatives
Lactulose
Saline cathartics (magnesium citrate, magnesium
    hydroxide, magnesium sulfate, magnesium
    phosphate, sodium phosphate)
Sorbitol
 	
Balanced Polyethylene Glycol (PEG)
PEG and isotonic salt solution
	Stimulants
	Bisacodyl
	Cascara sagrada
	Castor oil
	Senna
	
	Stool Softeners
	Docusate
	Glycerin
	Mineral oil

B. **Types of laxatives** (Box 21-5)
   1. Bulk-forming laxatives
      a. Examples
         • Psyllium
         • Methylcellulose
      b. Natural and semisynthetic polysaccharides
      c. Cellulose derivatives (similar to dietary fiber)
   2. Osmotic laxatives
      a. The osmotic effect of these laxatives increases water in the colon.
      b. Saline cathartics
         (1) Magnesium salts
         (2) Sodium phosphate
            • Used when prompt, complete evacuation is necessary.
      c. Other osmotic drugs
         (1) Lactulose
         (2) Sorbitol
   3. Balanced polyethylene glycol (PEG)
      • PEG plus isotonic salt solution
   4. Stimulant laxatives
      a. Examples
         (1) Castor oil
         (2) Cascara
         (3) Senna
         (4) Bisacodyl
      b. Castor oil, a primary irritant, increases intestinal motility.
      c. Cascara, senna, and bisacodyl are irritants found in many over-the-counter (OTC) preparations.
   5. Stool softeners
      a. Surfactants (e.g., docusate)
      b. Lubricants (e.g., mineral oil, glycerin)

PEG plus magnesium citrate and large quantities of fluids are use to cleanse the bowel prior to colonoscopy.

Irritant compounds from plant extracts found in many OTC laxatives.

Docusate widely used in hospitalized patients.

Chapter 22

IMMUNOSUPPRESSIVE DRUGS AND DRUGS USED IN THE TREATMENT OF RHEUMATIC DISORDERS AND GOUT

I. Immunosuppressive Drugs (Box 22-1)

A. Corticosteroids (see Chapter 23)
1. Examples
   a. Prednisone
   b. Methylprednisolone
2. Mechanism of action
   a. Decrease phospholipase A_2 (PLA_2) and cyclooxygenase 2 (COX-2) activity (see Chapter 23)
   b. This leads to inhibition of prostaglandin and leukotriene synthesis
   c. Cytotoxic to certain T-cell subpopulations (helper and suppressor)
   d. Suppress both cellular and humoral immunity
   e. Inhibition of leukocyte infiltration at site of inflammation
   f. Interference in the function of mediators of inflammatory response
   g. *Not* toxic to myeloid and erythroid progenitor cells
3. Use
   a. Acute episodes of rheumatoid arthritis
   b. Autoimmune diseases
   c. Bronchial asthma
4. Adverse effects
   • Predispose to infection; adrenal gland suppression; also see Chapter 23

B. Other immunosuppressive drugs
   • See Table 22-1 for sites of action
1. These drugs are used to suppress immune responses under a wide number of conditions where an overactive immune system contributes to pathogenesis (Table 22-2).
2. Azathioprine
   a. Pharmacokinetics
      (1) Well absorbed from gastrointestinal (GI) tract
      (2) Converted to 6-mercaptopurine (6-MP) by glutathione-S-transferases and then to 6-thiouric acid by xanthine oxidase
      (3) Reduce dose in patients with thiopurine methyltransferase (TPMT) deficiency
   b. Mechanism of action
      (1) Interferes with nucleic acid metabolism and synthesis, thus inhibiting cell proliferation
      (2) Toxic to proliferating lymphocytes following antigen exposure
   c. Adverse effects
      (1) Bone marrow suppression
         (a) Leukopenia
         (b) Anemia
         (c) Thrombocytopenia

Glucocorticoids increase the synthesis of lipocortin, which inhibits PLA_2.

Glucocorticoids are *not* toxic to myeloid or erythroid cell linage.

Azathioprine is converted to 6-MP.

Allopurinol decreases the metabolism of 6-MP and increases toxicity of azathioprine

BOX 22-1 IMMUNOSUPPRESSIVE DRUGS

Abatacept
Adalimumab
Antithymocyte globulin
Azathioprine
Basiliximab
Cyclophosphamide
Cyclosporine
Daclizumab
Etanercept

Infliximab
Methotrexate
Methylprednisolone
Muromonab-CD3 (OKT3)
Mycophenolate mofetil
Prednisone
Rho[D] immune globulin
Tacrolimus

Table 22-1. Sites of Action of Selected Immunosuppressive Agents on T-Cell Activation

DRUG	SITE OF ACTION
Glucocorticoids	Glucocorticoid response elements in DNA (regulate gene transcription)
Muromonab-CD3	T-cell receptor complex (blocks antigen recognition)
Cyclosporine	Calcineurin (inhibits phosphatase activity)
Tacrolimus	Calcineurin (inhibits phosphatase activity)
Azathioprine	Deoxyribonucleic acid (false nucleotide incorporation)
Mycophenolate Mofetil	Inosine monophosphate dehydrogenase (inhibits activity)
Daclizumab Basiliximab	Interleukin-2 receptor (block IL-2–mediated T-cell activation)
Sirolimus	Protein kinase involved in cell-cycle progression (mTOR) (inhibits activity)

Table 22-2. Clinical Uses of Immunosuppressive Agents

AUTOIMMUNE DISEASES	IMMUNOSUPPRESSIVE AGENTS
Idiopathic thrombocytopenic purpura	Prednisone, vincristine, occasionally mercaptopurine or azathioprine, high-dose gamma globulin, plasma immunoabsorption
Autoimmune hemolytic anemia	Prednisone cyclophosphamide, chlorambucil, mercaptopurine, azathioprine, high-dose gamma globulin
Acute glomerulonephritis	Prednisone mercaptopurine, cyclophosphamide
Acquired factor XII antibodies	Cyclophosphamide plus factor XII
Miscellaneous "autoreactive" disorders: Systemic lupus erythematosus, Wegener's granulomatosis, rheumatoid arthritis, chronic active hepatitis, inflammatory bowel disease	Prednisone, cyclophosphamide, azathioprine, cyclosporine, infliximab, etanercept, adalimumab, interferons
Isoimmune disease Hemolytic anemia of the newborn	Rho[D] immune globulin
Organ transplantation Renal Heart	Cyclosporine, azathioprine, prednisone, ALG, muromonab-CD3 monoclonal antibody, tacrolimus, basiliximab, daclizumab
Liver	Cyclosporine, prednisone, azathioprine, tacrolimus
Bone marrow (HLA-matched)	Cyclosporine, cyclophosphamide, prednisone, methotrexate, ALG, total body irradiation, donor marrow purging with monoclonal anti-T cell antibodies, immunotoxins

ALG, antilymphocytic globulin.

Azathioprine is the antipurine most often used as an immunosuppressive agent.

    (2) At high doses:
       (a) Skin rashes
       (b) Fever
       (c) Nausea and vomiting
       (d) Diarrhea and GI disturbances
    (3) Occasional liver dysfunction with mild jaundice
    (4) Increased by kidney disease and allopurinol (xanthine oxidase inhibitor)
  d. Uses
    (1) Kidney transplantation
    (2) Autoimmune diseases

3. Cyclophosphamide (see Chapter 29)
   a. Mechanism of action
      (1) Alkylates DNA
      (2) Most potent immunosuppressive agent
      (3) Destroys proliferating lymphoid cells in addition to some quiescent cells
   b. Uses
      (1) Organ transplantation
      (2) Autoimmune diseases
      (3) Anticancer drugs

> Cyclophosphamide causes hemorrhagic cystitis, treat with Mesna.

4. Methotrexate
   a. Mechanism of action
      (1) Its principal mechanism of action at the low doses used in the rheumatic diseases probably relates to inhibition of amino imidazolecarboxamide ribonucleotide (AICAR) transformylase and thymidylate synthetase
      (2) At higher doses, it inhibits dihydrofolate reductase, thus blocks folate-requiring reactions in the biosynthesis of nucleotides needed for cell proliferation
      (3) Cytotoxic to proliferating lymphocytes following antigen exposure
   b. Uses
      (1) Active rheumatoid arthritis (RA)
      (2) More effective when used in combination with other drugs, such as etanercept or infliximab
      (3) Prophylaxis for graft versus host syndrome for bone marrow transplantation in leukemia patients
      (4) Psoriasis

> Methotrexate plus anti-tumor necrosis factor-alpha (TNFα) agents are very effective in RA.

   c. Adverse effects
      (1) Macrocytic anemia (caused by folate deficiency)
      (2) Bone marrow suppression
      (3) Pulmonary fibrosis
      (4) Hepatotoxicity
      (5) Teratogenic activity

> Alcohol and methotrexate have synergistic hepatotoxicity.

5. Cyclosporine
   a. Pharmacokinetics
      (1) Administered orally and intravenously
         (a) After oral administration, roughly 20% to 50% is absorbed
         (b) High "first-pass" metabolism
      (2) Metabolized extensively in liver by cytochrome CYP3A4 to at least 25 metabolites, some of which are biologically active
      (3) Drugs that decrease clearance via inhibition of hepatic microsomal enzymes can cause cyclosporine toxicity (e.g., nephrotoxicity, seizures).
         • Examples: androgens, clarithromycin, diltiazem, erythromycin, estrogens, nefazodone, nicardipine, verapamil, and azole antifungal drugs
      (4) Drugs that increase clearance of cyclosporine by stimulating its metabolism may lead to graft rejection.
         • Examples: nafcillin, omeprazole; rifampin; and certain anticonvulsants such as carbamazepine, phenytoin, phenobarbital, primidone, and St. John's Wort

> Drug-drug interactions must be closely monitored with cyclosporine therapy.

   b. Mechanism of action
      (1) One of several polypeptide antibiotics produced by certain fungi that have immunosuppressive activity
      (2) Cyclosporine complexes with cyclophilin, which inhibits calcineurin (a phosphatase) and blocks production of cytokines (e.g., interleukin-2 [IL-2], interleukin-3 [IL-3], TNFα) by antigen-stimulated T-helper cells that otherwise stimulate T-cell growth and differentiation.
      (3) Cyclosporine does *not* affect suppressor T-cells or T-cell independent, antibody-mediated immunity.
      (4) Immunosuppressive actions involve inhibition of the production and/or release of various lymphokines including IL-1 and IL-2.
         • In turn, the actions of T-helper (inducer) lymphocytes, the agents of cellular immunity and tissue rejection, are impaired.
   c. Adverse effects
      (1) Nephrotoxicity is most common adverse effect, occurs in virtually all patients
         (a) Clonidine minimizes nephrotoxicity; decreases ischemic kidney

> Cyclosporine may produce nephrotoxicity in therapeutic doses; reduced by co-administration of clonidine.

(b) Additive nephrotoxicity occurs if cyclosporine is administered with other nephrotoxic agents:
- Amphotericin B
- Acyclovir
- Aminoglycosides
- Foscarnet
- Nonsteroidal anti-inflammatory drugs (NSAIDs)
- Vancomycin

(2) Hypertension
(3) Hyperglycemia
(4) Seizures
(5) Increased risk for squamous cell carcinoma of the skin

d. Used as an immunosuppressive agent:
(1) To prevent allograft rejection
(2) To treat autoimmune conditions such as:
(a) Uveitis
(b) Psoriasis
(c) Type I diabetes mellitus
(d) RA
(e) Inflammatory bowel disease
(f) Certain nephropathies

6. Tacrolimus
a. Macrolide derived from a fungus with similar pharmacokinetics to cyclosporine
b. Does *not* bind to cyclophilin, but inhibits calcineurin
c. Like cyclosporine, *but* is more effective in acute rejection than in chronic rejection and is a more potent immunosuppressant than cyclosporine
d. Overall adverse effects are greater than cyclosporine but kidney toxicity is less.
e. Oral and parenteral immunosuppressive agent approved for prophylaxis of hepatic allograft rejection *but* effective for other organ transplantations

7. Mycophenolate mofetil
a. Is a prodrug for the immunosuppressive agent mycophenolic acid (MPA)
b. MPA inhibits activity of inosine monophosphate dehydrogenase
c. MPA inhibits *de novo* purine synthesis.
d. Is used in combination with cyclosporine and corticosteroids for the prevention of rejection in patients with a renal allograft

8. Abatacept
a. A recombinant fusion protein composed of the extracellular domain of cytotoxic T-lymphocyte-associated antigen 4 (CTLA-4) fused to human IgG
b. CTLA-4 is a costimulatory molecule found on T cells that binds to CD80 and CD86 on antigen presenting cells.
c. Abatacept blocks activation of T cells by binding to CD80 or 86 so that CD28 on T cells *cannot* bind and stimulate the T cell and lead to cytokine release.
d. Abatacept is approved for patients with severe rheumatoid arthritis who have failed other disease-modifying antirheumatic drugs (DMARDS).
e. Individuals should *not* take other anti-TNFα drugs or anakinra while taking abatacept.

9. Anti-TNFα agents
a. All anti-TNFα drugs markedly increase opportunistic infections.
b. Etanercept
(1) Is a dimeric fusion protein produced by recombinant DNA technology that binds TNFα
(2) It is a soluble TNF receptor
(3) It is given by injection
(4) Is effective in the treatment of RA and works by decreasing the effects of TNFα
c. Infliximab
(1) A chimeric monoclonal antibody that binds TNFα
(2) Given by intravenous infusion and has a terminal $t_{1/2}$ of 8 to 12 days
(3) Given at week 0, 2, 6 and thereafter, every 4 to 8 weeks
(4) Often given with methotrexate for RA
(5) Use for Crohn's disease when conventional therapy fails

Cyclosporine can cause seizures at high doses.

Cyclosporine alone or with other immunosuppressive agents widely used to prevent transplant organ rejection.

Tacrolimus is *not* as nephrotoxic as cyclosporine.

Mycophenolate inhibits *de novo* purine synthesis.

Abatacept blocks T-cell activation.

Anti-TNFα agents markedly increase opportunistic infections.

Etanercept is *not* an antibody, it is a TNFα soluble circulating receptor.

d. Adalimumab
   (1) Neutralizes TNFα by binding to it and blocking its interaction with the p55 and p75 cell surface TNF receptors
   (2) Given SC every other week to patients who have had inadequate response to at least one other DMARD.
   (3) Methotrexate, glucocorticoids, salicylates, NSAIDs, or DMARDs may be continued during treatment.

   Etanercept; infliximab; adalimumab: anti-TNFα agents.

10. Antithymocyte globulin (ATG)
    a. Horse antibody against human T-lymphocytes also known as lymphocyte immune globulin
    b. Reduces number of circulating thymus-dependent lymphocytes, which alters T-cell function and ultimately affects cell-mediated immunity
    c. Manages allograft rejection in renal transplant patients and moderate to severe aplastic anemia in those unsuited for bone marrow transplants

11. Muromonab-CD3 (OKT3)
    a. Parenteral monoclonal antibody of murine origin that targets CD3/TCR receptor complex
    b. Treatment of acute allograft rejection in patients who have undergone one of the following transplantations
       (1) Kidney
       (2) Heart
       (3) Liver

    Muromonab-CD3 targets CD3/TCR receptor complex.

12. Chimeric (murine/human) monoclonal antibodies (IgG1)
    a. Daclizumab and basiliximab are chimeric (murine/human) monoclonal antibodies (IgG$_1$) produced by recombinant DNA technology.
    b. These drugs block the binding of IL-2 to its receptors.
    c. They are used prophylactically in combination with cyclosporine in patients undergoing renal transplantation.

    Daclizumab and basiliximab block IL-2 receptors.

13. Rh0[D] Immune Globulin
    a. Parenteral immune globulin used to prevent erythroblastosis fetalis in Rh0-negative women exposed to Rh-positive blood
    b. Also, indicated for idiopathic thrombocytopenic purpura (ITP)

C. **Therapeutic summary of selected immunosuppressive drugs:** (Table 22-3)

II **Antiarthritic Drugs** (Box 22-2): used to treat rheumatoid arthritis and act at various sites (Fig. 22-1).

A. **Nonsteroidal anti-inflammatory drugs (NSAIDs) and cyclooxygenase 2 (COX-2) inhibitors** (see Chapter 18)
   1. NSAIDs and COX-2 inhibitors primarily provide symptomatic relief in the initial therapy of rheumatoid arthritis, rheumatic fever, and other inflammatory joint conditions, as well as treatment of acute pain syndromes.

Table 22-3. **Therapeutic Summary of Selected Immunosuppressive Drugs**

DRUGS	CLINICAL APPLICATIONS	ADVERSE EFFECTS	CONTRAINDICATIONS
Mechanism: *Immunosuppressive glucocorticoids*			
Prednisone Methylprednisolone	Anti-inflammatory or immunosuppressant agents used in the treatment of a variety of diseases including hematologic, allergic, inflammatory, neoplastic, and autoimmune origin. Prevention and treatment of graft-versus-host disease following allogeneic bone marrow transplantation.	Iatrogenic Cushing's syndrome with long use Diabetes mellitus Hypertension Peptic ulcer disease Hypomania and psychosis Depression Adrenal insufficiency on abrupt cessation of therapy	Hypersensitivity Serious infectious
Mechanism: *Antagonizes purine metabolism and may inhibit synthesis of DNA, RNA, and proteins*			
Azathioprine	Adjunctive therapy in prevention of rejection of kidney and other organ transplants Active rheumatoid arthritis Fistulizing Crohn's disease Steroid-sparing agent for corticosteroid-dependent Crohn's disease Ulcerative colitis	Alopecia Bleeding Leukopenia Macrocytic anemia Pancytopenia Thrombocytopenia Hepatotoxicity	Hypersensitivity Pregnancy

(Continued)

Table 22-3. **Therapeutic Summary of Selected Immunosuppressive Drugs—Cont'd**

DRUGS	CLINICAL APPLICATIONS	ADVERSE EFFECTS	CONTRAINDICATIONS
Mechanism: *Alkylating agent that prevents cell division by cross-linking DNA strands*			
Cyclophosphamide	Treatment of several cancers Prophylaxis of rejection for kidney, heart, liver, and bone marrow transplants Severe rheumatoid disorders Nephrotic syndrome Wegener's granulomatosis Idiopathic pulmonary hemosideroses Myasthenia gravis Multiple sclerosis Systemic lupus erythematosus lupus nephritis Autoimmune hemolytic anemia Idiopathic thrombocytic purpura (ITP) Macroglobulinemia Antibody-induced pure red cell aplasia	Bladder cystitis Alopecia Bleeding Leukopenia Macrocytic anemia Pancytopenia Thrombocytopenia	Hypersensitivity Pregnancy
Mechanism: *Inhibition of production and release of interleukin 2 and inhibits interleukin-2-induced activation of resting T-lymphocytes*			
Cyclosporine Tacrolimus	Prophylaxis of rejection in organ transplants Severe, active rheumatoid arthritis Severe autoimmune diseases	Renal toxicity Hypertension Seizures	Hypersensitivity Renal disease Numerous drug-drug interactions
Mechanism: *A folate antimetabolite that inhibits DNA synthesis; inhibition of amino imidazolecarboxamide ribonucleotide (AICAR) transformylase and thymidylate synthetase at low doses*			
Methotrexate	Psoriasis Rheumatoid arthritis Cancers Crohn's disease	Hepatotoxicity GI toxicity Hematopoietic toxicity	Hypersensitivity Pregnancy Severe renal disease Severe liver disease

GI, gastrointestinal.

BOX 22-2   ANTIARTHRITIC DRUGS

Nonsteroidal Anti-inflammatory Drugs (NSAIDs)
Diclofenac
Diflunisal
Indomethacin
Oxaprozin
Piroxicam
Sulindac
Tolmetin

Cyclooxygenase-2 (COX-2) Inhibitor
Celecoxib

Corticosteroids
Prednisone
Methylprednisolone

Disease-Modifying Antirheumatic Drugs (DMARDs)
Antimetabolite
  Methotrexate

Immunologic Drugs
  Abatacept
  Adalimumab
  Anakinra
  Etanercept
  Infliximab
  Leflunomide
  Mycophenolate
Antimalarial Drug
  Hydroxychloroquine
Gold Salts
  Auranofin
  Gold sodium thiomalate
Chelator
  Penicillamine
Miscellaneous
  Sulfasalazine

Long-term use of all NSAIDs *except* aspirin increase cardiovascular events.

COX-2 inhibitors decrease the formation of prostaglandin PGI_2, producing adverse effects on vasculature and kidney.

2. Celecoxib, approved in 1998 for the treatment of rheumatoid arthritis and osteoarthritis, along with rofecoxib and valdecoxib, became widely used to treat inflammatory diseases.
3. After 2004, reports suggesting increased cardiovascular risk compared with placebo from long-term use of selective COX-2 inhibitors including rofecoxib, celecoxib, and valdecoxib, as well as the nonselective NSAID naproxen, have resulted in the removal of rofecoxib and valdecoxib from the market and much stronger warnings on the long-term use of all NSAIDs *except* aspirin.

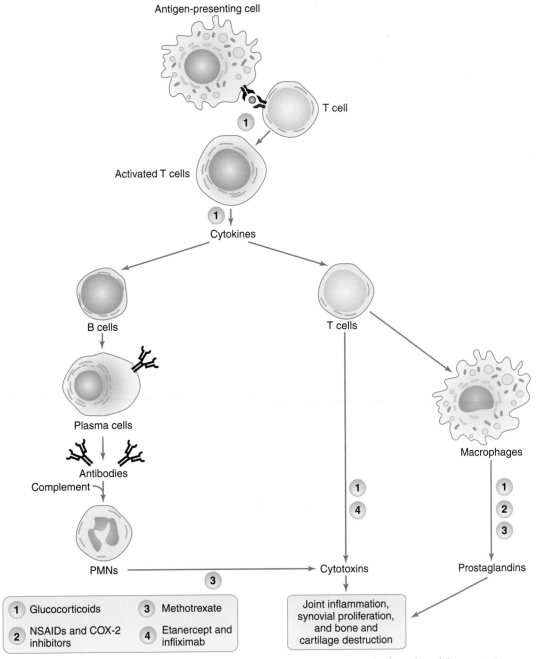

22-1: Pathogenesis of rheumatoid arthritis and sites of action of drugs. Etanercept and infliximab work by inactivating tumor necrosis factor. COX-2, cyclooxygenase-2; NSAID, nonsteroidal anti-inflammatory drug; PMNs, polymorphonuclear neutrophils.

B. Corticosteroids (see Chapter 23)
1. Examples
   a. Prednisone
   b. Methylprednisolone
2. Some corticosteroids are used short term in treating acute rheumatoid arthritis
3. Steroids result in dramatic improvement but do *not* arrest the disease process

C. Disease-modifying antirheumatic drugs (DMARDs)
1. Examples
   a. Methotrexate
   b. Immunosuppressive drugs
   c. Antimalarial drugs
   d. Gold salts
   e. Penicillamine

f. Infliximab
g. Anakinra
h. Abatacept
i. Mycophenolate
j. Leflunomide
2. General characteristics
   a. Suppress proliferation and activity of lymphocytes and polymorphonuclear neutrophils (PMNs)
   b. Counteract joint inflammation and destruction
   c. Slow progression of joint erosion in rheumatoid arthritis and systemic lupus erythematosus (SLE)
3. Methotrexate
   a. Mechanism of action
      • Inhibition of human folate reductase, lymphocyte proliferation, and production of cytokines and rheumatoid factor
   b. Widely used in rheumatoid arthritis usually in combination with other drugs
4. Immunosuppressive drugs
   a. Mechanism of action
      (1) Leflunomide suppresses mononuclear and T-cell proliferation.
         • Its active metabolite inhibits dihydroorotate dehydrogenase (DHODH), an important enzyme in *de novo* pyrimidine synthesis.
      (2) Etanercept, infliximab, and adalimumab inhibit TNFα
      (3) Anakinra targets interleukin-1 receptor (IL-1Ra).
      (4) Mycophenolate is converted to mycophenolic acid, which inhibits lymphocyte purine synthesis.
         • It is used to treat rheumatoid arthritis, *but* even more widely used to prevent allograft rejection.
5. Antimalarial drugs (see Chapter 28)
   a. Examples
      (1) Chloroquine
      (2) Hydroxychloroquine
   b. Mechanism of action (unclear)
      • May inhibit lymphocyte function and chemotaxis of PMNs
   c. Use (other than malaria prophylaxis and treatment)
      • Adjunct to NSAIDs in the treatment of rheumatoid arthritis, juvenile chronic arthritis, Sjögren's syndrome, and SLE
   d. Adverse effects
      (1) Retinal degeneration
      (2) Dermatitis
6. Gold compounds
   a. Examples
      (1) Aurothioglucose
      (2) Gold sodium thiomalate
   b. Mechanism of action
      • Alter morphology and function of macrophages, which may be a major mode of action
   c. Use
      • Early stages of adult and juvenile RA
   d. Adverse effects
      (1) Cutaneous reactions such as erythema and exfoliative dermatitis
      (2) Blood dyscrasias
      (3) Renal toxicity
7. Penicillamine
      • Oral chelating agent
   a. Mechanism of action
      (1) Chelates heavy metals
      (2) Penicillamine should *not* be used in combination with gold compounds to treat RA.
   b. Uses
      (1) Wilson's disease
      (2) Cystinuria
      (3) Resistant cases of rheumatoid arthritis

The beneficial effects from many DMARDs don't occur until after weeks or months of therapy.

Methotrexate is widely used to treat rheumatoid arthritis in combination with other DMARDs

Leflunomide inhibits pyrimidine synthesis.

Mycophenolate inhibits purine synthesis.

As better agents are becoming available, gold and antimalarials are used considerably less today.

Don't use penicillamine with gold salts.

        c. Adverse effects
            (1) Aplastic anemia
            (2) Renal disease (membranous glomerulonephritis)
        8. Sulfasalazine (see Chapter 21) is used to treat:
            a. RA
            b. Ankylosing spondylitis
            c. Ulcerative colitis
    D. Therapeutic summary of selected antiarthritic drugs: (Table 22-4)
III. Drugs Used in the Treatment of Gout (Box 22-3)
    A. Types of gout
        • Gout is a disorder of uric acid metabolism that results in deposition of monosodium urate in joints and cartilage (Fig. 22-2).
            1. Primary gout is caused by overproduction (increased purine metabolism) or underexcretion (e.g., diabetes, starvation states of uric acid.
            2. Secondary gout is caused by accumulation of uric acid due to one of the following factors:
                a. Disease, such as leukemia
                b. Drugs that interfere with uric acid disposition, such as diuretics (e.g., thiazides, furosemide, ethacrynic acid)
    B. Treatment of acute attacks
        1. Colchicine
            a. Mechanism of action
                • Binds to microtubule and inhibits leukocyte migration and phagocytosis, thereby blocking the ability to inflame the joint
            b. Colchicine is *not* an analgesic.
            c. Use
                • Reduction of pain and inflammation of acute attacks of gouty arthritis

Acidic drugs compete with uric acid active transport in the proximal tubules.

Table 22-4. Therapeutic Summary of Selected Antiarthritis Drugs

DRUGS	CLINICAL APPLICATIONS	ADVERSE EFFECTS	CONTRAINDICATIONS
Mechanism: *Reversible cyclooxygenase (COX) inhibitor; anti-inflammatory, analgesic; antipyretic*			
Diclofenac Diflunisal Indomethacin Oxaprozin Piroxicam Sulindac Tolmetin	Fever, acute rheumatic fever, headache, mild pain, dysmenorrhea Inflammatory conditions such as osteoarthritis and rheumatoid arthritis (RA) Closure of patent ductus arteriosus (indomethacin)	GI effects Bleeding Tinnitus Fluid retention Hypocalcemia	Hypersensitivity Pregnancy (especially third trimester)
Mechanism: *Selective COX-2 inhibitor: anti-inflammatory, analgesic; antipyretic*			
Celecoxib	Rheumatic arthritis Osteoarthritis Acute pain Dysmenorrhea	Hypertension Diarrhea GI distress	Hypersensitivity Sulfonamide allergies Pregnancy (especially third trimester)
Mechanism: *Anti-tumor necrosis factor-α (TNF$_\alpha$); proinflammatory cytokine*			
Adalimumab Etanercept Infliximab	Treatment of moderately- to severely-active rheumatoid arthritis Treatment of Crohn's disease Treatment of and maintenance of healing of ulcerative colitis	Headache GI distress Increased risk of infection	Hypersensitivity Congestive heart failure (NYHA Class III/IV)
Mechanism: *Selective costimulation modulator; inhibits T-cell function*			
Abatacept	Treatment of moderately- to severely-active adult rheumatoid arthritis Treatment of moderately- to severely-active juvenile idiopathic arthritis	Headache Upper respiratory tract infection Hypertension	Hypersensitivity Serious infections
Mechanism: *Antagonist of the interleukin-1 (IL-1) receptor*			
Anakinra	Treatment of moderately- to severely-active rheumatoid arthritis	Headache Infections Flu-like syndrome	Hypersensitivity Serious infections
Mechanism: *Inhibits pyrimidine synthesis*			
Leflunomide	Treatment of active rheumatoid arthritis	Headache Upper respiratory tract infection Hypertension	Hypersensitivity Pregnancy

COX, cyclooxygenase; GI, gastrointestinal; NYHA, New York Heart Association.

BOX 22-3	DRUGS USED IN THE TREATMENT OF GOUT

Acute Therapy
Colchicine
Indomethacin and other nonsteroidal anti-inflammatory drugs (NSAIDs)

Prevention
Allopurinol
Probenecid
Rasburicase

22-2: Sites of action of drugs that affect uric acid metabolism and excretion.

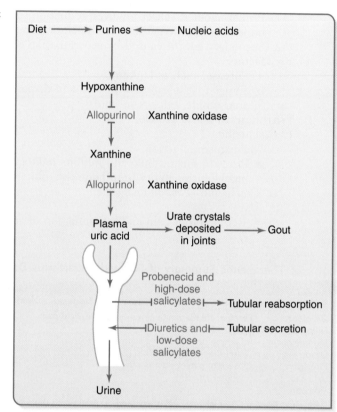

d. Adverse effects
(1) Diarrhea
(2) Nausea and vomiting

Don't use aspirin to treat gout.

2. Indomethacin and other NSAIDs (see Chapter 18)
a. All these drugs are effective in the relief of pain and inflammation due to acute gouty arthritis (see Chapter 18).
b. Additional uses for indomethacin
(1) Ankylosing spondylitis and osteoarthritis of the hip
(2) Closure of patent ductus arteriosus

C. **Prevention of acute attacks**
• The goal is to prevent gouty attacks by decreasing the serum concentration of uric acid (see Fig. 22-2).
1. Uricosuric drugs
a. Drugs that block active reabsorption of uric acid in the proximal tubule, increasing urinary excretion of uric acid
b. Probenecid
• Only oral uricosuric agent used today
(1) Mechanism of action
• Uricosuric; also inhibits the renal excretion of penicillins and other weak organic acids

(2) Uses

    (a) Hyperuricemia associated with chronic gout or drug-induced hyperuricemia

    (b) Chronic gouty arthritis with frequent attacks (in combination with colchicine)

    (c) Probenecid is *not* effective in the treatment of acute attacks of gout.

2. Allopurinol

    a. Mechanism of action

      • Inhibits xanthine oxidase and thus inhibits synthesis of uric acid

    b. Use

      • Prevention of primary and secondary gout

    c. Adverse effects

      (1) Maculopapular rash

      (2) Toxic epidermal necrolysis

      (3) Vasculitis

3. Rasburicase

    • Recombinant form of nonhuman urate oxidase

    a. Mechanism of action

      • Converting uric acid to allantoin, which is effectively excreted by the kidneys

    b. Uses

      • Patients with hematologic malignancies (children) or solid tumors who are at particular risk for tumor lysis syndrome (TLS)

    c. Adverse reactions

      • Severe hypersensitivity reactions including anaphylactic shock and anaphylactoid reactions

D. Therapeutic summary of selected drugs used to treat gout: (Table 22-5)

> Probenecid can aggravate inflammation from gout if administered during the initial stages of an acute attack.
>
> Allopurinol potentiates the effects of 6-mercaptopurine and azathioprine.
>
> Allopurinol should *not* be used in acute attacks of gout; it exacerbates symptoms.
>
> Probenecid and allopurinol may provoke acute gout symptoms at the beginning of therapy, concomitant colchicine can prevent it
>
> Rasburicase is a recombinant urate oxidase used to metabolize uric acid.

Table 22-5. **Therapeutic Summary of Selected Drugs used to Treat Gout**

DRUGS	CLINICAL APPLICATIONS	ADVERSE EFFECTS	CONTRAINDICATIONS
Mechanism: *Decreases leukocyte motility, decreases phagocytosis in joints and lactic acid production, reducing the deposition of urate crystals that trigger the inflammatory response*			
Colchicine	Treatment of acute gouty arthritis attacks Prevention of recurrences of acute gouty arthritis attacks	GI distress Alopecia	Hypersensitivity Pregnancy Cardiac disorders Liver disease Renal disease Blood dyscrasias GI disorders
Mechanism: *Reversible cyclooxygenase (COX) inhibitor; anti-inflammatory, analgesic; antipyretic*			
Indomethacin Naproxen **Other NSAIDs but not aspirin**	Fever, acute rheumatic fever, headache, mild pain, dysmenorrhea Inflammatory conditions such as osteoarthritis and rheumatoid arthritis (RA) Closure of patent ductus arteriosus (indomethacin)	GI effects Bleeding Tinnitus Fluid retention Hypocalcemia	Hypersensitivity Pregnancy (especially third trimester)
Mechanism: *Uricosuric agent*			
Probenecid	Prevention of hyperuricemia associated with gout or gouty arthritis Prolongation and elevation of β-lactam plasma levels	Flushing GI distress Hepatic necrosis Alopecia Anemia	Hypersensitivity Children <2 years of age High-dose aspirin therapy Blood dyscrasias
Mechanism: *Recombinant urate-oxidase enzyme*			
Rasburicase	Management of uric acid levels in pediatric patients with leukemia, lymphoma, and solid tumor malignancies receiving anticancer therapy	Fever GI distress Neutropenia	Hypersensitivity Glucose-6-phosphatase dehydrogenase (G6PD) deficiency

GI, gastrointestinal; NSAIDs, nonsteroidal anti-inflammatory drugs.

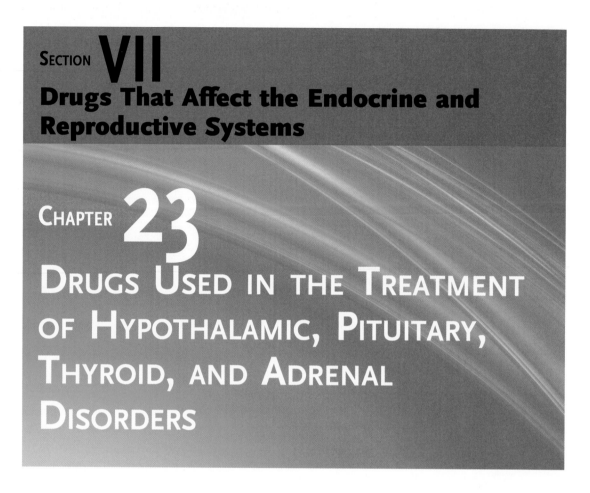

Drugs That Affect the Endocrine and Reproductive Systems

CHAPTER **23**

DRUGS USED IN THE TREATMENT OF HYPOTHALAMIC, PITUITARY, THYROID, AND ADRENAL DISORDERS

I. General Considerations

A. Overview

1. A hormone is a substance secreted by one tissue or gland that is transported via the circulation to a site where it exerts its effects on different tissues.
2. See Endocrine Physiology section of Rapid Review Physiology for a review of hormone signaling pathways and physiological mechanisms.

B. Uses for hormones and synthetic analogues

1. Diagnostic tools in endocrine disorders
2. Replacement therapy in endocrine disorders
3. Treatment of non-endocrine disorders

C. Review hypothalamic/pituitary/target organ interactions: (Table 23-1 and Fig. 23-1)

II. Hypothalamic Hormones and Related Drugs (Box 23-1)

A. Sermorelin (growth hormone-releasing hormone)

1. Mechanism of action
   • Causes rapid elevation of growth hormone in the blood
2. Uses
   a. Assessment of responsiveness
   b. Treatment of growth hormone deficiency

B. Somatostatin (growth hormone-inhibiting hormone)

1. Octreotide
   • Synthetic analogue used as a drug
2. Mechanism of action
   a. Inhibits release of pituitary hormones
   b. Inhibits the release of gastrointestinal hormones
3. Uses
   a. Symptomatic treatment of hormone-secreting tumors
      (1) Pituitary tumors
      (2) Carcinoid tumors
      (3) Insulinomas
      (4) Vasoactive intestinal peptide tumors (VIPomas)

Hormone is a substance secreted by one tissue but has actions at remote tissues.

Understand the negative feedback principle of the hypothalamic/pituitary/ target organ axis.

The ending -relin indicates a hypothalamus-related hormone.

TABLE 23-1. **Relationships Among Hypothalamic, Pituitary, and Target Gland Hormones**

HYPOTHALAMIC	PITUITARY	TARGET ORGAN	TARGET ORGAN HORMONES
GHRH (+), SRIH (–), CRH (+)	GH (+)	Liver	Somatomedins
	ACTH (+)	Adrenal cortex	Glucocorticoids Mineralocorticoids Androgens
TRH (+)	TSH (+)	Thyroid	T_4, T_3
GnRH or LHRH (+)	FSH (+) LH (+)	Gonads	Estrogen Progesterone Testosterone
Dopamine (–), PRH (+)	Prolactin (+)	Breast	—

+, stimulant; –, inhibitor; ACTH, adrenocorticotropic hormone; CRH, corticotropin-releasing hormone; FSH, follicle-stimulating hormone; GH, growth hormone; GHRH, growth hormone–releasing hormone; GnRH, gonadotropin-releasing hormone; LHRH, luteinizing hormone-releasing hormone; LH, luteinizing hormone; PRH, prolactin-releasing hormone; SRIH, somatotropin-releasing inhibiting hormone; TRH, thyrotropin-releasing hormone; TSH, thyroid-stimulating hormone.

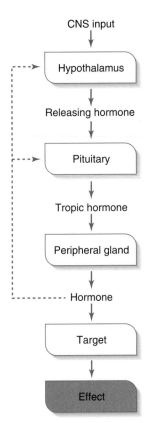

23-1: Regulation of hormone synthesis and secretion. A negative feedback mechanism is an example of a negative effect. CNS, central nervous system.

BOX 23-1   HYPOTHALAMIC HORMONES AND RELATED DRUGS

Corticorelin (CRH)
Gonadorelin (GnRH)
Goserelin
Histrelin
Leuprolide
Nafarelin
Octreotide

Protirelin (TRH)
Sermorelin
Somatostatin
Triptorelin
GnRH antagonists
Ganirelix
Cetrorelix

Octreotide used to treat various peptide secreting tumors; pituitary tumors, carcinoid tumors, insulinomas, vasoactive intestinal peptide tumors (VIPomas), ZE, glucagonoma

          (5) Glucagonoma
          (6) Zollinger-Ellison (ZE) syndrome
    b. Esophageal varices
      • Octreotide reduces portal vein blood flow
  4. Adverse effects
    a. Abdominal pain
    b. Diarrhea
    c. Nausea and vomiting

C. Protirelin (thyrotropin-releasing hormone; TRH)
  1. Mechanism of action
    • Stimulates synthesis and release of thyrotropin and prolactin from the anterior pituitary
  2. Uses
    a. Assessment of thyroid function in patients with pituitary or hypothalamic dysfunction

TRH levels are useful in diagnosing thyroid and prolactin disorders.

    b. Detection of defective control of prolactin secretion

D. Corticotropin-releasing hormone (CRH; corticorelin)
  1. Mechanism of action
    • Stimulates release of corticotropin and β-endorphin from the anterior pituitary
  2. Uses
    a. Diagnostic test in distinguishing causes of Cushing's syndrome (pituitary, ectopic, adrenal)
      (1) Further increase in plasma adrenocorticotropic hormone (ACTH) in pituitary Cushing's
      (2) *No* effect in ectopic Cushing's (tumor production of ACTH)
      (3) ACTH is suppressed due to increase cortisol production in adrenal Cushing's.

CRH levels are useful in diagnosing adrenocorticoid disorders.

    b. Differentiate hypothalamic from pituitary dysfunction as a cause of hypocortisolism
      • Delayed increase in plasma ACTH with hypothalamic dysfunction but *no* increase with hypopituitarism

E. Gonadotropin-releasing hormone (GnRH)-related preparations
  1. Examples
    a. Gonadorelin
    b. Goserelin
    c. Histrelin
    d. Leuprolide
    e. Nafarelin
    f. Triptorelin
  2. Mechanism of action
    a. Stimulate secretion of follicle-stimulating hormone (FSH) and luteinizing hormone (LH)
      • Pulsatile intravenous administration every 1 to 4 hours
    b. Inhibit gonadotropin release
      • Continuous administration of longer-lasting synthetic analogues
  3. Uses

Pulsatile administration of GnRH increases but continuous administration inhibits gonadotropin release from pituitary.

    a. Shorter-acting preparations (gonadorelin)
      (1) Treatment of delayed puberty
      (2) Induction of ovulation in women with hypothalamic amenorrhea
      (3) Stimulation of spermatogenesis in men with hypogonadotropic hypogonadism (infertility)
    b. Longer-acting GnRH analogues
      (1) Examples
        (a) Goserelin
        (b) Histrelin
        (c) Leuprolide
        (d) Nafarelin
        (e) Triptorelin

GnRH analogues used to treat both prostate and breast cancer.

GnRH analogues produce a transient initial increase of testosterone levels, prevented by concomitant flutamide

      (2) Suppression of FSH and LH in polycystic ovary syndrome
      (3) Endometriosis
      (4) Precocious puberty
      (5) Prostate cancer
      (6) Leuprolide for anemia caused by uterine leiomyomata (fibroids)
      (7) Breast cancer, premenopausal ovarian ablation (unlabeled use of leuprolide)

c. Stimulation test to distinguish hypothalamic from pituitary dysfunction in patients with decreased FSH and LH
   (1) *No* increase in serum FSH and LH in pituitary dysfunction (e.g., hypopituitarism)
   (2) Delayed increase in serum FSH and LH in hypothalamic dysfunction (e.g., Kallmann's syndrome)
4. Adverse effects
   a. Menopausal symptoms
   b. Amenorrhea
   c. Testicular atrophy
5. GnRH antagonist
   a. Examples
      (1) Ganirelix
      (2) Cetrorelix
   b. Uses
      (1) To prevent premature surges of LH during controlled ovarian hyperstimulation
      (2) May be effective in endometriosis, uterine fibrinoids in women, and prostate cancer in men.

> GnRH antagonists are now available to prevent ovulation until the follicles are of adequate size.

F. **Therapeutic summary of selected hypothalamic hormone related drugs** (Table 23-2)

III. **Anterior Pituitary Hormones and Related Drugs** (Box 23-2)
   A. **Growth hormone-related preparations**
      1. Physiology (Fig. 23-2)
         a. Human growth hormone (GH)
            (1) Stimulates normal growth in children and adolescents
            (2) Controls metabolism in adults
            (3) Stimulates uptake of amino acids in muscle

> Drugs that end in -tropin are related to the pituitary hormones.

TABLE 23-2. **Therapeutic Summary of Selected Hypothalamic Hormone Related Drugs**

DRUGS	CLINICAL APPLICATIONS	ADVERSE EFFECTS	CONTRAINDICATIONS
Mechanism: *Somatostatin analogue that inhibits the secretion of gastrin, VIP, insulin, glucagon, secretin, motilin, and pancreatic polypeptide; decreases growth hormone and IGF-1 in acromegaly*			
Octreotide	Treatment of acromegaly Symptomatic treatment of hormone-secreting tumors 　Pituitary tumors 　Carcinoid tumors 　Insulinomas 　Vasoactive intestinal peptide tumors (VIPomas) 　Treatment of esophageal varices	Bradycardia Pruritus Hyperglycemia GI distress Headache	Hypersensitivity
Mechanism: *Stimulates synthesis and release of thyrotropin and prolactin from the anterior pituitary*			
Protirelin	Adjunct in the diagnostic assessment of thyroid function Used to detect defective control of prolactin secretion	Headache Flushing Dry mouth Urge to urinate	Hypersensitivity
Mechanism: *Stimulates adrenocorticotropic hormone (ACTH) release from anterior pituitary*			
Corticorelin	Diagnostic test in ACTH-dependent Cushing's syndrome; differentiates between pituitary and ectopic production of ACTH	Flushing Metallic taste Dyspnea	Hypersensitivity
Mechanism: *Stimulate secretion of follicle-stimulating hormone (FSH) and luteinizing hormone (LH); Inhibit gonadotropin release with continuous administration of longer-lasting synthetic analogues*			
Gonadorelin Goserelin Histrelin Leuprolide Nafarelin Triptorelin	**Shorter-acting preparations** (gonadorelin) Treatment of delayed puberty Induction of ovulation in women with hypothalamic amenorrhea Stimulation of spermatogenesis in men with hypogonadotropic hypogonadism (infertility) **Longer-acting GnRH analogues** (leuprolide, nafarelin, goserelin, histrelin, triptorelin) Suppression of FSH and LH in polycystic ovary syndrome Endometriosis Precocious puberty Advanced prostate cancer Leuprolide for anemia caused by uterine leiomyomata (fibroids) Breast cancer, premenopausal ovarian ablation (unlabeled use of leuprolide)	Edema Vaginal bleeding Headache Hot flashes GI distress Vaginitis Testicular atrophy	Hypersensitivity Abnormal vaginal bleeding Pregnancy Breast-feeding
Mechanism: *GnRH antagonists that suppress gonadotropin secretion and luteinizing hormone (LH) secretion, preventing ovulation until the follicles are of adequate size*			
Ganirelix Cetrorelix	Used to inhibit premature LH surges in women undergoing controlled ovarian hyperstimulation	Headache Ovarian hyperstimulation syndrome Pelvic pain	Hypersensitivity Pregnancy

GI, gastrointestinal; GnRH, gonadotropin releasing hormone; IGF-1, insulin-like growth factor 1; VIP, vasoactive intestinal peptide.

BOX 23-2 ANTERIOR PITUITARY HORMONES AND RELATED DRUGS

Corticotropin (ACTH)
Cosyntropin (ACTH)
Chorionic gonadotropin (human); (LH)
Chorionic gonadotropin (recombinant); (LH)
Follitropin alfa (FSH)
Follitropin beta (FSH)
Lutropin alfa (LH)

Mecasermin
Menotropins (FSH & LH)
Pegvisomant
Prolactin
Somatropin (recombinant human growth hormone)
Thyrotropin (TSH)
Urofollitropin (FSH)

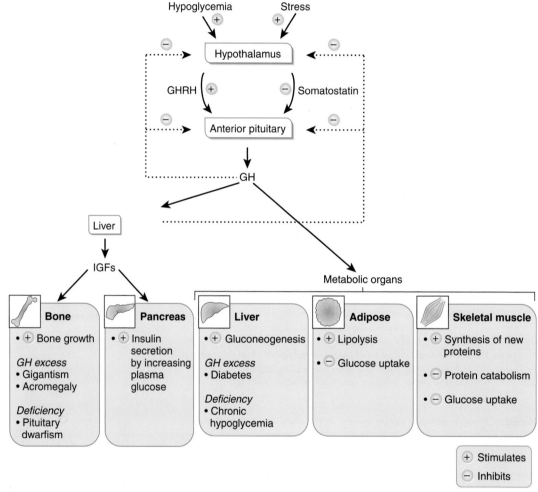

23-2: Physiologic actions of growth hormone. GH, growth hormone; GHRH, growth hormone-releasing hormone; IGF, insulin-like growth factor. *(From Brown TA: Rapid Review Physiology. Philadelphia, Mosby, 2007, Figure 3-17.)*

    (4) Stimulates erythropoietin (increases red blood cell mass)
    (5) Has insulin-like and diabetogenic effects (stimulates gluconeogenesis)
    (6) Enhances transmucosal transport of water, electrolytes, and nutrients across
        the gut
    (7) Stimulates the liver to secrete insulin-like growth factor-1 (IGF-1); anabolic
        actions include:
        • Stimulates growth of bone (linear, lateral), cartilage, soft tissue, and organs
  2. Pathology
    a. Disorders of excess of GH
      (1) Gigantism (*before* puberty)

(2) Acromegaly (*after* fusion of epiphyseal plates of the long bones)
  b. Disorders of deficiency of GH
    • Dwarfism
3. Pharmacology
  a. Somatropin
    • Recombinant human growth hormone (rhGH)
      (1) Mechanism of action
        (a) Increase production of somatomedins, such as IGF-1, in the liver and other tissues
        (b) Oppose the actions of insulin
      (2) Uses in children with growth failure:
        (a) Inadequate endogenous growth hormone secretion
        (b) Born small for gestational age and who fail to manifest catch-up growth by 2 years of age
      (3) Uses in children with short stature; examples include:
        (a) Turner syndrome
        (b) Noonan syndrome
        (c) Idiopathic (non-growth hormone-deficient)
        (d) Homeobox gene (SHOX) deficiency
      (4) Used in children with Prader-Willi syndrome
      (5) Uses in adults:
        (a) HIV patients with wasting or cachexia with concomitant antiviral therapy
        (b) Endogenous growth hormone deficiency who meet appropriate criteria
        (c) Short-bowel syndrome
          • Malabsorption due to surgical removal of small bowel
      (6) Adverse effects
        (a) Arthralgia
        (b) Edema
        (c) Impaired glucose tolerance may develop over long periods.
        (d) Adverse effects are less in children than adults.
          • *Only* use synthetic GH (Creutzfeldt-Jakob disease resulted from the use of cadaveric GH).
  b. Mecasermin
    (1) Mechanism of action
      • IGF-1 produced by using recombinant DNA technology
    (2) Uses
      (a) Growth failure in children with severe primary IGF-1 deficiency
      (b) Treatment of patients with GH gene deletions who have developed neutralizing antibodies to GH
    (3) Adverse effects
      (a) Cardiac murmur
      (b) Hyper/hypoglycemia
      (c) Iron-deficiency anemia
  c. Pegvisomant
    (1) Mechanism of action
      (a) A protein of recombinant DNA origin covalently bound to polyethylene glycol (PEG) polymers
      (b) GH analogue that selectively binds GH receptors
        • Blocks the binding of endogenous GH
        • Leads to decreased serum concentrations of IGF-1 and other GH-responsive proteins
    (2) Use
      • Acromegaly (patients resistant to or unable to tolerate other therapies)
    (3) Adverse effects
      (a) Pain
      (b) Abnormal liver function tests
B. Thyrotropin (thyroid-stimulating hormone; TSH)
  1. Mechanism of action
    a. Stimulates growth of thyroid gland
    b. Stimulates the synthesis and release of thyroid hormones

Don't administer growth hormone products to children after epiphyseal plate closure.

Excess growth hormone production results in gigantism and acromegaly; deficiency results in dwarfism.

Growth hormone increases production of IGF-1.

Growth hormone has been misused by athletes.

Mecasermin is a recombinant IGF-1 product that promotes growth.

Pegvisomant is a GH antagonist useful in the treatment of acromegaly.

2. Use
   a. Diagnosis of hypothyroidism
      (1) Increased in primary hypothyroidism
      (2) Decreased in secondary hypothyroidism
   b. Diagnosis of thyrotoxicosis (decreased)

C. **Adrenocorticotropin (ACTH; corticotropin)-related preparations**
   1. Examples
      a. Corticotropin
      b. Cosyntropin
   2. Regulation of secretion
      a. ACTH levels undergo daily cyclic changes (circadian rhythms).
      b. Peak plasma levels (6:00 AM); lowest levels occur about midnight (see Fig. 23-7)
      c. Stress increases the release of ACTH.
   3. Mechanism of action
      a. Stimulate growth of the adrenal gland
      b. Stimulate the production and release adrenocorticoids from adrenal glands
         (1) Glucocorticoids
            • 11-Deoxycortisol and cortisol
         (2) Mineralocorticoids
            • All mineralocorticoids except aldosterone, which requires angiotensin II conversion of corticosterone to aldosterone
         (3) Androgens
            (a) 17-Ketosteroids dehydroepiandrosterone and androstenedione
            (b) Testosterone and dihydrotestosterone (peripheral conversion by 5-α-reductase)
   4. Used to differentiate between adrenocortical insufficiencies
      a. Primary (adrenal malfunction)
         • ACTH is increased
      b. Secondary (pituitary malfunction)
         • ACTH is decreased
   5. Adverse effects (corticotropin or glucocorticoids) known as Cushing's syndrome
      a. General
         (1) Weight gain
         (2) Cushing's appearance ("moon face")
         (3) Sodium retention
         (4) Edema
      b. Musculoskeletal
         (1) Osteoporosis
         (2) Myopathy
         (3) Growth retardation (children)
      c. Ophthalmic
         (1) Cataracts
         (2) Glaucoma
      d. Miscellaneous
         (1) Diabetes mellitus
         (2) Peptic ulcer disease
         (3) Psychosis
         (4) Decreased resistance to infection

D. **Follicle-stimulating hormone (FSH)**
   1. Examples
      a. Urofollitropin
      b. Follitropin alfa
      c. Follitropin beta
   2. Sources
      a. Urofollitropin is a preparation of
         • Highly purified FSH extracted from the urine of postmenopausal women
      b. Follitropin alfa and follitropin beta
         • Recombinant preparations of FSH
   3. Mechanism of action
      a. Stimulates ovarian follicle growth (females)
         • Also stimulates granulosa cell synthesis of aromatase for conversion of testosterone synthesized in the theca interna to estradiol.
      b. Stimulates spermatogenesis (males)

TSH kevels are the best indicator of thyroid status.

ACTH and glucocorticoid levels undergo daily circadian changes.

Stress markedly affects multiple hormonal systems.

ACTH and glucocorticoids cause iatrogenic Cushing's syndrome.

Patients with Cushing's syndrome can be recognized by their appearance: "moon facies" and "buffalo hump."

4. Uses
   a. Infertility
   b. Polycystic ovarian syndrome
5. Adverse effects
   a. Multiple births
   b. Ovarian enlargement

E. **Luteinizing hormone (LH)**
   1. Examples and sources
      a. Menotropins
         • Extracted from urine of postmenopausal women (both FSH and LH activity)
      b. Chorionic gonadotropin (human)
         • LH obtained from the urine of pregnant women
      c. Chorionic gonadotropin (recombinant)
         • LH analogue produced by recombinant DNA techniques
      d. Lutropin alfa
         • LH prepared using Chinese hamster cell ovaries
   2. Mechanism of action
      a. Increases follicular estradiol secretion
      b. Required for FSH induced follicular development
   3. Uses
      a. Menotropins
         (1) In conjunction with chorionic gonadotropins (human) to induce ovulation and pregnancy in infertile women
         (2) Stimulation of multiple follicle development in ovulatory patients as part of an assisted reproductive technology (ART)
         (3) Stimulation of spermatogenesis in primary or secondary hypogonadotropic hypogonadism in males
      b. Lutropin
         (1) Stimulation of follicular development in infertile hypogonadotropic hypogonadal women with profound LH deficiency
         (2) Given in combination with follitropin alfa
      c. Chorionic gonadotropin (recombinant)
         (1) As part of an ART program, induces ovulation in infertile females who have been pretreated with FSH
         (2) To induces ovulation and pregnancy in infertile females when the cause of infertility is functional

F. **Prolactin and related preparations**
   1. Prolactin
      a. Regulation of secretion (Fig. 23-3)
         (1) Stimulus of release
            (a) Stress
            (b) Suckling
            (c) Dopamine antagonists (phenothiazines; haloperidol)
            (d) TRH
         (2) Inhibitors of release
            (a) Dopamine tonically inhibits the release of prolactin in the central nervous system (CNS) (see Table 23-1)
            (b) Dopamine agonists (bromocriptine, cabergoline)
      b. Mechanism of action
         • Stimulates milk production
      c. Use
         • *Not* available for clinical use
   2. Inhibitors of prolactin release
      a. Examples
         (1) Bromocriptine
         (2) Cabergoline
      b. Uses
         (1) Prevention of breast tenderness and engorgement in women who are *not* breastfeeding
         (2) Inhibition of lactation
         (3) Treatment of amenorrhea and galactorrhea associated with hyperprolactinemia due to pituitary adenomas

Multiple preparations with FSH, LH, or both activities are available to use in programs designed to increase fertility.

Preparations containing FSH and LH activity are used in various fertility paradigms.

Prolactin stimulates milk production; Oxytocin stimulates milk letdown

Bromocriptine or cabergoline used to decrease prolactin release

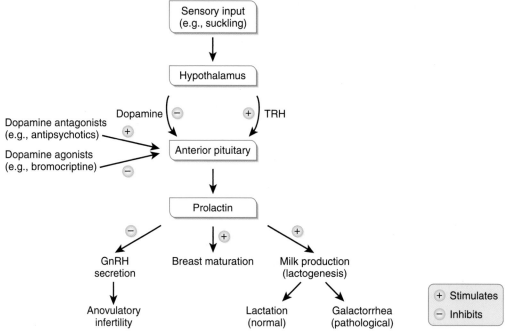

23-3: Physiologic actions of prolactin. TRH, thyrotropin-releasing hormone. *(From Brown TA: Rapid Review Physiology. Philadelphia, Mosby, 2007, Figure 3-16.)*

G. **Therapeutic summary of selected anterior pituitary hormone related drugs**
(Table 23-3)

IV. **Posterior Pituitary Hormones and Related Drugs**

- These hormones are produced in the hypothalamus and are transported to the posterior pituitary (neurohypophysis), where they are stored and released into the circulation (Box 23-3).

> Posterior pituitary hormones are synthesized in the hypothalamus

A. **Vasopressin (antidiuretic hormone [ADH])**
1. General considerations
   a. Desmopressin is the synthetic analogue
   b. Disorders from an absence of ADH
      - Diabetes insipidus (increased thirst, polyuria, hypernatremia)
   c. Disorders from an excess of ADH; syndrome of inappropriate antidiuretic hormone (SIADH)
      (1) Water retention producing severe dilutional hyponatremia
      (2) Most commonly due to small cell carcinoma of lung ectopically secreting ADH
      (3) Other causes:
         (a) Drugs that enhance ADH effect
            - Chlorpropamide, cyclophosphamide, phenothiazines, narcotics
         (b) CNS injury, lung infections (e.g., tuberculosis)
2. Regulation of secretion
   a. Increases in plasma osmolality (e.g., dehydration) result in increased secretion of ADH.
   b. Decreases in blood pressure (e.g., due to hemorrhage) increase ADH secretion.
3. Mechanism of action
   a. Activation of V_2 vasopressin receptor
      (1) This effect is mediated by an increase in cyclic adenosine monophosphate (cAMP).
      (2) Modulates renal tubular reabsorption of water, increasing permeability of the distal tubule and collecting ducts to water by insertion of water channels (aquaporin 2)

> V_2 is cAMP pathway

   b. Activation of V_1 vasopressin receptor
      (1) This effect occurs via the stimulation of the polyphosphoinositide pathway.
      (2) Causes vasoconstriction at high concentrations
         - Helps maintain blood pressure during hemorrhage

> V_1 is polyphosphoinositide pathway

4. Uses (desmopressin)
   a. By injection

TABLE 23-3. **Therapeutic Summary of Selected Anterior Pituitary Hormone Related Drugs**

DRUGS	CLINICAL APPLICATIONS	ADVERSE EFFECTS	CONTRAINDICATIONS
Mechanism: *Increase production of somatomedins, such as insulin-like growth factor 1 (IGF-1), in the liver and other tissues*			
Somatropin	**Children:** Growth failure or Short stature with: Turner syndrome Prader-Willi syndrome Chronic renal insufficiency Idiopathic short stature Homeobox gene (SHOX) deficiency Noonan syndrome **Adults:** HIV patients with wasting or cachexia with concomitant antiviral therapy Endogenous growth hormone deficiency who meet appropriate criteria Short-bowel syndrome	Arthralgia Edema Impaired glucose tolerance may develop over long periods	Hypersensitivity Patients with closed epiphyses Acute critical illness
Mechanism: *Recombinant protein; insulin-like growth factor (IGF-1) activity*			
Mecasermin	Treatment of growth failure in children with severe primary IGF-1 deficiency Treatment of patients with growth hormone (GH) gene deletions who have developed neutralizing antibodies to GH	Cardiac murmur Hyper/hypoglycemia Iron-deficiency anemia	Hypersensitivity Patients with closed epiphyses Neoplasia
Mechanism: *Growth hormone antagonist*			
Pegvisomant	Treatment of acromegaly	GI distress Abnormal liver function tests Hypertension	Hypersensitivity
Mechanism: *Stimulates growth of the adrenal gland; stimulates the production and release of glucocorticoids, mineralocorticoids, and androgens from the adrenal cortex*			
Corticotropin Cosyntropin	Diagnostic test to differentiate primary adrenal from secondary (pituitary) adrenocortical insufficiency	Cushing's syndrome	Hypersensitivity
Mechanism: *Products with follicle-stimulating hormone(FSH) or luteinizing hormone (LH) activity*			
Chorionic gonadotropin (human) Chorionic gonadotropin (recombinant) Follitropin alfa Follitropin beta Lutropin alfa Menotropins Urofollitropin	Used as part of an assisted reproductive technology (ART) Treatment of infertility Polycystic ovary disease	Headache Flushing Multiple births Ovarian enlargement Hot flashes Ectopic pregnancy	Hypersensitivity Sex hormone-dependent tumors of the reproductive tract and accessory organs Pregnancy
Mechanism: *Dopamine antagonist; inhibits prolactin release*			
Bromocriptine Cabergoline	Treatment of hyperprolactinemia Treatment of prolactin-secreting adenomas Treatment of acromegaly Treatment of Parkinson's disease (bromocriptine)	Somnolence Orthostatic hypotension Arrhythmias Psychosis Dyskinesia	Concomitant use with other sedatives

GI, gastrointestinal; HIV, human immunodeficiency virus.

BOX 23-3 　 POSTERIOR PITUITARY HORMONES AND RELATED DRUGS

Desmopressin
Oxytocin

(1) Treatment of central (neurogenic) diabetes insipidus
(2) Maintenance of hemostasis and control of bleeding by increasing release of factor VIII: coagulant and von Willebrand's factor from endothelial cells
    (a) Mild hemophilia A
    (b) Mild-to-moderate classic von Willebrand's disease (type 1)
  b. Nasal solutions
    • Treatment of central (neurogenic) diabetes insipidus
  c. Nasal spray
    • Maintenance of hemostasis and control of bleeding in mild hemophilia A and mild to moderate classic von Willebrand's disease (type 1)

Desmopressin treats neurogenic diabetes insipidus.

d. Tablets
(1) Treatment of central (neurogenic) diabetes insipidus
(2) Primary nocturnal enuresis
e. Note: Thiazide diuretics are used to treat peripheral (nephrogenic) diabetes insipidus
• They cause a reduction in the polyuria of patients with diabetes insipidus by causing volume depletion, hence reducing glomerular filtration rate and volume of urine.

Thiazide diuretics treat nephrogenic diabetes insipidus.

5. Adverse effects
a. Overhydration
b. Hypertension
6. Drugs that increase the secretion or action of ADH
a. Diuretics
b. Carbamazepine
c. Morphine
d. Tricyclic antidepressants
e. Chlorpropamide
f. Cyclophosphamide
7. Agents that decrease the secretion or action of ADH
a. Ethanol (decreased secretion)
b. Lithium and demeclocycline
(1) Reduce the action of ADH at the collection ducts of the nephron
(2) Used to treat SIADH
(3) Because of its nephrotoxicity, demeclocycline is generally reserved for treating SIADH in patients with small cell carcinoma of the lungs; water restriction is *not* necessary.

Excess ADH results in SIADH, water retention, hyponatremia, and cerebral edema; absence of ADH results in diabetes insipidus.

Lithium and demeclocycline treat SIADH.

B. Oxytocin
1. This substance is secreted by the supraoptic and paraventricular nuclei in the hypothalamus.
2. It is used to induce labor and stimulate uterine contractions (see Chapter 26).

V. Thyroid Hormones and Related Drugs (Box 23-4)
A. General considerations (Fig. 23-4)
1. Functions of thyroid hormone
a. Control of total energy expenditure
b. Growth and maturation of tissue
c. Turnover of hormones and vitamins
d. Cell regeneration
2. Pathology
a. Excess
• Hyperthyroidism (thyrotoxicosis)
b. Deficiency
• Hypothyroidism due to hypothalamic/pituitary dysfunction or primary thyroid gland dysfunction (e.g., Hashimoto's thyroiditis)

Graves' disease causes hyperthyroidism.

c. Common causes
(1) Stimulatory autoantibody in Graves' disease
• IgG antibody against the TSH receptor on the thyroid causes increased thyroid hormone secretion with concomitant suppression of TRH and TSH levels
(2) Inhibitory IgG autoantibody directed against TSH receptor and thyroidal peroxidase; plus destruction of thyroid in Hashimoto's disease by cytotoxic T cells

---

BOX 23-4   THYROID HORMONES AND RELATED DRUGS

β-Adrenergic receptor antagonists	Methimazole
Iodinated contrast media (iohexol; diatrizoate)	Potassium iodide
Levothyroxine (T_4)	Propylthiouracil
Liothyronine (T_3)	Sodium iodine I^{131}

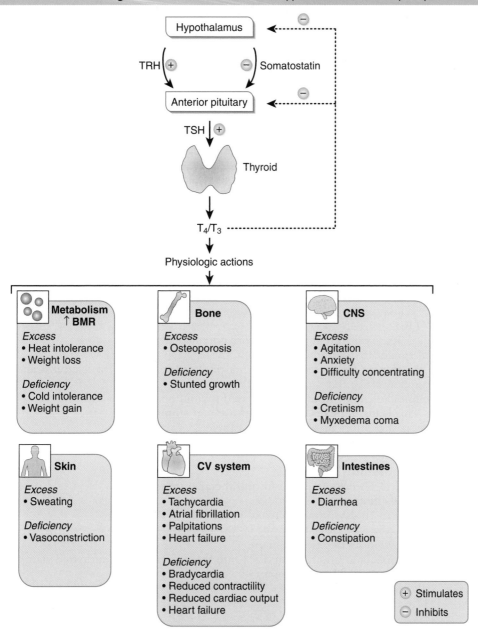

23-4: Thyroid regulation, physiology, and pathophysiology. BMR, basal metabolic rate; CNS, central nervous system; CV, cardiovascular; T_3, triiodothyronine; T_4, thyroxine; TRH, thyrotropin-releasing hormone; TSH, thyroid-stimulating hormone. *(From Brown TA: Rapid Review Physiology. Philadelphia, Mosby, 2007, Figure 3-12.)*

    (a) Causes decreased thyroid hormone secretion
    (b) Decreased thyroid hormone production with concomitant increase in serum TRH and TSH

B. Thyroid hormone synthesis, release and actions
  1. Iodide (I^-) is taken up by thyroid follicular cells
    a. Via a membrane Na^+/I^- transporter
    b. TSH-mediated
  2. I^- is converted to organic iodine
    • By thyroidal peroxidase
  3. Organic iodide is coupled to tyrosine residues on the thyroglobulin molecule (iodide organification)
    a. Forming monoiodotyrosine (MIT) and diiodo-tyrosine (DIT)
    b. TSH-mediated
  4. Thyroidal peroxidase also catalyzes the coupling
    a. Two molecules of DIT to form thyroxine (T_4)
    b. One molecule each of MIT and DIT to form triiodothyronine (T_3)

Hashimoto's disease causes hypothyroidism.

Thyroid peroxidase oxidizes inorganic iodide to organic iodine.

Trapping, organification, proteolysis are TSH-mediated

5. Thyroglobulin is stored as a colloid in the lumen.
6. TSH signals to hydrolyze thyroglobulin to free MIT, DIT, T_3 and T_4 (proteolysis)
   • Regulated by TSH
7. MIT and DIT are deiodinated to recycle while T_3 and T_4 are released by exocytosis.
8. Plasma T_3 and T_4 are reversibly bound to thyroxine-binding globulin (TBG)
   • Plasma transport form.

T_4 (prohormone) is converted to T_3 by outer ring deiodinase in peripheral tissues.

9. T_4 (a prohormone) is converted to T_3 in peripheral tissues (active hormone)
   • By 5'-diodinase (outer ring deiodinase).
10. T_3 acts on intracellular thyroid hormone receptors (TRs) located in all cells of the body.
11. TR monomers interact with retinoic acid X receptor (RXR) to form heterodimers.
12. In the absence of T_3,
    • The TR:RXR heterodimer associates with a co-repressor complex that binds to DNA to inhibit gene expression.

The thyroid receptor functions as an "On/Off" switch for gene expression; when co-repressor is bound, it is off ; when co-activator is bound, it is on.

13. In the presence of T_3,
    • The co-repressor complex dissociates, and coactivators bind the complex to stimulate gene expression.
C. **Thyroxine (T_4)- and triiodothyronine (T_3)-related preparations**
   1. General
      a. T_3 is less tightly bound than T_4 to the transport protein.
         • TBG
      b. T_3 is approximately four times more potent than T_4.
   2. Regulation of thyroid function
      a. Thyrotropin (TSH) from the anterior pituitary stimulates the synthesis and secretion of T_4 and T_3.
      b. Iodine deficiency results in decreased thyroid hormone synthesis.
         • This leads to increased TSH release and goiter.
      c. Drugs that affect thyroid function (Table 23-4)
   3. Levothyroxine (T_4)
      a. Pharmacokinetics
         (1) Slow-acting
            • 1 to 3 weeks required for full therapeutic effect
         (2) Half-life ($t_{1/2}$)
            • 9 to 10 days in hypothyroid patients
      b. Uses

Goal is to bring TSH into the normal range (euthyroid state)

         (1) Thyroid replacement therapy
            • Goal is to bring serum TSH into the normal range (euthyroid state)
         (2) Pituitary TSH suppression

Hyperthyroidism speeds and hypothyroidism slows many biological processes.

      c. Adverse effects
         (1) Cardiotoxicity

TABLE 23-4. Drugs That Affect Thyroid Function

DRUGS	EFFECT ON THYROID GLAND
Amiodarone	Contains iodide causing hypothyroidism (inhibits thyroid peroxidase- Wolff-Chaikoff effect) or hyperthyroidism in patients with preexisting multinodular goiter (Jod-Basedow effect)
Androgens	Decreased TBG, causing decrease in serum T_4 but normal free T_4 and TSH
Carbamazepine	Induced cytochrome P450 system, causing hypothyroidism ($\uparrow$ degradation T_4)
Estrogens	Increased TBG, causing increase in serum T_4 but normal free T_4 and TSH
Glucocorticoids	Decreased TBG, causing decrease in serum T_4 but normal free T_4 and TSH Decreased release of TSH causing hypothyroidism
Iodides	Altered thyroid synthesis, causing hypothyroidism (Wolff-Chaikoff effect) or hyperthyroidism if preexisting multinodular goiter (Jod-Basedow effect)
Levodopa	Prevents release of TSH, causing hypothyroidism
Lithium	Altered thyroid hormone synthesis and release, causing hypothyroidism
Phenobarbital	Induced cytochrome P450 system, causing hypothyroidism ($\uparrow$ metabolism of T_4)
Phenytoin	Induced cytochrome P450 system, causing hypothyroidism ($\uparrow$ metabolism of T_4)
Propranolol	Inhibited 5'-deiodinase, causing euthyroid sick syndrome ($\downarrow$ serum T_3/T_4, normal/$\downarrow$ serum TSH)
Rifampin	Induced cytochrome P-450 system, causing hypothyroidism ($\uparrow$ metabolism of T_4)
Salicylates	Displaced from TBG, causing thyrotoxicosis
Tamoxifen	Increased TBG, causing increase in serum T_4 but normal free T_4 and TSH

T_4, thyroxine; TBG, thyroxine-binding globulin; TSH, thyroid stimulating hormone.

(2) Excessive thermogenesis
(3) Increased sympathetic activity
(4) Insomnia
(5) Anxiety
4. Triiodothyronine (T_3)
  • Liothyronine (synthetic T_3)
    a. General
      (1) Faster acting than T_4
        (a) *Not* usually used because T_4 is converted to T_3 in the body
        (b) Thyroxine (T_4) is a prodrug to T_3
    b. Uses
      Given IV to treat myxedema coma or precoma

D. Antithyroid agents
1. Thioamides
  a. Examples
    (1) Propylthiouracil
    (2) Methimazole
  b. Mechanism of action
    • Inhibits the synthesis of T_3 and T_4
      (1) Prevents oxidation of iodide to iodine
      (2) Inhibits coupling of two iodotyrosine residues (iodinated tyrosine molecules) to form T_3 or T_4
      (3) Propylthiouracil also inhibits conversion of peripheral T_4 to T_3.
  c. Uses
    (1) Treat hyperthyroidism
      (a) Use beta-blockers to control adrenergic symptoms of the disease
      (b) Use thionamides to decrease synthesis of the hormone
        • Methimazole is longer acting than propylthiouracil; so it is favored for long term therapy
  d. Adverse effects
    (1) Hypothyroidism
    (2) Hepatotoxicity
    (3) Leukopenia
    (4) Granulocytosis
    (5) Teratogenicity
      • Propylthiouracil less than methimazole
      • Should be used in caution during pregnancy and nursing
2. Iodide compounds
  a. Sodium or potassium iodide
    • Intravenous or oral
  b. Iodinated contrast media
    (1) Iohexol
      • IV or oral
    (2) Diatrizoate
      • Oral
  c. Mechanism of action
    (1) Rapidly inhibits release of T_3 and T_4
      • Pharmacologic doses inhibit the proteolysis of thyroglobulin
    (2) Effects are transient
      • Thyroid gland "escapes" the block after a few weeks
    (3) Iodinated contrast media (diatrizoate by mouth, or iohexol; IV or oral), though *not* approved by the U.S. Food and Drug Administration (FDA), act by inhibiting conversion of T_4 to T_3 in liver, kidney, pituitary, and brain
  d. Uses
    (1) Preparation for surgical thyroidectomy
      • Decreases size and vascularity of gland
    (2) Treatment of thyrotoxicosis
  e. Adverse effects
    (1) Uncommon, but include
      (a) Acneiform rash
      (b) Swollen salivary glands
      (c) Mucous membrane ulceration
      (d) Conjunctivitis

Thyroid hormone may cause hyperthyroid symptoms and allergic skin reactions.

Thionamides inhibit organification of iodide.

Propylthiouracil also inhibits conversion of peripheral T_4 to T_3.

Propylthiouracil is less likely to cross the placenta than methimazole.

Potassium iodide decreases release of thyroid hormones by inhibiting proteolysis; thus, useful for initial treatment in thyrotoxicosis.

Diatrizoate and iohexol inhibit 5'-deiodonase and thereby block the conversion of T_4 to T_3.

(e) Rhinorrhea

(f) Metallic taste

(g) Drug fever

(h) Bleeding disorders

(i) Anaphylaxis

(j) Thyroid storm

• Tachyarrhythmias, hyperpyrexia, shock, coma

   (2) Potassium iodide should be avoided if therapy with radioactive iodine is necessary.

• Blocks its uptake

  3. Radioactive iodine (^{131}I)

    a. ^{131}I, the radioactive isotope of iodine

• Administered orally as sodium iodide ^{131}I

    b. Mechanism of action

     (1) Trapped by the thyroid gland and incorporated into thyroglobulin

     (2) Emission of beta radiation destroys the cells of the thyroid gland.

    c. Uses

     (1) Ablation of the thyroid in hyperthyroidism if non-responsive to thionamides and beta blockers

     (2) Uptake and scan to identify "cold" (non-functional) from "hot" (functional) nodules

     (3) Differentiate thyrotoxicosis due to taking excess hormone or acute thyroiditis versus hyperthyroidism (increased gland synthesis of thyroid hormone)

      (a) Decreased uptake in taking excess thyroid hormone or acute thyroiditis

      (b) Increased uptake in hyperthyroidism

    d. Adverse effects

     (1) Bone marrow suppression

     (2) Angina

     (3) Radiation sickness

  4. β-Adrenergic receptor antagonists (see Chapter 5)

    a. Reduce the adrenergic symptoms of hyperthyroidism

    b. β-Adrenergic symptoms include:

     (1) Tremor

     (2) Palpitations

     (3) Anxiety

     (4) Heat intolerance

     (5) Sinus tachycardia

E. Therapeutic summary of selected thyroid hormone related drugs (Table 23-5)

VI. Adrenocorticosteroids (Box 23-5; Tables 23-6 and 23-7)

 A. General considerations

  1. Endogenous adrenocortical hormones (Fig. 23-5)

• Steroid molecules produced and secreted from the adrenal cortex

  2. The adrenal cortex has three functionally discrete compartments (Fig. 23-5)

• Secrete distinctly different hormones (Fig. 23-6).

    a. Outer zona glomerulosa

     (1) Secretes the mineralocorticoids such as aldosterone

     (2) Secretion is regulated mainly by extracellular K^+ through angiotensin receptors.

    b. Middle zona fasciculata

     (1) Secretes the glucocorticoids → cortisol

     (2) Synthesis and secretion regulated by ACTH

     (3) Catalyzed by three enzymes

      (a) 17α-hydroxylase (P-45017a)

      (b) 21-hydroxylase (P-450c21)

      (c) 11β-hydroxylase (P-45011β)

    c. Inner zona reticularis

     (1) Secretes adrenal androgens → dehydroepiandrosterone (DHEA) and androstenedione, which are 17-ketosteroids

     (2) Androstenedione is converted to testosterone by an oxidoreductase reaction.

     (3) Testosterone is peripherally converted to dihydrotestosterone (DHT) by 5-α-reductase.

Margin notes:

Radioactive iodine (^{131}I) destroys (ablates) the thyroid gland.

Give beta-blockers first in thyroid storm.

GFR: **G**lomerulosa, **F**asciculata, **R**eticularis. Zona glomerulosa produces mineralocorticoids.

21-hydroxylase deficiency is the most common cause of adrenal insufficiency.

Zona fasciculata produces glucocorticoids (11-deoxycortisol and cortisol).

Zona reticularis produces androgens (17-ketosteroids, testosterone).

TABLE 23-5. **Therapeutic Summary of Selected Thyroid Hormone Related Drugs**

DRUGS	CLINICAL APPLICATIONS	ADVERSE EFFECTS	CONTRAINDICATIONS
Mechanism: *Thyroid hormone activity*			
Levothyroxine (T_4) Liothyronine (T_3)	Replacement or supplemental therapy in hypothyroidism Pituitary TSH suppression	Cardiotoxicity Excessive thermogenesis Increased sympathetic activity Insomnia Anxiety Tension	Hypersensitivity Recent MI or thyrotoxicosis Uncorrected adrenal insufficiency
Mechanism: *Inhibits iodide organification and thyroid hormone synthesis; thyroid peroxidase inhibitor*			
Methimazole Propylthiouracil	Palliative treatment of hyperthyroidism prior to surgery or radioactive iodine therapy Management of thyrotoxic crisis	Hypothyroidism Hepatotoxicity Leukopenia Granulocytosis Teratogenic: methimazole > propylthiouracil	Hypersensitivity Should be used in caution during pregnancy and nursing
Mechanism: *Rapidly inhibits organic binding of iodide (inhibits thyroid peroxidase) in pharmacologic doses (Wolff-Chaikoff effect) for 24 to 50 hours*			
Potassium iodide	Preparation for surgical thyroidectomy (decreases size and vascularity of gland) Treatment of thyrotoxicosis Block thyroidal uptake of radioactive isotopes of iodine in a radiation emergency	Acneiform rash Swollen salivary glands Mucous membrane ulceration Conjunctivitis Rhinorrhea Metallic taste Drug fever Bleeding disorders Thyroid storm if preexisting multinodular goiter (Jod-Basedow effect)	Hypersensitivity Hyperkalemia Pulmonary edema Impaired renal function Hyperthyroidism Iodine-induced goiter Dermatitis herpetiformis Hypocomplementemic vasculitis
Mechanism: *Accumulates in and destroys the thyroid gland*			
Sodium iodine ^{131}I	For diagnostic use with the radioactive iodide uptake test to evaluate thyroid function Treatment of hyperthyroidism Select cases of thyroid cancer Scan for "hot" vs "cold" nodules	Tachycardia Alopecia Thrombocytopenia Blood dyscrasia Acute leukemia	Hypersensitivity Concurrent antithyroid medication Pregnancy
Mechanism: *Contrast dyes that inhibit the conversion of T_4 to T_3 in peripheral tissues*			
Iohexol Diatrizoate	Management of hyperthyroidism	Similar to potassium iodide	Hypersensitivity
Mechanism: *Beta receptor blocker; thyroid hormones act synergistically with catecholamine*			
Propranolol	Initial treatment of thyrotoxicosis along with thionamides	See Chapter 5	See Chapter 5

BOX 23-5   ADRENAL HORMONES AND RELATED DRUGS

Glucocorticoids
Short- to Medium-Acting
  Cortisone
  Hydrocortisone (cortisol)
  Prednisolone
  Prednisone
Intermediate-Acting
  Fluprednisolone
  Methylprednisolone
  Triamcinolone
Long-Acting
  Betamethasone
  Dexamethasone

Mineralocorticoids
Desoxycorticosterone
Fludrocortisone

Glucocorticoid Antagonists and Synthesis Inhibitors
Aminoglutethimide
Ketoconazole
Metyrapone
Mifepristone
Mitotane

Mineralocorticoid Antagonists
Spironolactone
Eplerenone

TABLE 23-6. Nonadrenal Disorders Treated with Corticosteroids

NATURE OF THE CONDITION	DISORDER
Allergic reactions	*Angioedema, anaphylaxis*
Bone and joint disorders	Rheumatoid arthritis, systemic lupus erythematosus
Collagen vascular disorders	Systemic lupus erythematosus
Eye diseases	Iritis, keratitis, chorioretinitis
Gastrointestinal disorders	Crohn's disease, ulcerative colitis
Hematologic disorders	Idiopathic cytopenic purpura
Neurologic disorders	Acute spinal cord injury, multiple sclerosis flare, increased intracranial pressure
Organ transplantations	Kidney transplant
Pulmonary diseases	Chronic obstructive pulmonary disease or asthma flares
Renal disease	Glomerulopathies (Goodpasture's syndrome; minimal change disease)
Skin disorders	Psoriasis, dermatitis, eczema
Thyroid diseases	Malignant exophthalmos, subacute thyroiditis

TABLE 23-7. The Relative Potencies of Various Steroids Compared to Cortisol (Arbitrary Value = 1.0)

DRUGS	RGP	RMP	DURATION OF ACTION (hr)
Short-Acting			
Cortisol (hydrocortisone)	1.0	1.0	8–12
Cortisone	0.8	0.8	8–12
Intermediate-Acting			
Prednisone	4.0	0.3	12–36
Prednisolone	5.0	0.3	12–36
Methylprednisolone	5.0	0	12–36
Triamcinolone	5	0	24–36
Long-Acting			
Betamethasone	25–40	0	>48
Dexamethasone	30	0	>48
Mineralocorticoids			
Fludrocortisone	10	125	
Deoxycortisone	0	20	
Aldosterone	0.3	3000	

RGP, relative glucocorticoid potency (liver glycogen deposition, or anti-inflammatory activity); RMP, relative mineralocorticoid potency (sodium retention).

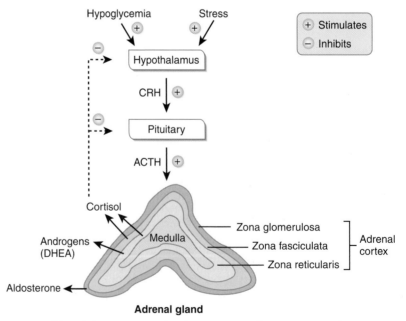

Adrenal gland

23-5: Main determinants of hypothalamic-pituitary-adrenal axis. ACTH, adrenocorticotropic hormone; CRH, corticotropin-releasing hormone; DHEA, dehydroepiandrosterone. *(From Brown TA: Rapid Review Physiology. Philadelphia, Mosby, 2007, Figure 3-5.)*

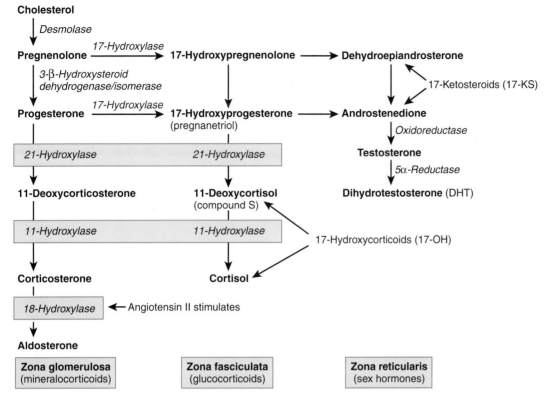

23-6: Pathways of adrenal steroidogenesis. *(From Goljan EF: Rapid Review Pathology, 2nd ed. Philadelphia, Mosby, 2007, Figure 22-7.)*

3. Adrenocorticoid receptors
   a. Two types
      (1) Type I - mineralocorticoid receptor
         • Expressed mainly in organs of excretion such as kidney, colon, salivary glands, sweat glands
      (2) Type II - glucocorticoid receptor
         • Broad tissue distribution
   b. Adrenocorticoid receptors
      • Cytoplasmic as oligomeric complexes with two bound molecules of heat shock proteins (Hsp90).
      (1) Free steroid enters cell cytoplasm to release the receptor from Hsp90
      (2) The steroid-receptor complex then enters the nucleus
      (3) Binds to the glucocorticoid response element (GRE)
      (4) Regulates transcription by RNA polymerase and other factors
      (5) mRNA is edited and exported to cytoplasm to form protein.

B. **Pathology** (See Rapid Review Pathology)
   1. Adrenocorticoid hypofunction (primary hypocorticalism)
      a. Acute adrenocorticoid insufficiency
         • Examples: abrupt withdrawal of exogenous corticosteroids; Waterhouse-Friderichsen's syndrome
      b. Chronic adrenal insufficiency (Addison's disease)
         • Most common cause is autoimmune destruction
      c. Adrenogenital syndrome (See Fig. 23-6 for location of enzymes)
         (1) 21-Hydroxylase deficiency (most common type)
         (2) 11-Hydroxylase deficiency
         (3) 17-Hydroxylase deficiency
   2. Adrenocorticoid hyperfunction
      a. Cushing's syndrome

Both Type I and Type II receptors are found in the brain and contribute to stress-induced brain dysfunction.

Glucocorticoids affect the gene expression of most cells in the body

Addison's disease: decreased mineralocorticoids, glucocorticoids, sex hormones; increased serum ACTH

(1) Prolonged corticosteroid therapy
  • Overall most common cause of Cushing's syndrome
(2) Pituitary Cushing's syndrome
  (a) Most common pathologic cause of Cushing's syndrome
  (b) ACTH-secreting pituitary adenoma
(3) Ectopic Cushing's syndrome
  (a) Most often due to small cell carcinoma of lung
  (b) Ectopic production of ACTH by tumor
(4) Adrenal Cushing's syndrome
  (a) Most often due to benign adrenal adenoma in zona fasciculata
  (b) Increased synthesis of cortisol
b. Hyperaldosteronism
  (1) Primary (Conn's syndrome)
    • Zona glomerulosa benign adenoma
  (2) Secondary
    • Compensatory increase due to increased renin secretion from decreased renal blood flow (e.g., decreased cardiac output)

C. **Glucocorticoids**
  1. Examples
    a. Cortisone
    b. Hydrocortisone
    c. Methylprednisolone
    d. Dexamethasone
  2. Synthesis and secretion
    a. Synthesized from cholesterol (see Fig. 23-6)
      • Adrenocorticosteroids are *not* stored by the adrenal gland but are released as soon as they are produced
    b. Regulated by ACTH
      • Exhibits a similar circadian rhythm (Fig. 23-7)
  3. Biological actions of glucocorticoids
    a. Have widespread effects on all tissues and organs
    b. Have both direct and "permissive" actions
    c. Metabolic actions (Fig. 23-8)
      (1) These effects contribute to supply adequate glucose to the brain in the fasting state by:
        (a) Increasing glucose from gluconeogenesis
        (b) Increasing amino acids from muscle catabolism
          • Amino acids are used as substrates for gluconeogenesis
        (c) Inhibiting peripheral glucose uptake
        (d) Stimulating lipolysis
          • Released glycerol is taken up by the liver, converted to glycerol 3-phosphate, which is then used as a substrate for gluconeogenesis

23-7: Diurnal secretion of adrenocorticotropic hormone and cortisol. ACTH, adrenocorticotropic hormone. *(From Brown TA: Rapid Review Physiology. Philadelphia, Mosby, 2007, Figure 3-6.)*

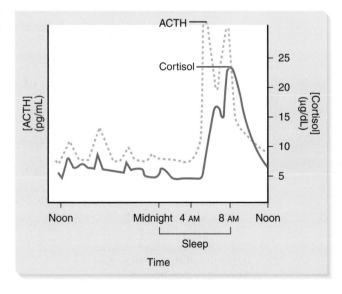

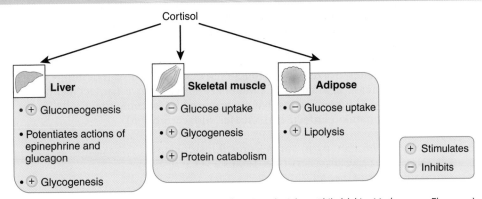

23-8: Metabolic actions of cortisol. *(From Brown TA: Rapid Review Physiology. Philadelphia, Mosby, 2007, Figure 3-7.)*

(2) These changes are generally beneficial.
  • But can also cause serious adverse effects even when therapeutic doses are used
  d. Catabolic and anti-anabolic actions
    (1) Occur in lymphoid and connective tissues, muscle, fat, and skin
    (2) Supraphysiologic amounts
      Reduce muscle mass causing weakness and skin thinning
    (3) Bone effects cause osteoporosis in Cushing's syndrome.
      Limit long-term therapeutic use of corticosteroids
    (4) Reduced growth in children
      Partly prevented with high doses of growth hormone
  e. CNS actions
    (1) Marked slowing of electroencephalograph (EEG) alpha rhythm and depression
    (2) Behavioral disturbances
      • Initially insomnia and euphoria followed by depression or psychosis
    (3) Large does may increase intracranial pressure
      • Pseudotumor cerebri
    (4) Suppressed pituitary release of ACTH, GH, TSH, and LH
      • Cause multiple endocrine effects
  f. Anti-inflammatory and immunosuppressive
    (1) Manifestations of inflammation are dramatically reduced
      (a) Increases circulating neutrophils (neutrophilic leukocytosis)
        • Inactivates neutrophil adhesion molecules causing marginating pool (pool normally adhering to endothelium) to become part of circulating pool
      (b) Decreases certain circulating hematopoietic cells by acting as a signal for apoptosis
        • Lymphocytes, monocytes, eosinophils, basophils
      (c) Suppresses cytokines, chemokines, lipid and glucolipid molecules, which are mediators of inflammation
      (d) Reduces synthesis of prostaglandins and leukotrienes
        • Increases the synthesis of lipocortin, which inhibits phospholipase A_2 suppressing the release of arachidonic acid from phospholipids and decreases cytokine driven cyclooxygenase-2 (COX-2) expression
      (e) Suppresses mast cell degranulation
        • Reduces histamine release; this decreases capillary permeability
    (2) These changes are responsible for *not* only for their major therapeutic use but also for serious adverse effects.
  g. Miscellaneous actions
    (1) Development of peptic ulcer
      • Suppresses local immune response to *Helicobacter pylori*
    (2) Promote fat redistribution
      (a) Increase visceral, facial, nuchal (nape), and supraclavicular fat
      (b) Hyperglycemia increases insulin, which increases fat deposition in these areas.
    (3) Antagonize Vitamin D effect on calcium absorption

Glucocorticoids are important for adequate glucose levels in brain.

Glucocorticoid excess cause muscle wasting and skin thinning (bruise easily).

Anti-inflammatory actions: decreased neutrophil adhesion (increased circulating count); cytopenias (lymphocytes, monocytes, eosinophils, basophils); decreased prostaglandins/leukotrienes

Glucocorticoids increase synthesis of lipocortin which decreases phospholipase A_2 and decreases arachidonic acid levels.

Arachidonic acid is a substrate for both cyclooxygenases and lipoxygenases; thus, glucocorticoids reduce inflammatory prostanoids and leukotrienes.

Glucocorticoids produce "moon face" and "buffalo hump"

(4) Increase numbers of circulating platelets and erythrocytes

(5) Cortisol deficiency impairs renal function and augments vasopressin secretion

(a) Results in an inability to excrete a water load normally

(b) May result in mild hyponatremia

(6) Stimulates structural and functional development of fetal lungs

- Increase production of pulmonary surface-active (surfactant) materials by type II pneumocytes that are required for keeping the distal airways open on expiration (surfactant decreases surface tension)

4. Uses

a. Substitution therapy in adrenocortical insufficiency

b. Non-endocrine disorders (see Tables 23-3 and 23-4)

c. Asthma (see Chapter 20)

d. Immunosuppressive therapy (see Chapter 22)

e. Diagnostic functions

(1) Dexamethasone in high doses

(a) Suppress ACTH release from pituitary adenomas

(b) Does *not* suppress ACTH from ectopic tumors or cortisol from adrenal tumors

(2) Urine levels of steroid metabolites are of diagnostic value in identifying hypofunction and hyperfunction conditions.

5. Adverse effects

a. Adrenal suppression due to negative feedback mechanisms

(1) The degree of suppression is a function of the dose and length of therapy.

(2) When therapy is discontinued, the dose must be tapered.

b. Iatrogenic Cushing's syndrome

c. Metabolic effects

(1) Hypokalemic metabolic alkalosis due to increased mineralocorticoids.

(2) Hyperglycemia due to increase in gluconeogenesis

(3) Hirsutism in women (androgen effect)

d. Hypertension due to Na^+ retention

e. Secondary cause of diabetes mellitus due to increased gluconeogenesis

f. Increased susceptibility to infection

g. Peptic ulcer disease

h. Musculoskeletal effects

(1) Myopathy with skeletal muscle weakness

(2) Osteoporosis from increased breakdown of mineral and organic components of bone

i. Behavioral disturbances

(1) Psychosis

(2) Euphoria

(3) Insomnia

(4) Restlessness

j. Ophthalmic effects

(1) Permanent visual impairment

(2) Cataracts

D. Mineralocorticoids

1. General information

a. Aldosterone is the most important naturally occurring hormone.

b. Fludrocortisone is an oral synthetic adrenocorticosteroid with both mineralocorticoid and glucocorticoid activity (only mineralocorticoid effects at clinically used doses).

2. Synthesis and secretion

a. Angiotensin II (Ang II) is the primary stimulus for aldosterone secretion.

b. Ang II activates 18-hydroxylase, which converts corticosterone to aldosterone.

3. Mechanism of action (see Chapter 15)

a. Increase the retention of Na^+ and water

- Excess mineralocorticoids produce hypertension.

b. Increase the excretion of K^+ and H^+

- Excess mineralocorticoids produce hypokalemia and metabolic alkalosis.

Margin notes:

Cortisol increases fetal surfactant synthesis

Glucocorticoids: taper doses on discontinuation; danger of acute adrenal insufficiency

Long-term use of glucocorticoids causes osteoporosis and cataracts.

Angiotensin II regulates aldosterone secretion.

Excess mineralocorticoids produce hypertension, hypokalemia and metabolic acidosis.

4. Uses
- Fludrocortisone
    a. Partial replacement therapy for primary and secondary adrenocortical insufficiency in Addison's disease
    b. Treatment of salt-losing adrenogenital syndrome (21-hydroxylase deficiency)
    c. Usually given with hydrocortisone in adrenal insufficiency disorders

E. **Antagonists of adrenocortical agents**
1. Glucocorticoid antagonists and synthesis inhibitors
    a. Metyrapone
        (1) Mechanism of action
            (a) Inhibits 11β-hydroxylase
            (b) This inhibits production of cortisol, which should increase plasma ACTH and 11-deoxycortisol, which is proximal to the enzyme block.
        (2) Uses
            (a) Diagnostic test for the production of ACTH by the pituitary and the production of 11-deoxycortisol by the adrenal cortex
                - Patients with hypopituitarism would have a decrease in plasma ACTH and 11-deoxycortisol; patient with Addison's would have an increase in plasma ACTH and a decrease in 11-deoxycortisol.
            (b) Treatment of Cushing's syndrome
                - Available only for compassionate use
    b. Aminoglutethimide
        (1) Mechanism of action
            (a) Inhibits enzymatic conversion of cholesterol to pregnenolone
            (b) This leads to reduced synthesis of all adrenocortical hormones.
            (c) Also, an aromatase inhibitor
                - Inhibits the conversion of testosterone to estrogen
        (2) Use
            - Cushing's syndrome
    c. Ketoconazole (antifungal agent)
        (1) Mechanism of action
            - Inhibits mammalian synthesis of glucocorticoids and steroid hormones by inhibiting the cytochrome P450 system and 11β-hydroxylase
        (2) Uses
            (a) Cushing's syndrome
            (b) Treatment of prostate cancer (androgen synthesis inhibitor)
    d. Mifepristone (RU 486)
        - Glucocorticoid receptor antagonist and progesterone antagonist (see Chapter 26)
    e. Mitotane
        (1) Adrenocortical cytotoxic antineoplastic agent
        (2) Used to treat adrenal carcinoma
2. Mineralocorticoid antagonists (see Chapter 15)
    a. Examples
        (1) Spironolactone
        (2) Eplerenone
    b. Mechanism of action
        - Competitive inhibitor of aldosterone
    c. Uses
        (1) Hypertension (in combination with thiazide diuretics as a potassium-sparing diuretic)
        (2) Primary hyperaldosteronism (treatment and diagnosis)
        (3) Hirsutism (women)
            - Spironolactone
        (4) Ascites associated with cirrhosis
        (5) Severe congestive heart failure

F. **Therapeutic summary of selected adrenocorticoid related drugs** (Table 23-8)

Metyrapone: inhibits 11-hydroxlase (normally converts 11-deoxycortisol to cortisol)

Aminoglutethimide inhibits the conversion of cholesterol to pregnenolone and testosterone to estrogen.

The antifungal drug, ketoconazole, also inhibits steroidogenesis and is used to treat Cushing's syndrome.

The aldosterone antagonists, spironolactone and eplerenone, are potassium-sparing diuretics

TABLE 23-8. **Therapeutic Summary of Selected Adrenocorticoid Related Drugs**

DRUGS	CLINICAL APPLICATIONS	ADVERSE EFFECTS	CONTRAINDICATIONS
Mechanism: *Short-acting glucocorticoids; glucocorticoid and mineralocorticoid activity*			
Cortisone Hydrocortisone	Management of adrenocortical insufficiency Relief of inflammation of corticosteroid-responsive dermatoses (*not* cortisone) Adjunctive treatment of ulcerative colitis	Cushing's syndrome Adrenal suppression Euphoria Depression Peptic ulcers Osteoporosis Cataracts	Hypersensitivity Serious infections Viral, fungal, or tuberculous skin lesions
Mechanism: *Intermediate-acting glucocorticoids; glucocorticoid and mineralocorticoid activity*			
Prednisone Prednisolone	Treatment of : Adrenocortical insufficiency Hypercalcemia Rheumatologic and collagen disorders Respiratory disorders Gastrointestinal and neoplastic diseases Organ transplantation Immunological and inflammatory diseases	Cushing's syndrome Adrenal suppression Euphoria Depression Peptic ulcers Osteoporosis Cataracts Neutrophilic leukocytosis Lymphopenia, eosinopenia Poor wound healing	Hypersensitivity Serious infections Viral, fungal, or tuberculous skin lesions
Mechanism: : *Intermediate-acting glucocorticoids; only glucocorticoid activity*			
Methylprednisolone Triamcinolone	Adrenocortical insufficiency Rheumatic disorders Allergic states Respiratory diseases Systemic lupus erythematosus (SLE) Diseases requiring anti-inflammatory or immunosuppressive effects	Cushing's syndrome without mineralocorticoid effects Adrenal suppression Euphoria Depression Peptic ulcers Osteoporosis Cataracts Neutrophilic leukocytosis Lymphopenia, eosinopenia Poor wound healing	Hypersensitivity Serious infections Viral, fungal, or tuberculous skin lesions
Mechanism: *Intermediate-acting glucocorticoids; only glucocorticoid activity*			
Betamethasone Dexamethasone	Used as an anti-inflammatory or immunosuppressant agent in the treatment of a variety of disease listed above Used in management of cerebral edema, septic shock, chronic swelling Used as a diagnostic agent for diagnosis of Cushing's syndrome Antiemetic Dexamethasone suppression test; an indicator consistent with depression and/or suicide Betamethasone used in premature labor (26–34 weeks gestation) to stimulate fetal lung maturation by increasing surfactant synthesis	Cushing's syndrome without mineralocorticoid effects Adrenal suppression Euphoria Depression Peptic ulcers Osteoporosis Cataracts Neutrophilic leukocytosis Lymphopenia, eosinopenia Poor wound healing	Hypersensitivity Serious infections Viral, fungal, or tuberculous skin lesions
Mechanism: *Only mineralocorticoid activity at therapeutic doses*			
Fludrocortisone	Replacement therapy with hydrocortisone for primary and secondary adrenocortical insufficiency in Addison's disease Treatment of salt-losing adrenogenital syndrome (21-hydroxylase deficiency)	Edema Hypertension Congestive heart failure Hypokalemic, metabolic alkalosis Peptic ulcer	Hypersensitivity Systemic fungal infections
Mechanism: *An aldosterone antagonist at the distal renal tubules, increasing sodium chloride and water excretion while conserving potassium and hydrogen ions*			
Spironolactone Eplerenone	**Spironolactone** Management of edema from excessive aldosterone excretion Hypertension Congestive heart failure Primary hyperaldosteronism Hypokalemia Ascites in cirrhosis of liver Female acne and hirsutism **Eplerenone** Treatment of hypertension Treatment of heart failure	Hyperchloremic metabolic acidosis Hyperkalemia Gynecomastia (spironolactone)	Hypersensitivity Renal disorders Hyperkalemia Pregnancy

DRUGS USED IN THE TREATMENT OF DIABETES MELLITUS AND ERRORS OF GLUCOSE METABOLISM

I. **General Considerations** (Table 24-1)
A. **Types of diabetes mellitus (DM)** (see Rapid Review Pathology)
1. Type 1
a. Autoimmune disease associated with destruction of pancreatic β-islet cells
b. Absolute insulin deficiency
2. Type 2
a. Decreased number of insulin receptors
• Down-regulation of receptor synthesis related to increased adipose
b. Postreceptor dysfunction
• Examples: dysfunction of tyrosine kinase; glucose transport unit dysfunction
c. Relative insulin deficiency
3. Secondary causes
a. Drugs
(1) Glucocorticoids
(2) Thiazide diuretics
(3) Interferon-α
(4) Pentamidine
b. Some endocrine diseases
• Examples: Cushing's syndrome; glucagonoma; acromegaly
c. Some genetic diseases
• Examples: hemochromatosis; metabolic syndrome; maturity onset DM
d. Insulin-receptor deficiency
• Acanthosis nigricans is a phenotypic marker
e. Some infections
• Examples: mumps; cytomegalovirus in acquired immune deficiency syndrome (AIDS)
4. Impaired glucose tolerance
5. Gestational diabetes
B. **Regulation of insulin secretion and physiological actions**
1. Endocrine pancreas
a. α Cells secrete
• Glucagon
b. β cells secrete
(1) Insulin
(2) C-peptide
(3) Amylin
c. δ cells secrete
• Somatostatin

Type 1 DM: autoimmune destruction of β-islet cells in pancreas; absolute insulin deficiency.

Type 2 DM: insulin resistance due to ↓ insulin receptor synthesis and postreceptor abnormalities; relative insulin deficiency.

Acanthosis nigricans is a phenotypic marker of insulin-receptor deficiency.

Pancreatic cells; α cells secrete glucagon; β cells secrete insulin; δ cells secrete somatostatin

TABLE 24-1. **Characteristics of Type 1 and Type 2 Diabetes Mellitus**

CHARACTERISTIC	TYPE 1	TYPE 2
Age of onset	Usually <25 yr	Usually >40 yr
Acuteness of onset	Usually sudden	Usually gradual
Presenting features	Polyuria, polydipsia, polyphagia, acidosis	Often asymptomatic
Body habitus	Often thin	Usually overweight
Control of diabetes	Difficult	Easy
Ketoacidosis	Frequent	Seldom, unless under stress
Insulin requirement	Always	Often unnecessary
Control by oral agents	Never	Frequent
Control by diet alone	Never	Frequent
Complications	Frequent	Frequent

Use C peptide levels to differentiate between exogenous insulin (overdose) and endogenous insulin (overproduction/insulinoma).

2. Insulin structure and storage
   a. Proinsulin is hydrolyzed to:
      (1) Insulin (51 amino acids)
         • Insulin molecule stored in secretory cells
      (2) C-peptide (endogenous marker of insulin synthesis)
3. Insulin release (Fig. 24-1)
   a. Glucose partially depolarizes β cells
      (1) Glucose enters via GLUT-2 transporter
      (2) Metabolism of glucose yields adenosine triphosphate (ATP)
      (3) Increased ATP/ADP (adenosine diphosphate) ratio closes the SUR1 ($K_{IR}6.2$) K^+ channel
         • SUR = Sulfonylurea receptor
      (4) Decreased K^+ permeability, which leads to partial depolarization of β cells
      (5) Open voltage gated Ca^{2+} channels
      (6) Increased Ca^{2+} stimulates exocytosis of insulin

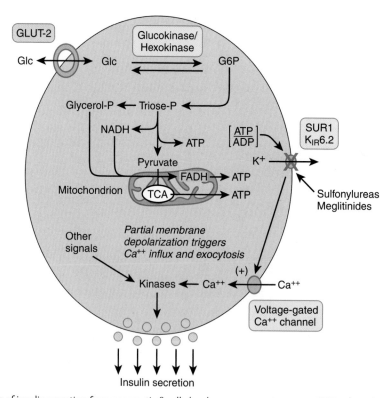

24-1: Mechanism of insulin secretion from pancreatic β cells by glucose or secretagogues. ADP, adenosine diphosphate; ATP, adenosine triphosphate; FADH, flavin adenine dinucleotide; Glc, glucose; GLUT-2, glucose transporter; G6P, glucose 6-phosphate; NADH, nicotinamide-adenine dinucleotide; SUR1r ($K_{IR}6.2$), K^+ channel; TCA, tricarboxylic acid cycle. *(From Wecker L, et al.: Brody's Human Pharmacology, 5th ed. Philadelphia, Mosby, 2010, Figure 43-3.)*

  b. Secretagogues, also, depolarize β cells
   (1) They bind to and close SUR1 ($K_{IR}6.2$) K^+ channel
   (2) This causes insulin release by mechanism above
  c. Effect of serum K^+
   (1) Hypokalemia inhibits insulin secretion
   (2) Hyperkalemia stimulates insulin secretion
 4. Insulin actions (Fig. 24-2)
  a. Translocation of GLUT-4 transporter to the cell surface
  b. Promotion of glucose uptake by
   (1) Muscle
   (2) Adipose
  c. Major role of insulin is to maintain plasma glucose levels and, to a lesser extent, serum K^+ levels

C. Complications
 1. Chronic hyperglycemia
  a. Glucose combines with amino groups in proteins.
  b. Produces advanced glycosylation end (AGE) products
   • Assessed by measuring glycosylated HbA_{1c}
 2. Protein glycosylation and osmotic changes contributes to many diseases
  a. Neuropathy (osmotic damage of Schwann cells from sorbitol)
  b. Retinopathy (osmotic damage to pericytes by sorbitol)
  c. Nephropathy
  d. Peripheral vascular disease
  e. Coronary artery disease
  f. Lacunar strokes

> Most important actions of insulin are in liver, skeletal muscle, and adipose tissue.

> Insulin promotes uptake of glucose in muscle and adipose via GLUT-4.

> Diabetes causes neuropathy, retinopathy, nephropathy, peripheral vascular disease, strokes, coronary artery disease.

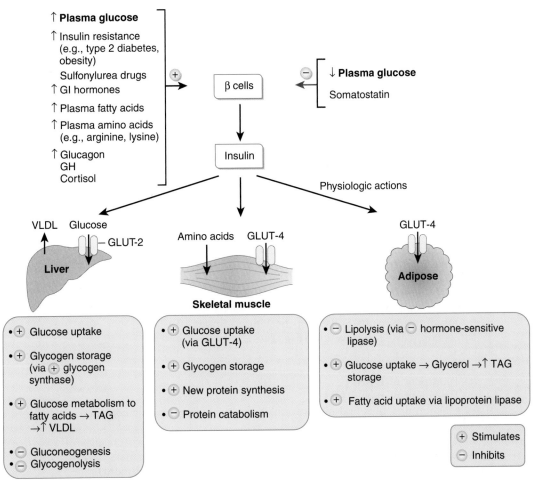

24-2: Regulation of insulin secretion and physiologic actions of insulin. GH, growth hormone; GI, gastrointestinal; GLUT, glucose transporter; TAG, triacylglycerides; VLDL, very low density lipoprotein. *(From Brown TA: Rapid Review Physiology. Philadelphia, Mosby, 2007, Figure 3-18.)*

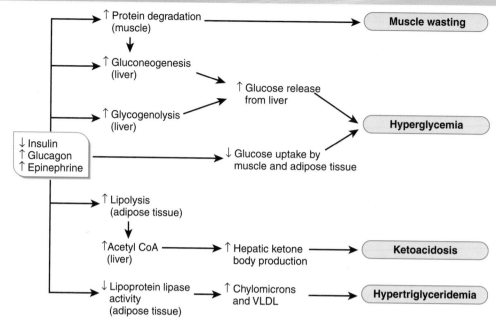

24-3: Mechanisms of metabolic changes in untreated type 1 diabetes mellitus (DM). VLDL, very low-density lipoprotein. *(From Pelley JW and Goljan EF: Rapid Review Biochemistry, 2nd ed. Philadelphia, Mosby, 2007, Figure 9-5.)*

3. Diabetic ketoacidosis (type 1 diabetes)
   a. Produces severe volume depletion and coma
   b. Multiple metabolic changes (Fig. 24-3)

II. Antidiabetic Agents (Box 24-1)

A. Insulins

1. Different insulin preparations (Table 24-2)
   a. Rapid-acting insulin
      (1) Insulin aspart
      (2) Insulin glulisine
      (3) Insulin inhalation (limited availability)
      (4) Insulin lispro
   b. Short-acting insulin
      • Regular insulin
   c. Intermediate-acting insulin
      • Neutral protamine Hagedorn (NPH); NPH insulin
   d. Combination insulin
      (1) Insulin aspart protamine and insulin aspart
      (2) Insulin lispro protamine and insulin lispro
      (3) Insulin NPH and insulin regular
   e. Long-acting insulin (peakless)
      (1) Insulin glargine
      (2) Insulin detemir
2. Human insulin produced by recombinant DNA technology
   • Only human insulin is used in the United States
3. Effects on plasma glucose use (Fig. 24-4).
4. Uses
   a. Treatment of type 1 DM
   b. Treatment of DKA
   c. Treatment of type 2 DM
      • When diet plus oral medications fail to provide glycemic control
5. Adverse effects
   a. Hypoglycemia (most common complication)
   b. Signs of severe hypoglycemia or insulin overdose
      (1) Neuroglycopenic (central nervous system [CNS] impairment)
         (a) Mental confusion
         (b) Bizarre behavior
         (c) Convulsions or coma

Regular insulin is the only intravenous preparation for treating diabetic ketoacidosis (DKA).

Insulin is always used in type 1 diabetes; sometimes in type 2.

BOX 24-1 DRUGS USED IN THE TREATMENT OF DIABETES MELLITUS

Insulins
Rapid-acting
  Insulin aspart
  Insulin glulisine
  Insulin inhalation (limited availability)
  Insulin lispro
Short-acting
  Regular insulin
Intermediate-acting
  Neutral protamine Hagedorn (NPH) insulin
Combination insulin
  Insulin aspart protamine and insulin aspart
  Insulin lispro protamine and insulin lispro
  Insulin NPH and insulin regular
Long-acting
  Insulin glargine
  Insulin detemir

Sulfonylureas
First generation
  Chlorpropamide
  Tolazamide
  Tolbutamide
Second generation
  Gliclazide
  Glimepiride
  Glipizide
  Glyburide

Meglitinides
Nateglinide
Repaglinide

Biguanide
Metformin

α-Glucosidase inhibitors
Acarbose
Miglitol

Thiazolidinediones
Pioglitazone
Rosiglitazone

Amylinomimetic
Pramlintide

Incretin-based
Exenatide
Sitagliptin

TABLE 24-2. Therapeutic Time Course of Selected Insulin Preparations

Preparation	Onset of Action	Duration of Action	Peak Effect
Rapid-Acting Insulin			
Insulin lispro, aspart, and glulisine	0–15 min	<5 hr	30–90 min
Short-Acting Insulin			
Insulin injection (regular insulin)	30–45 min	5–7 hr	2–4 hr
Intermediate-Acting Insulin			
NPH insulin (neutral protamine Hagedorn insulin)	1–4 hr	18–24 hr	6–14 hr
Long-Acting Insulin			
Insulin glargine	1.5 hr	>24 hr	No peak

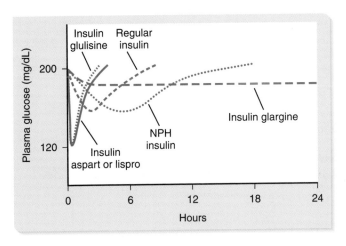

24-4: Effects of various insulin preparations on plasma glucose levels in a fasting individual.

Insulin-induced hypoglycemia activates both the sympathetic and parasympathetic systems.

Beta-blockers may mask the symptoms of approaching hypoglycemia and delay recovery.

Treat severe hypoglycemia with intravenous glucose or glucagon.

(2) Autonomic hyperactivity
    (a) Sympathetic (tachycardia, palpitations, sweating, tremors)
    (b) Parasympathetic (nausea, hunger)
(3) Rapidly relieved by giving:
    (a) Glucose
       • Patients who can swallow
       • Orange juice or any sugar-containing food or beverage
    (b) IV 50% glucose (unconscious patients)
    (c) Glucagon (IM, IV, or SC)
  c. Lipodystrophy (change in the subcutaneous fat at the site of injections)

B. Oral agents
  1. Sulfonylureas (secretagogues)
    a. First-generation drugs
      (1) Chlorpropamide
      (2) Tolazamide
      (3) Tolbutamide
    b. Second-generation drugs
      (1) Gliclazide
      (2) Glipizide
      (3) Glyburide
      (4) Glimepiride
    c. Comparisons
      (1) Second-generation drugs most used in the United States
        (a) Fewer adverse effects
        (b) Fewer drug interactions
      (2) Tolbutamide preferred in elderly
        • Less potent leads to fewer hypoglycemic episodes

Tolbutamide preferred for elderly; less likely to cause severe hypoglycemia.

    d. Mechanism of action
      (1) Bind to ATP-sensitive potassium-channel (SUR1) receptors on the β cells
        (a) Depolarizing the membrane
        (b) Calcium-dependent exocytoses of insulin
      (2) Stimulate the release of insulin from the functional β cells of the pancreas
      (3) Orally effective hypoglycemic agents

Sulfonylureas increases pancreatic secretion of insulin.

    e. Use
      • Treatment of type 2 DM
    f. Adverse effects
      (1) Hypoglycemia

Endogenous hormones that counter-regulate insulin: glucagon, cortisol, epinephrine

Chlorpropamide noted for its disulfiram-like actions with alcohol.

      (2) Disulfiram-like reaction after ingestion of ethanol
        (a) Most prominent with chlorpropamide
        (b) Ethanol also inhibits gluconeogenesis; thus, hypoglycemia can occur more readily in patients receiving oral hypoglycemic drugs when consuming alcohol.
      (3) Allergic response in patients with sulfonamide allergies

Sulfonamide hypersensitivity: cross-hypersensitivity with sulfonamide antimicrobials, thiazides, furosemide, celecoxib

      (4) Syndrome of inappropriate antidiuretic hormone (SIADH)
        • Most prominent with chlorpropamide
  2. Meglitinides (secretagogues)
    a. Examples
      (1) Nateglinide
      (2) Repaglinide
    b. Mechanism of action
      (1) Binds to a site on the β cells and closes ATP-dependent potassium channels (SUR1)
      (2) Similar to the sulfonylureas

Meglitinides increase pancreatic secretion of insulin.

      (3) Unique in that it has a rapid onset and short duration
      (4) When taken just prior to meals, replicates physiologic insulin profiles
    c. Uses
      (1) Adjunct to diet and exercise in the treatment of type 2 DM

Repaglinide can be used in patients with sulfonamide hypersensitivity.

      (2) No sulfur in structure; can be given to patients with sulfonamide allergies
  3. Biguanide
    a. Example
      • Metformin

  b. Mechanism of action
  (1) Does *not* stimulate insulin release (euglycemic)
  (2) Improves glucose tolerance
    (a) Activates AMP-activated protein kinase (AMPK)
    (b) Reduces hepatic gluconeogenesis
    (c) Increases peripheral utilization of glucose
    (d) Direct stimulation of tissue glycolysis
    (e) Reduces gastrointestinal (GI) glucose absorption
    (f) Reduces plasma glucagon
  (3) Does *not* induce weight gain
  (4) Reduce macrovascular complications of type 2 DM
  c. Use
  (1) Treatment of type 2 DM
  (2) Treatment of gestational DM (unlabeled use)
  (3) Treatment of polycystic ovary syndrome (unlabeled use)
  d. Adverse effects
  (1) Lactic acidosis
    • Especially in patients who have cardiac/respiratory, renal, or hepatic disease and in chronic alcoholics
  (2) GI distress
  (3) Decreased vitamin B_{12} levels
4. Thiazolidinediones ("insulin sensitizers")
  a. Examples
  (1) Rosiglitazone
  (2) Pioglitazone
    • Troglitazone removed from the market because of hepatotoxicity
  b. Mechanism of action
  (1) Act via the peroxisome proliferator-activated receptor-γ (PPAR-γ)
    • A nuclear receptor that alters a number of gene products involved in glucose and lipid metabolism
  (2) Decrease hepatic gluconeogenesis
  (3) Enhance uptake of glucose by skeletal muscle cells
  c. Use
  (1) Treatment of type 2 DM
  (2) Especially in patients with insulin resistance
  d. Adverse effects
  (1) Elevated hepatic enzymes
    • Rare hepatic failure
  (2) Edema
  (3) Heart failure
    • Boxed warning in the United States: Thiazolidinediones may cause or exacerbate congestive heart failure.
5. α-Glucosidase inhibitors
  a. Examples
  (1) Acarbose
  (2) Miglitol
  b. Mechanism of action
  (1) Inhibitor of α-glucosidases in enterocytes of the small intestine
  (2) Results in delayed carbohydrate digestion
  (3) Delays and reduces absorption of glucose
    • α-Glucosidase inhibitors effectively lower postprandial serum glucose but have minimal effects on fasting glucose.
  c. Use
    • Treatment of type 2 DM
  d. Adverse effects
  (1) Abdominal pain
  (2) Diarrhea
  (3) Flatulence

C. Amylinomimetic
1. Example
  • Pramlintide is a synthetic analogue of amylin given by subcutaneous injection.

Metformin reduces hepatic gluconeogenesis.

Metformin often causes weight loss whereas secretagogues and insulin often promote weight gain in type 2 diabetics.

Metformin may cause lactic acidosis.

Note common ending -glitazone.

Thiazolidinediones decrease hepatic gluconeogenesis and insulin resistance in peripheral tissues.

Glitazones are "insulin sensitizers."

Glitazones are reported to exacerbate congestive heart failure.

α-Glucosidase inhibitors delay intestinal reabsorption of glucose.

2. Mechanism of action
  a. Amylin secretion
    (1) Absent in patients with type 1 DM
    (2) Decreased in patients with type 2 diabetes mellitus
  b. Amylin affects glucose concentrations
    (1) Slows gastric emptying
      • Without affecting absorption of nutrients
    (2) Suppresses postprandial glucagon secretion
    (3) Reduces appetite leading to decreased caloric intake
3. Uses
  a. Adjunct treatment of type 1 DM
    • Patients who use mealtime insulin therapy and who have failed to achieve desired glucose control despite optimal insulin therapy
  b. Adjunct treatment of type 2 DM
    (1) Patients who use mealtime insulin therapy
    (2) Who have failed to achieve desired glucose control despite optimal insulin therapy
    (3) With or without a concurrent sulfonylurea agent and/or metformin
  c. Adverse effects
    (1) Hypoglycemia
    (2) Nausea
    (3) Cause weight loss rather than weight gain

D. Incretin-based therapy
  1. Exenatide
    a. Given by subcutaneous injection
    b. Mechanism of action
      (1) An incretin mimetic
        (a) A 39-amino acid glucagon-like peptide-1 (GLP-1) agonist
          • Isolated from the salivary gland venom of the lizard *Heloderma suspectum* (Gila monster)
        (b) Endogenous incretins improve glycemic control once released into the circulation via the gut.
        (c) Exenatide mimics the enhancement of glucose-dependent insulin secretion and other antihyperglycemic actions of incretins.
    c. Use
      • Adjunctive treatment of type 2 DM
    d. Adverse effects
      (1) Hypoglycemia
      (2) GI distress
      (3) Decreased appetite
      (4) Pancreatitis
        • The U.S. Food and Drug Administration (FDA) issued information on reports of acute pancreatitis occurring in patients taking exenatide.
  2. Sitagliptin
    a. Orally effective dipeptidyl-peptidase-IV (DPP-IV) inhibitor
    b. Mechanism of action
      (1) Potentiates the effects of the incretin hormones by inhibiting their breakdown by DPP-IV
        (a) Glucagon-like peptide-1 (GLP-1)
        (b) Glucose-dependent insulinotropic peptide (GIP)
      (2) Decreases glucagon secretion from pancreatic α cells
    3. Use
      a. Type 2 diabetes mellitus with metformin in naïve patients
      b. Adjunctive treatment of type 2 diabetes mellitus
        (1) Add-on therapy to a sulfonylurea
        (2) Add-on therapy to a sulfonylurea plus metformin
    4. Adverse effects
      a. GI distress
      b. Nasopharyngitis
      c. Hypoglycemia

E. Therapeutic summary of selected drugs used to treat diabetes mellitus: (Table 24-3)

Pramlintide promotes weight loss in obese diabetics and inhibits glucagon secretion and gastric emptying.

Exenatide enhances glucose-dependent insulin secretion from pancreas.

Exenatide reported to cause acute pancreatitis.

Exenatide and sitagliptin mimic the actions of incretin hormones.

TABLE 24-3. **Therapeutic Summary of Selected Drugs Used to Treat Diabetes Mellitus**

DRUGS	CLINICAL APPLICATIONS	ADVERSE EFFECTS	CONTRAINDICATIONS
Mechanism: *Insulin replacement*			

Rapid-acting
  Insulin aspart
  Insulin glulisine
  Insulin lispro
Short-acting
  Regular insulin
Intermediate-acting
  NPH insulin
Long-acting
  Insulin glargine
  Insulin detemir
	Treatment of type 1 diabetes mellitus
	Adjunctive therapy for type 2 diabetes mellitus
		Hypoglycemia
		Lipodystrophy
			Hypersensitivity

Mechanism: *Stimulates insulin secretion from the pancreatic β cells; secretagogue*			

Sulfonylureas
First generation
  Chlorpropamide
  Tolazamide
  Tolbutamide
Second generation
  Gliclazide
  Glimepiride
  Glipizide
  Glyburide
	Treatment of type 2 diabetes mellitus	Hypoglycemia
		Disulfiram-like reaction with ethanol
		Allergies in patients with sulfonamide
		  hypersensitivity
		SIADH (particularly chlorpropamide)
			Hypersensitivity
			Patients with sulfonamide
			  allergies

Mechanism: *Stimulates insulin secretion from the pancreatic β cells; secretagogue*			
Nateglinide Repaglinide	Management of type 2 diabetes mellitus; alone or with other agents	Hypoglycemia Upper respiratory tract infection Hepatotoxicity	Hypersensitivity Diabetic ketoacidosis Type 1 diabetes mellitus
Mechanism: *Inhibits hepatic gluconeogenesis plus other mechanisms to provide euglycemic control*			

Metformin	Treatment of type 2 diabetes mellitus
	Treatment of gestational diabetes mellitus
	  (unlabeled use)
	Treatment of polycystic ovary syndrome
	  (unlabeled use)
		Lactic acidosis
		GI distress
		Decreased vitamin B_{12} levels
			Hypersensitivity
			Diabetic ketoacidosis
			Severe renal disease
			Severe liver disease
			Acute or chronic metabolic
			  acidosis
			Severe cardio/respiratory
			  disease

Mechanism: *Stimulate peroxisome proliferator-activated receptor-γ (PPAR-γ) to promote insulin sensitivity*			
Pioglitazone Rosiglitazone	Treatment of type 2 diabetes mellitus Especially in patients with insulin resistance	Elevated hepatic enzymes Rare hepatic failure Edema Heart failure	Hypersensitivity NYHA Class III/IV heart failure
Mechanism: *α-Glucosidases inhibitor; delays and reduces the absorption of glucose*			
Acarbose Miglitol	Treatment of type 2 diabetes mellitus	Abdominal pain Diarrhea Flatulence	Hypersensitivity Diabetic ketoacidosis Bowel disorders
Mechanism: *Mimics the action of endogenous amylin*			

Pramlintide	Adjunctive treatment in type 1 and type 2 diabetes
	  mellitus
	Especially useful in obese patients
		Hypoglycemia
		Nausea
		Cause weight loss rather than weight gain
			Hypersensitivity
			Gastroparesis
			Hypoglycemia
			  unawareness

Mechanism: *Analogue of the incretin (glucagon-like peptide 1; GLP-1) which increases insulin secretion*			
Exenatide	Adjunctive treatment in type 2 diabetes mellitus	Hypoglycemia GI distress Decreased appetite Pancreatitis	Hypersensitivity Diabetic ketoacidosis
Mechanism: *Potentiates the effects of the incretin hormones by inhibiting their breakdown*			
Sitagliptin	Adjunctive treatment in type 2 diabetes mellitus	GI distress Nasopharyngitis Hypoglycemia	Hypersensitivity Diabetic ketoacidosis
Mechanism: *↑ cAMP; Counter regulatory hormone to insulin; raises plasma glucose*			
Glucagon	Treat severe hypoglycemia Diagnostic uses Treat beta blocker overdose	Hyperglycemia GI distress	Hypersensitivity Insulinoma Pheochromocytoma

cAMP, cyclic adenosine monophosphate; GI, gastrointestinal; NPH, neutral protamine Hagedorn; NYHA, New York Heart Association; SIADH, syndrome of inappropriate antidiuretic hormone.

III. Hyperglycemic Agent
- Glucagon
  #### A. Regulation of secretion
  - Glucagon is synthesized by the α cells of the pancreas.
    1. Stimulators of release
        a. α-Adrenergic agents
        b. Amino acids
    2. Inhibitors of release
        a. Glucose
        b. Incretins (GLP-1)
        c. Somatostatin
        d. Free fatty acids
  #### B. Physiologic actions
  1. Glucagon increases blood glucose by stimulating liver.
      a. Glycogenolysis
      b. Gluconeogenesis
  2. Actions oppose insulin
      a. Hyperglycemia
      b. Gluconeogenesis
  #### C. Uses
  1. Severe hypoglycemia in unconscious patients (emergency use)
  2. Diagnostic uses
      a. Radiologic and contrast procedures (reduction of GI spasms)
      b. Glycogen storage disease
      c. Pheochromocytoma and insulinoma
      d. Growth hormone dysfunction
  3. Treat overdoses of beta blockers

Insulin produces hypoglycemia; Glucagon produces hyperglycemia.

Beta blocker overdose treated with glucagon

CHAPTER 25
DRUGS USED IN THE TREATMENT OF BONE AND CALCIUM DISORDERS

I. General Considerations

- Parathyroid hormone (PTH) and vitamin D play a role in the regulation of calcium and phosphorus (Fig. 25-1; and Table 25-1); See Rapid Review Pathology

A. Parathyroid hormone

1. Regulation of secretion
   a. Stimulated by hypocalcemia
   b. Stimulated by hyperphosphatemia
   c. Inhibited by hypercalcemia
   d. Inhibited by hypophosphatemia
2. Functions
   a. Increases calcium reabsorption in the early distal tubule
   b. Decreases bicarbonate reclamation in the proximal tubule
   c. Decreases phosphorus reabsorption in the proximal tubule
   d. Maintains ionized calcium level in blood
      - Increases bone resorption and renal reabsorption of calcium
   e. Increases synthesis of 1-α-hydroxylase in proximal renal tubule
      (1) Increases synthesis of 1,25(OH)$_2$D (dihydroxycholecalciferol; calcitriol)
      (2) Inhibits 24 hydroxylase in proximal tubule, which normally converts 25-hydroxycholecalciferol synthesized in the liver to *inactive* 24,25-(OH)$_2$D.
3. Use
   a. *No* therapeutic use of PTH
   b. Teriparatide, a PTH analogue, is used clinically.

B. Disorders of parathyroid function

1. Hypoparathyroidism
   a. Causes
      (1) Previous thyroid surgery (most common cause)
      (2) Autoimmune hypothyroidism
      (3) DiGeorge syndrome
         - Absent third and fourth pharyngeal pouch; no thymus or parathyroid glands
      (4) Hypomagnesemia
         (a) Magnesium is a cofactor for adenylyl cyclase.
         (b) Cyclic adenosine monophosphate (cAMP) is required for PTH activation.
   b. Clinical findings
      (1) Tetany
      (2) Calcification of basal ganglia
      (3) Cataracts
2. Hyperparathyroidism
   a. Primary hyperparathyroidism
      (1) Causes
         (a) Adenoma (85% of cases)
         (b) Primary hyperplasia
         (c) Carcinoma (rare)

Regulators of calcium and phosphorus: PTH, vitamin D, calcitonin.

PTH: ↑renal calcium reabsorption; ↓ renal phosphorus, bicarbonate reabsorption.

PTH: hypocalcemia/hyperphosphatemia ↑ PTH; hypercalcemia/hypophosphatemia ↓ PTH

Pulsatile administration of a PTH analogue increases calcium deposition in the bones

Hypoparathyroidism leads to a decrease in serum calcium and an increase in serum phosphate.

Primary hyperparathyroidism: may be seen with adenomas (most common), hyperplasia, or carcinomas of the gland.

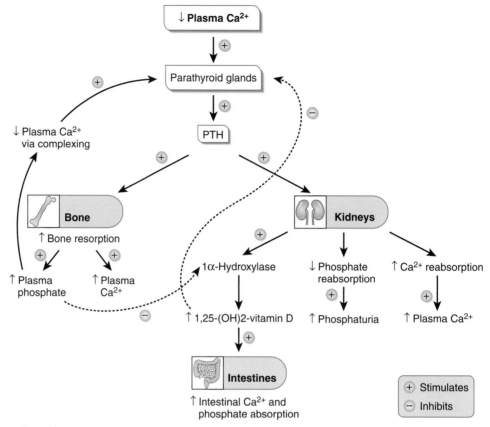

25-1: Parathyroid hormone (PTH) overview. *(From Brown TA. Rapid Review Physiology. Philadelphia, Mosby, 2007, Figure 3-20.)*

TABLE 25-1. **Actions of Parathyroid Hormone and Vitamin D on Intestine, Kidney, and Bone**

AREA OF ACTION	PARATHYROID HORMONE	VITAMIN D
Intestine	↑ Calcium and phosphate absorption by ↑synthesis of 1, 25-$(OH)_2$D	↑ Calcium and phosphate absorption
Kidney	↓ Calcium excretion ↑ Phosphate excretion	Calcium and phosphate excretion may be ↓ by 25-(OH)D and 1,25-$(OH)_2$D*
Bone	↑ Calcium and phosphate resorption in high doses Low doses may ↑bone formation	↑ Calcium and phosphate resorption by 1,25-$(OH)_2$D Bone formation may be ↑by 24,25-$(OH)_2$D (stimulates alkaline phosphatase)
Net effect on serum levels	↑ Serum calcium ↓ Serum phosphate	↑ Serum calcium ↑ Serum phosphate

*Direct effect; Vitamin D often ↑ urine calcium due to ↑ calcium absorption from the intestine and resulting ↓ PTH.

(2) Clinical findings
    (a) Renal stones
       • Most common presentation
    (b) Nephrocalcinosis
       • Calcification of collecting tubule basement membrane due to hypercalcemia
    (c) Peptic ulcer disease
       • Calcium stimulates gastrin release, which increases gastric acidity.
    (d) Cystic and hemorrhagic bone lesions
    (e) Diastolic hypertension
    (f) Band keratopathy in the limbus of the eye
  b. Secondary hyperparathyroidism
    • A compensatory mechanism when chronic hypocalcemia (malabsorption, vitamin D deficiency) is present

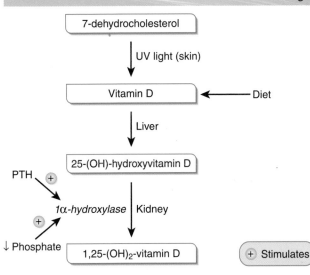

25-2: Vitamin D synthesis. PTH, parathyroid hormone; UV, ultraviolet. *(From Brown TA: Rapid Review Physiology. Philadelphia, Mosby, 2007, Figure 3-21.)*

C. Vitamin D
- Vitamin D deficiency causes rickets in children and osteomalacia in adults.
1. Sources and formation
   a. Dehydrocholesterol in the skin is photoconverted by sunlight to ergocalciferol (vitamin D_2) and cholecalciferol (vitamin D_3) in the skin.
      (1) Vitamin D_2 derivatives from plants
      (2) Vitamin D_3 derivatives from animals
      (3) Dihydrotachysterol (ergocalciferol analogue)
   b. Reabsorbed vitamin D precursors are first metabolized in the liver by the cytochrome P-450 system to 25-hydroxyvitamin D or 25-(OH)D (calcidiol), which is converted to metabolically active 1, 25-(OH)$_2$D$_3$ (calcitriol)by 1-α-hydroxylase in the proximal renal tubule cells (Fig. 25-2; see also Table 25-1).
      (1) Calcitriol: 1,25-(OH)$_2$D$_3$
         - Active form
      (2) Secalcifediol: 24,25-(OH)$_2$D$_3$
         - Inactive form
2. Vitamin D disorders
   a. Vitamin D deficiency
      (1) Causes
         (a) Decreased intake of vitamin D
         (b) Decreased exposure to sun light
            - Decreased conversion of 7-dehyrocholesterol to precursor vitamin D
         (c) Renal failure (most common cause of deficiency)
            - Decreased 1-α-hydroxylation
         (d) Chronic liver disease
            - Decreased 25-hydroxylation
         (e) Fat malabsorption
            - Decreased reabsorption of vitamin D
         (f) Increased metabolism
            - Cytochrome P-450 inducers increase conversion of 25-(OH)D to an inactive metabolite
   b. Excess vitamin D administration
      - May cause hypercalcemia with suppression of PTH
D. Calcitonin
1. Produced by the parafollicular cells of the thyroid gland.
2. Regulation of secretion
   - Hypercalcemia stimulates release
3. Mechanism of action (see Table 25-2)
   a. Inhibits bone resorption by osteoclasts
   b. Increases kidney excretion of:
      (1) Calcium
      (2) Phosphorus
   c. Lowers serum calcium and phosphate levels

Vitamin D_2 from plants.

Vitamin D_3 from animals.

Vitamin D deficiency: rickets (children) and osteomalacia (adults)

Calcitonin actions antagonize the effects of PTH on bone resorption.

II. **Drugs That Affect Calcium Levels** (Box 25-1)
   A. **Calcium salts**
      1. Calcium citrate (many other salts)
         a. Uses (given orally)
            (1) Antacid
            (2) Treatment and prevention of calcium deficiency or hyperphosphatemia
               (a) Osteoporosis
               (b) Osteomalacia
               (c) Mild/moderate renal insufficiency
               (d) Hypoparathyroidism
               (e) Postmenopausal osteoporosis
               (f) Rickets (type of osteomalacia in children)
         b. Adverse effects
            (1) Hypercalcemia
            (2) Constipation
      2. Calcium gluconate
         a. Uses (mostly given IV)
            (1) Treatment and prevention of hypocalcemia
            (2) Treatment of tetany
            (3) Treatment of cardiac disturbances of hyperkalemia
            (4) Treatment of hypocalcemia
            (5) Calcium supplementation
         b. Adverse effects
            (1) Arrhythmia
            (2) Hypotension
            (3) Constipation
   B. **Teriparatide** (a PTH analogue)
      1. Uses
         a. Osteoporosis in postmenopausal women at high risk of fracture
         b. Primary or hypogonadal osteoporosis in men at high risk of fracture
      2. Adverse effects
         a. Hypercalcemia
         b. Hyperuricemia
         c. Arthralgia
         d. Respiratory effects
   C. **Vitamin D analogues**
      1. Examples
         a. Calcitriol
         b. Cholecalciferol
         c. Dihydrotachysterol
         e. Doxercalciferol
         f. Ergocalciferol
         g. Paricalcitol

Calcium citrate given orally.

Calcium gluconate given intravenously.

Teriparatide, a PTH analogue, is given subcutaneously.

BOX 25-1   DRUGS THAT AFFECT CALCIUM LEVELS

Drugs That Increase Calcium Levels
Calcium citrate (many other salts)
Calcium gluconate
Teriparatide
Vitamin D Analogues
  Calcitriol
  Cholecalciferol
  Dihydrotachysterol
  Doxercalciferol
  Ergocalciferol
  Paricalcitol

Drugs That Decrease Calcium Levels
Bisphosphonates
  Alendronate

Calcitonin
Cinacalcet
Clodronate
Estrogens and raloxifene
Etidronate
Gallium nitrate
Ibandronate
Pamidronate
Phosphate
Risedronate
Tiludronate
Zoledronic acid

2. Uses
   a. Treatment of vitamin D deficiency
   b. Prophylaxis against vitamin D deficiency
   c. Rickets prevention
      • Given with calcium to supplement the diet of infants
   d. Hypoparathyroidism (with calcium supplements)
   e. Osteoporosis
      • Prevention and treatment
   f. Chronic renal disease
      (1) Calcitriol
      (2) Paricalcitol (Oral and IV)
3. Hypervitaminosis D
   a. Hypercalcemia
   b. Hyperphosphatemia
   c. Nephrocalcinosis
      • Calcification of collecting tubule basement membrane
   d. Calcification of soft tissues (e.g., skin)

D. Calcitonin
1. Uses
   a. Administered parenterally to treat hypercalcemia
   b. Paget's disease of bone
   c. Postmenopausal osteoporosis (intranasal)
2. Adverse effects
   a. Rhinitis
   b. Flushing
   c. Back pain

E. Cinacalcet
1. Mechanism of action
   a. Increases the sensitivity of the calcium-sensing receptor on the parathyroid gland
   b. This lowers serum calcium levels
2. Uses
   a. Treatment of secondary hyperparathyroidism in patients with chronic kidney disease on dialysis
   b. Treatment of hypercalcemia in patients with parathyroid carcinoma
3. Adverse effects
   a. Hypocalcemia
   b. GI distress
   c. Myalgia
   d. Hypertension
   e. Muscle weakness

F. Bisphosphonates
1. Mechanism of action
   • Bind to hydroxyapatite in bone, inhibiting osteoclast activity
2. Uses
   a. Postmenopausal bone loss
      (1) Alendronate (oral; once a week)
      (2) Risedronate (oral; once a week)
   b. Osteoporosis and compression fractures
      (1) Alendronate (oral; once a week)
      (2) Risedronate (oral; once a week)
      (3) Ibandronate (oral; once a month)
      (4) Zoledronic acid (IV; once a year)
   c. Hypercalcemia due to malignancy
      (1) Clodronate
      (2) Etidronate
      (3) Tiludronate
      (4) Zoledronic acid
   d. Paget's disease
      (1) Clodronate
      (2) Etidronate
      (3) Tiludronate
      (4) Zoledronic acid

Calcitriol is the preferred drug for management of hypocalcemia in dialysis-dependent renal failure patients.

Hypervitaminosis D: hypercalcemia, hyperphosphatemia, nephrocalcinosis, calcification of soft tissues

Calcitonin is given intranasally for treatment of osteoporosis.

Cinacalcet increases calcium-sensing by the parathyroid gland.

Alendronate and risedronate are given once a week to prevent osteoporosis.

Ibandronate is given once a month to prevent osteoporosis.

Zoledronic acid is infused once a year to prevent osteoporosis.

Note common ending -dronate for all bisphosphonates.

Bisphosphonates irritate
the stomach and
esophagus.

3. Adverse effects
   a. Reflux esophagitis (gastroesophageal reflux disease; GERD) when taken orally;
      avoid this by:
      (1) Taking these drugs on an empty stomach, with at least 8 oz water, immediately
          upon awakening
      (2) Remaining in an upright position for at least 30 minutes after taking the drug
      (3) Avoiding food or drink for 30 minutes after taking the drug
   b. Musculoskeletal pain
   c. Hypocalcemia
   d. Hypophosphatemia
   e. Osteonecrosis (jaw)

G. Estrogen or hormonal replacement therapy (HRT, see Chapter 26)

No evidence that
"natural" estrogens are
more or less efficacious or
safe than "synthetic"
estrogens when given at
equi-estrogenic doses.

   • Evidence-based medicine states that overall health risks from HRT in postmenopausal
     women appear to exceed the possible benefits.
   1. Mechanism of action
      • Reduces bone resorption
   2. Uses
      a. Postmenopausal osteoporosis (reduces bone loss)
      b. *Cannot* restore bone
   3. Adverse effects

When prescribing
estrogens solely for the
prevention of
osteoporosis, use only for
women at significant risk
of osteoporosis;
nonestrogen drugs should
always be considered as
alternatives.

      a. Similar to oral contraceptives but to a lesser extent because of lower estrogen content
      b. The Women's Health Initiative (WHI) Trial reported an increase in the incidence of
         strokes in both the estrogen-alone and the estrogen-progestin subgroups as
         compared with placebo groups.
      c. Thromboembolism

H. Raloxifene
   1. Selective estrogen receptor modulator (SERM)
      a. Agonist in bone
      b. Antagonist in breast
      c. Antagonist in uterus

Drugs used in the
prevention and treatment
of postmenopausal
osteoporosis: estrogens
with or without
progestins,
bisphosphonates,
raloxifene, calcium,
fluoride

   2. Uses
      a. Prevention and treatment of osteoporosis in postmenopausal women
      b. Risk reduction for invasive breast cancer in postmenopausal women with
         osteoporosis
      c. Risk reduction in postmenopausal women with high risk for invasive breast cancer
   3. Adverse effects

Raloxifene increases risk
of thromboembolism.

      a. Thromboembolism
      b. Peripheral edema
      c. Hot flashes
      d. Headache
      e. Depression
      f. Vaginal bleeding

Gallium nitrate inhibits
osteoclasts.

I. Gallium nitrate
   1. Mechanism of action
      • Inhibits bone resorption by inhibiting osteoclast function.
   2. Uses
      • Treatment of symptomatic cancer-related hypercalcemia.
   3. Adverse effects
      a. Edema
      b. Hypotension
      c. Tachycardia
      d. Hypophosphatemia
      e. Bicarbonate loss
      f. Hypocalcemia

J. Phosphate
   • Quickly lowers serum calcium levels when given intravenously

K. Therapeutic summary of selected drugs used to affect calcium levels: (Table 25-2)

TABLE 25-2. **Therapeutic Summary of Selected Drugs Used to Affect Calcium Levels**

DRUGS	CLINICAL APPLICATIONS	ADVERSE EFFECTS	CONTRAINDICATIONS
Mechanism: *Increase availability of calcium; given orally*			
Calcium citrate	Treatment and prevention of calcium deficiency Antacid	Constipation Hypercalcemia	Hypersensitivity Hypercalcemia Renal calculi Ventricular fibrillation
Mechanism: *Increase availability of calcium; given intravenously*			
Calcium gluconate	Treatment and prevention of hypocalcemia Treatment of tetany Treatment of cardiac disturbances of hyperkalemia Treatment of hypocalcemia	Arrhythmia Hypotension Constipation	Hypersensitivity Hypercalcemia Renal calculi Ventricular fibrillation with digoxin
Mechanism: *Parathyroid hormone analogue*			
Teriparatide	Osteoporosis in postmenopausal women at high risk of fracture Primary or hypogonadal osteoporosis in men at high risk of fracture	Hypercalcemia Hyperuricemia Arthralgia Respiratory effects	Hypersensitivity
Mechanism: *Increase calcium absorption from gastrointestinal tract; increase calcium resorption from bone; decrease calcium excretion in the kidney*			
Vitamin D analogues Calcitriol Cholecalciferol Dihydrotachysterol Doxercalciferol Ergocalciferol Paricalcitol	Treatment of vitamin D deficiency Prophylaxis against Vitamin D deficiency Rickets prevention Hypoparathyroidism Osteoporosis Chronic renal disease (calcitriol, paricalcitol)	Hypercalcemia Nephrocalcinosis	Hypersensitivity Evidence of vitamin D toxicity Hypercalcemia
Mechanism: *Antagonizes the effects of parathyroid hormone by inhibiting osteoclast activity*			
Calcitonin	Treatment of: Hypercalcemia Paget's disease of bone Postmenopausal osteoporosis (intranasal)	Rhinitis Flushing Back pain	Hypersensitivity
Mechanism: *Increases the sensitivity of the calcium-sensing receptor on the parathyroid gland*			
Cinacalcet	Treatment of secondary hyperparathyroidism in patients with chronic kidney disease on dialysis Treatment of hypercalcemia in patients with parathyroid carcinoma	Hypocalcemia GI distress Myalgia Hypertension Muscle weakness	Hypersensitivity
Mechanism: *Bind to hydroxyapatite in bone, inhibiting osteoclast activity*			

Bisphosphonates
Alendronate
Clodronate
Etidronate
Ibandronate
Pamidronate
Risedronate
Tiludronate
Zoledronic acid
	Osteoporosis
	Hypercalcemia due to malignancy
	Paget's disease of bone
		Esophageal
		    erosions
		Musculoskeletal
		    pain
		Hypocalcemia
		Hypophosphatemia
		Osteonecrosis
		    (jaw)
			Hypersensitivity
			Hypocalcemia
			Abnormalities of the
			    esophagus

Mechanism: *Selective estrogen receptor modulator (SERM)*			
Raloxifene	Osteoporosis in postmenopausal women (controversial) Breast cancer prevention	Thromboembolism Peripheral edema Hot flashes Headache Depression Vaginal bleeding	Thromboembolic disorders Pregnancy Breast-feeding

CHAPTER 26
DRUGS USED IN REPRODUCTIVE ENDOCRINOLOGY

I. Drugs That Act on the Uterus (Box 26-1)

   A. Oxytocin

      1. General considerations

         a. Peptide hormone

            (1) Synthesized in the hypothalamus

            (2) Transported to the posterior pituitary by nerves (neurohypophysis)

            (3) Stored in the posterior pituitary

            (4) Released as needed

         b. Has a facilitatory role in parturition

         c. Essential element in the milk-ejection reflex

           • Suckling stimulates oxytocin release, which leads to milk "let-down."

         d. Involved in several behaviors

             (1) Mating

            (2) Parental

            (3) Social

            (4) Emotional bond between mother and child

         e. Oxytocin may have a protective role against stress-related diseases.

      2. Mechanism of action

         a. Stimulates contraction of uterine muscle

         b. Stimulates smooth muscles of mammary glands

      3. Uses

         a. Induction of labor (IV infusion)

         b. Control of postpartum hemorrhage (IM or IV infusion)

         c. Prevent bleeding post D & C (dilation and curettage) procedure (IM or IV infusion)

         d. Treatment of incomplete, inevitable, or elective abortion (IV infusion; less common use)

         e. Stimulate milk letdown reflex (intranasal)

      4. Adverse effects

         a. Fetus or neonate

             (1) Arrhythmia

            (2) Permanent brain damage

            (3) Retinal damage

            (4) Fetal death

         b. Mother

             (1) Uterine rupture

            (2) Arrhythmia

            (3) Hypertension

      5. Contraindications

         a. Fetal distress

         b. Prematurity

         c. When vaginal delivery is contraindicated

             (1) Abnormal fetal presentation

            (2) Cephalopelvic disproportion

Oxytocin is referred to as an anti-stress hormone.

Oxytocin is used to induce labor and to manage postpartum bleeding.

Oxytocin is used in contraction stress tests.

BOX 26-1 **DRUGS THAT ACT ON THE UTERUS**

Drugs That Cause Contraction
Ergot alkaloids: ergonovine, methylergonovine
Oxytocin
Prostaglandins: dinoprostone (PGE_2), carboprost ($PGF_{2\alpha}$), misoprostol (PGE_1 analogue)

Drugs That Cause Relaxation
β_2-Adrenoceptor agonists: terbutaline, ritodrine
Magnesium sulfate
Nifedipine
Nonsteroidal anti-inflammatory drugs (NSAIDs)

      (3) Invasive cervical cancer
      (4) Active genital herpes
      (5) Prolapse of the cord
B. Prostaglandins
  1. Examples
    a. Dinoprostone (PGE_2)
    b. Carboprost ($PGF_{2\alpha}$)
    c. Misoprostol (PGE_1 analogue)
  2. Mechanism of action
    a. Potent stimulation of uterine contractions
    b. PGE_2 plays an important role in cervical ripening.
  3. Uses
    a. Induction of abortion
      (1) Dinoprostone (PGE_2): intravaginal
      (2) Carboprost ($PGF_{2\alpha}$): IM
      (3) Misoprostol (PGE_1 analogue): oral and intravaginal
    b. Softening of the cervix (cervical ripening) before induction of labor (administered intravaginally)
    c. Facilitation of delivery of intrauterine fetus (especially immature fetus)
  4. Adverse effects
    a. Prolonged vaginal bleeding
    b. Severe uterine cramps
    c. Gastrointestinal (GI) distress (systemic administration)
    d. Carboprost is contraindicated in asthma
C. Ergot alkaloids and related compounds
  1. Examples
    a. Ergonovine
    b. Methylergonovine
  2. Mechanism of action
    a. Increases motor activity of the uterus
    b. Results in forceful, prolonged contractions
  3. Use to treat
    a. Postpartum bleeding
    b. Hemorrhage after miscarriage
    c. Hemorrhage after D & C procedure
  4. Adverse effects
    a. Hypertension/hypotension
    b. Bradycardia/tachycardia
    c. Nausea and vomiting
    d. Abdominal pain
    e. Prolactin suppression
    f. Acute myocardial infarction
  5. Contraindication
    a. Hypertension
    b. Toxemia
    c. Pregnancy

Don't use oxytocin if vaginal delivery is contraindicated.

Prostaglandins used for cervical ripening

Carboprost contraindicated in asthma

Ergot alkaloids should *only* be used post partum.

Don't use ergot alkaloids in hypertensive patients.

D. Other drugs that affect the uterus

1. Nonsteroidal anti-inflammatory drugs (NSAIDs)
   a. Mechanism of action
      - Inhibit prostaglandin synthesis
   b. Use
      (1) Relief of cramps associated with menstruation (dysmenorrhea)
      (2) Blocks endometrial synthesis of prostaglandins during menstruation
         - NSAIDs are contraindicated in late second and all of third trimester; close ductus arteriosus necessary for fetal circulation.

Don't administer NSAIDs during late second or third trimester of pregnancy; premature closure of ductus arteriosus.

2. β₂-Adrenoceptor agonist (see Chapter 5)
   a. Examples
      (1) Terbutaline (actually used)
      (2) Ritodrine (approved by the U.S. Food and Drug Administration [FDA])
   b. Mechanism of action
      (1) Increases cyclic adenosine monophosphate (cAMP) via activation of β₂-adrenoceptors
      (2) Relaxes uterine smooth muscle
   c. Uses
      (1) Prevention of premature labor (controversial)
      (2) Relax hyper-stimulated (tetanic contraction) uterus
      (3) Relax uterus for external version breech (turning of fetus)

Terbutaline blocks hyper-stimulated uterus.

3. Magnesium sulfate
   a. Mechanism of action
      (1) Required for movement of calcium, sodium and potassium out of cells
      (2) Relaxes uterine muscle
      (3) Reduces transmitter release
   b. Uses
      (1) Prevention of premature labor (tocolytic agent)
      (2) Prevention and treatment of seizures in severe preeclampsia or eclampsia
      (3) Treatment and prevention of hypomagnesemia
      (4) Treatment of pediatric acute nephritis
      (5) Treatment of torsade de pointes
      (6) Treatment of cardiac arrhythmias ([VT/VF]) caused by hypomagnesemia
      (7) Short-term treatment of constipation
   c. Adverse effects (magnesium toxicity)
      - Reversed with calcium gluconate
         (1) Hypertension
         (2) Shock
         (3) Myocardial infarction
         (4) Nausea and vomiting
         (5) Pulmonary edema
         (6) Cardiovascular collapse
         (7) Hypotonia (muscle weakness)
            - Myasthenia gravis is an absolute contraindication

Magnesium toxicity reversed with calcium gluconate

Myasthenia gravis is an absolute contraindication for magnesium sulfate.

4. Nifedipine (see Chapter 14)
   a. Mechanism of action
      (1) Calcium channel antagonist
      (2) Relaxes vascular smooth muscles (e.g., uterus)
   b. Use
      (1) Prevent preterm labor (IV administration)
      (2) Cardiovascular uses (see Chapters 12–14)
   c. Adverse effects
      (1) Hypotension
      (2) Flushing
      (3) Headache
      (4) Dizziness
      (5) Nausea
      (6) Nervousness
      (7) Nasal congestion
   d. Contraindication
      (1) Aortic stenosis
      (2) Congestive heart failure
      (3) *Don't* use with magnesium sulfate; masks magnesium toxicity

Intravenous nifedipine used to prevent preterm labor

Don't use nifedipine with magnesium sulfate.

E. **Therapeutic summary of selected uterine drugs** (Table 26-1)

II. **Estrogens and Related Drugs** (Box 26-2)

    A. **Estrogens**

        1. Synthesis and secretion (Fig. 26-1)

            a. Synthesized in ovarian follicles

                • Aromatase conversion of testosterone to estradiol in granulosa cells

            b. Controlled by follicle-stimulating hormone (FSH)

                • FSH increases aromatase synthesis in granulosa cells.

            c. Major secretory product of the ovary is estradiol

        2. Physiologic actions

            a. Necessary for the normal maturation of females

            b. Important for the proliferation of endometrial tissue

            c. Required for normal menstrual cycling (Fig. 26-2)

Table 26-1. Therapeutic Summary of Selected Uterine Drugs

DRUGS	CLINICAL APPLICATIONS	ADVERSE EFFECTS	CONTRAINDICATIONS
Mechanism: *Produces rhythmic uterine contractions characteristic of the delivery process*			

Oxytocin	Induction of labor
	Control of postpartum hemorrhage
		Fetus or neonate
		Arrhythmia
		Permanent brain damage
		Retinal damage
		Fetal death
		Mother
		Uterine rupture
		Postpartum hemorrhage
		  Arrhythmia
		Hypertension
			Hypersensitivity
			Significant cephalopelvic
			  disproportion
			Unfavorable fetal positions
			Fetal distress
			Hypertonic or hyperactive
			  uterus
			When vaginal delivery is
			  contraindicated

Mechanism: *Stimulates uterine contractions and produces cervical ripening similar to those seen during natural labor*			

Dinoprostone (PGE₂)
Carboprost (PGF2α)
Misoprostol
  (PGE₁ analogue)
	Induction of abortion
	Cervical ripening
	Induction of tissue passage for demised fetus
		Prolonged vaginal bleeding
		Severe uterine cramps
		GI distress (systemic
		  administration)
			Hypersensitivity
			Significant cephalopelvic
			  disproportion
			Unfavorable fetal positions
			Fetal distress
			Hypertonic or hyperactive uterus
			Active herpes genitalia
			When vaginal delivery is
			  contraindicated

Mechanism: *Increases motor activity of the uterus; produces forceful and prolonged contractions*			
Ergonovine Methylergonovine	Prevention and treatment of postpartum and post- abortion hemorrhage	Nausea and vomiting Abdominal pain Prolactin suppression	Hypersensitivity With potent inhibitors of CYP3A4 Induction of labor Threatened spontaneous abortion Hypertension Pregnancy
Mechanism: *Increases cAMP via activation of β₂-adrenoceptors; relaxes uterine smooth muscle*			

Terbutaline (actually
  used)
Ritodrine (FDA
  approved)
	Prevention of premature labor	Tremors
		Nervousness
		Xerostomia
		Tachycardia
		Hypertension
			Hypersensitivity
			Cardiac arrhythmias

Mechanism: *Relaxes smooth muscles including uterine muscle; reduces transmitter release*			

Magnesium sulfate	Prevention of premature labor (tocolytic agent)
	Prevention and treatment of seizures in severe pre-
	  eclampsia or eclampsia
	Treatment and prevention of hypomagnesemia
	Treatment of pediatric acute nephritis
	Treatment of torsade de pointes
	Treatment of cardiac arrhythmias (VT/VF) caused by
	  hypomagnesemia
	Short-term treatment of constipation
		Hypertension
		Shock
		Myocardial infarction
		Nausea and vomiting
			Hypersensitivity
			Heart block
			Myocardial damage

Mechanism: *Inhibit prostaglandin synthesis*			

NSAIDs
  Aspirin
  Ibuprofen
  Naproxen
	Relief of cramps associated with menstruation
	  (dysmenorrhea)
		GI effects
		Bleeding
		Tinnitus
		Fluid retention
		Hypocalcemia
			Hypersensitivity
			Bleeding
			Thrombocytopenia
			Coagulation defects
			Necrotizing enterocolitis
			Significant renal dysfunction

cAMP, cyclic adenosine monophosphate; FDA, U.S. Food and Drug Administration; GI, gastrointestinal; VT, ventricular tachycardia; VF, ventricular fibrillation.

BOX 26-2   GONADAL HORMONES AND INHIBITORS

Estrogen Derivatives
Estradiol
Estrogens (conjugated A/synthetic)
Estrogens (conjugated B/synthetic)
Estrogens (conjugated/equine)
Estrogens (esterified)
Estropipate

Estrogen and Progestin Combinations
Drospirenone and estradiol (HRT; oral)
Estradiol and levonorgestrel (HRT; patch)
Estradiol and norethindrone (HRT; patch)
Estradiol and norgestimate (HRT; oral)
Estrogens (conjugated/equine) and
medroxyprogesterone (HRT; oral)
Estrogens (esterified) and methyltestosterone (HRT;
oral)
Ethinyl estradiol and desogestrel (OC)
Ethinyl estradiol and drospirenone (OC)
Ethinyl estradiol and ethynodiol diacetate (OC)
Ethinyl estradiol and etonogestrel (VRC)
Ethinyl estradiol and levonorgestrel (OC)
Ethinyl estradiol and norelgestromin (PC)
Ethinyl estradiol and norethindrone (OC)
Ethinyl estradiol and norgestimate (OC)
Ethinyl estradiol and norgestrel (OC)
Mestranol and norethindrone (OC)

**Selective Estrogen Receptor Modulators
(SERMs)**
Clomiphene
Raloxifene
Tamoxifen
Toremifene

Progestins
Etonogestrel
Levonorgestrel
Medroxyprogesterone
Megestrol
Norethindrone
Progesterone

Antiprogestins
Danazol
Mifepristone

Androgens
Danazol
Fluoxymesterone
Methyltestosterone
Nandrolone
Oxandrolone
Testolactone
Testosterone

Antiandrogens
Androgen receptor blockers
    Bicalutamide
    Flutamide
    Nilutamide
5 α-Reductase inhibitors
    Dutasteride
    Finasteride

GnRH Analogues
Goserelin
Leuprolide

HRT, hormonal replacement therapy; OC, oral contraceptive; VRC, vaginal ring contraceptive; PC, patch contraceptives

3. Pharmacokinetics
   a. Metabolized by the liver
      • High first-pass metabolism
   b. Enterohepatic cycling contributes to increased protein synthesis responsible for adverse effects.
      (1) Clotting factors (e.g., fibrinogen, V, VIII)
      (2) Angiotensinogen (renin substrate)
         • Most common cause of hypertension in young women
      (3) Steroid hormone transport proteins
         (a) Thyroid-binding globulin (TBG)
            • Increases total serum thyroxine (T_4) without increasing free (unbound) T_4 or serum thyroid stimulating hormone (TSH)
         (b) Corticosteroid-binding globulin (CBG)
            • Increases total serum cortisol without increasing free (unbound) cortisol or serum adrenocorticotropic hormone (ACTH)
         (c) Sex hormone-binding globulin (SHBG)
            • Decreases free testosterone levels; useful in treating hirsutism.
         (d) Transdermal and intravaginal preparations may reduce these effects.
4. Uses
   a. Oral contraception
   b. Estrogen replacement therapy (ERT)
      (1) Primary hypogonadism
      (2) Postmenopausal women (reduces vasomotor symptoms)
   c. Osteoporosis

Enterohepatic cycling of estrogens contributes to increased protein synthesis responsible for many adverse effects.

Estrogen increases synthesis of angiotensinogen; most common cause of hypertension in young women.

Estrogen increases synthesis of TBG and CBG without affecting free hormone levels

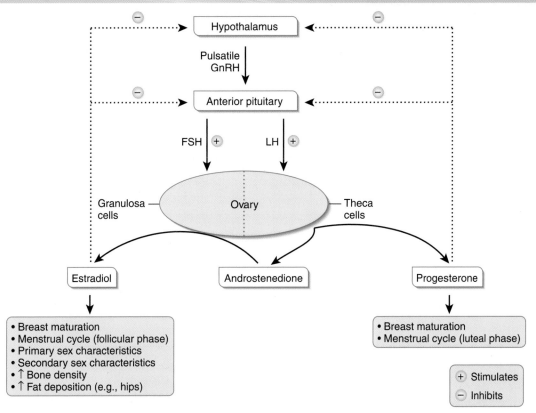

26-1: Female axis. FSH, follicle-stimulating hormone; GnRH, gonadotropin-releasing hormone; LH, luteinizing hormone. *(From Brown TA: Rapid Review Physiology. Philadelphia, Mosby, 2007, Figure 3-14.)*

      (1) Prevention and treatment
      (2) Usually should consider alternative treatments (See Chapter 25)
   d. Treatment of vulvar and vaginal atrophy
   e. Treat postmenopausal urogenital symptoms of the lower urinary tract (urinary urgency, dysuria)
   f. Suppression of ovulation in women with intractable dysmenorrhea or excessive ovarian androgen secretion
  5. Adverse effects
   a. Postmenopausal bleeding during ERT
   b. Nausea
   c. Breast tenderness
   d. Increased incidence of:
      (1) Migraine headaches
      (2) Intrahepatic cholestasis
      (3) Hypertension
        • Due to increase in angiotensinogen
      (4) Cholesterol gallstones
        • Due to increased mobilization of cholesterol in peripheral tissue to the liver by high-density lipoprotein (synthesis increased by estrogen)
      (5) Thrombophlebitis
      (6) Deep vein thrombosis with thromboembolism
        (a) Due to increase in synthesis of clotting factors and decreased synthesis of antithrombin III
        (b) Causes blood clots, heart attack and stroke
        (c) Markedly increased risk in smokers
          • Oral contraceptives are contraindicated in smokers.
        (d) Increased in family history of blood clots
      (7) Increased platelet aggregation
      (8) Accelerated blood clotting

Hormonal replacement therapy no longer considered appropriate choice to prevent osteoporosis in postmenopausal women.

Oral contraceptives are thrombogenic; contraindicated in smokers.

Conditions associated with thromboembolism are the greatest risk of estrogen-containing preparations.

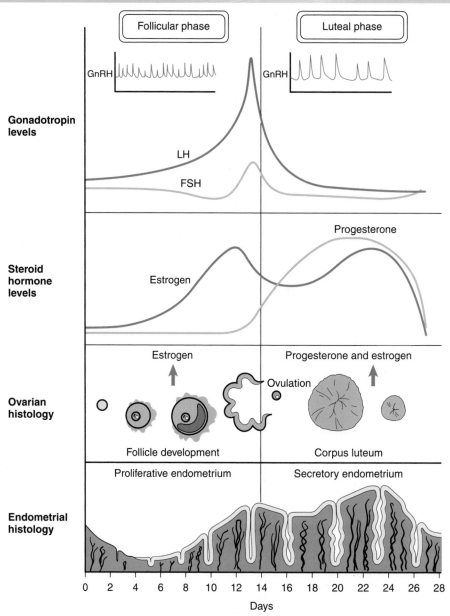

26-2: Hormonal secretion during the human menstrual cycle. FSH, follicle-stimulating hormone; GnRH, gonadotropin-releasing hormone; LH, luteinizing hormone. *(From Brenner G and Stevens C: Pharmacology, 3rd ed. Philadelphia, Saunders, 2010, Figure 34-2.)*

6. Contraindications
   a. Estrogen-dependent neoplasms (e.g., endometrial carcinoma)
   b. Known or suspected carcinoma of the breast
   c. Liver disease
   d. History of thromboembolic disorders
   e. Smoking
   f. Pregnancy
   g. Undiagnosed abnormal vaginal bleeding
   h. Porphyria

7. Boxed warnings
   a. The risk of dementia may be increased in postmenopausal women.
   b. Adequate diagnostic measures, including endometrial sampling, if indicated, should be performed to rule out malignancy in all cases of undiagnosed abnormal vaginal bleeding.
      (1) Unopposed estrogens (lack of progestin) may increase the risk of endometrial carcinoma in postmenopausal women with an intact uterus.
      (2) Oral contraceptives with progestin protect against developing endometrial carcinoma.

Women who smoke should not use estrogens.

Unopposed estrogen therapy should not be used in women with an intact uterus.

    c. Estrogens with or without progestin should *not* be used to prevent coronary heart disease.

    d. Estrogens with or without progestin should be used for shortest duration possible at the lowest effective dose consistent with treatment goals.

B. Selective estrogen receptor modulators (SERMs)
1. General considerations
   a. Agonists in some tissues
   b. Antagonists in other tissues
   c. SERMs are partial agonists
2. Clomiphene
   a. Mechanism of action
      (1) Blocks estrogen negative feedback
      (2) Causing an increase in FSH and luteinizing hormone (LH)
   b. Use
      • Stimulate ovulation in the treatment of infertility
   c. Adverse effects
      (1) Ovarian enlargement
      (2) Multiple pregnancies (incidence 5–10%)
      (3) Hot flashes
3. Tamoxifen and toremifene
   a. Mechanism of action
      (1) Estrogen receptor antagonist in the breast
      (2) Estrogen receptor agonist in the uterus
         • Because it is an agonist in the uterus, it is associated with an increased risk of endometrial hyperplasia and cancer.
      (3) Estrogen receptor agonist in the bone
   b. Uses
      (1) Treatment of metastatic (female and male) breast cancer
      (2) Adjuvant treatment of breast cancer
      (3) Reduce risk of invasive breast cancer in women with ductal carcinoma *in situ* (DCIS)
      (4) Reduce the incidence of breast cancer in women at high risk
   c. Adverse effects
      (1) Hot flashes (flushes)
      (2) Nausea and vomiting (incidence 25%)
      (3) Hypertension
      (4) Peripheral edema
      (5) Fluid retention
      (6) Vaginal bleeding
      (7) Endometrial hyperplasia and cancer
4. Raloxifene (see Chapter 25)
   a. Mechanism of action
      (1) Partial agonist in bone but does not stimulate the endometrium or breast
      (2) Does increase risk of deep vein thrombosis and thromboembolic events
   b. Uses
      (1) Prevention and treatment of osteoporosis in postmenopausal women
      (2) Risk reduction for invasive breast cancer in postmenopausal women with osteoporosis and in postmenopausal women with high risk for invasive breast cancer

C. Progestins
1. General considerations
   a. Progesterone is the most important progestin in humans (see Fig. 26-1 and Fig. 26-2)
   b. The newer third-generation progestins have less androgenic effects.
      (1) Norgestimate
      (2) Desogestrel
2. Synthesis and secretion
   a. Sites of synthesis
      (1) Ovary
      (2) Testes
      (3) Adrenal cortex
      (4) Placenta
   b. LH regulates synthesis and secretion.
   c. LH stimulates the corpus luteum of pregnancy.

The Women's Health Initiative (WHI) Trial reported an increase in the incidence of strokes in both the estrogen-alone and the estrogen-progestin subgroups as compared with placebo groups.

Clomiphene noted for causing multiple births.

Tamoxifen is an estrogen antagonist in the breast but an agonist in the uterus and bone.

Tamoxifen causes endometrial hyperplasia and increased incidence of endometrial cancer.

SERMs increase risk of thromboembolic disease.

3. Physiologic actions
   a. Contributes to the development of a secretory endometrium in the normal cycle and pregnancy
4. Uses
   a. Hormonal contraception
   b. Down-regulate endometrial lining to treat endometrial hyperplasia or cancer (non-surgical candidates)
      • Glands undergo atrophy
   c. Dysmenorrhea, endometriosis, uterine bleeding disorders
   d. Hirsutism
   e. Hormonal replacement therapy (estrogens and progestins)
   f. Acne vulgaris
      • Norgestimate/ethinyl estradiol

Norgestimate/ethinyl estradiol reduces acne vulgaris in young women.

5. Adverse effects
   a. Increased risk of breast cancer
   b. Bone mineral density loss
   c. Risk of dementia in postmenopausal women
   d. Weight gain (mild mineralocorticoid activity); stimulates appetite
      • This may be beneficial in anorexic patients
6. Boxed warnings

Long-term use of progestins causes a loss of bone mineral density.

   a. Prolonged use of medroxyprogesterone contraceptive injection may result in a loss of bone mineral density
   b. Long-term use (i.e., >2 years) should be limited to situations where other birth control methods are inadequate

D. **Antiprogestins**
   1. Mifepristone (RU 486)
      a. Medical termination of intrauterine pregnancy, through day 49 of pregnancy.
      b. Patients may need misoprostol and possibly surgery to complete therapy.

Mifepristone is used to terminate pregnancy.

   2. Danazol
      a. Mechanism of action
         (1) Decreases secretion of FSH and LH
         (2) Has weak progestational, androgenic, and glucocorticoid actions
      b. Uses
         (1) Endometriosis
         (2) Fibrocystic disease of the breast
         (3) Hereditary angioedema
      c. Adverse effects
         (1) Androgenic effects
         (2) Alopecia (male pattern baldness)
         (3) Edema
         (4) Hirsutism
         (5) Seborrhea
         (6) Weight gain

III. **Contraceptives**
   A. **Types**
      1. Oral estrogen-progestin combination contraceptives
         a. Estrogen components
            (1) Ethinyl estradiol
            (2) Mestranol
         b. Progestin component
            (1) Desogestrel
            (2) Drospirenone
            (3) Ethynodiol diacetate
            (4) Levonorgestrel
            (5) Norethindrone
            (6) Norgestimate
            (7) Norgestrel
         c. Monophasic combination tablets

Oral estrogen-progestin combination contraceptives are the most common form of contraception.

            • Same combination of estrogen and progestin given for 21 days and stopped for 7 days each month

d. Biphasic combination tablets
- Same estrogen dose for 21 days, with a higher progestin dose in the last 10 days of each month

e. Triphasic combination tablets
- Generally the same estrogen dose for 21 days, with a varying progestin dose over the 3 weeks of administration

f. 24 Day pill regimen
- Loestrin® 24 Fe; Ethinyl estradiol 0.02 mg and norethindrone acetate 1 mg for 24 days and ferrous fumarate for 4 days

g. Extended cycle oral contraceptives
   (1) One active tablet/day for 84 consecutive days, followed by 1 inactive tablet/day for 7 days
   (2) If all doses have been taken on schedule and one menstrual period is missed, pregnancy should be ruled out prior to continuing therapy.

> Extended cycle oral contraceptives gaining in popularity.

2. Vaginal ring estrogen-progestin contraceptive
   a. Ethinyl and etonogestrel
   b. Procedure
      (1) Ring inserted vaginally; left in place for 3 consecutive weeks
      (2) Then removed for 1 week
      (3) New ring inserted 7 days later; even if bleeding is *not* complete
      (4) New ring should be inserted at approximately the same time of day the old ring was removed

3. Transdermal (patch) estrogen-progestin contraceptive
   a. Ethinyl estradiol and norelgestromin
   b. Procedure
      (1) Apply one patch each week for 3 weeks (21 total days).
      (2) Then one week patch-free
      (3) Apply each patch on the same day each week.
      (4) *Only* one patch should be worn at a time.
      (5) *No* more than 7 days patch-free interval
   c. FDA posted concerns that use of the ethinyl estradiol and norelgestromin transdermal patch may increase the risk of blood clots in some women.

> The contraceptive patch may increase blood clots in some women since the area-under-the curve (AUC) is high in some women due to more extensive dermal absorption.

4. Continuous progestins
   a. Daily progestin (norethindrone) tablets
   - For patients in whom estrogen administration is undesirable
   b. Etonogestrel implantation
   - Implant 1 rod in the inner side of the upper arm; remove *no* later than 3 years after the date of insertion.

> Continuous progestins are preferred as contraceptives in women who should *not* take estrogens (e.g., heavy smokers).

5. Intrauterine device (IUD)
   a. Two types used in the United States
      (1) Copper (TCu-380A) IUD
         (a) T-shaped device produces sterile inflammatory reaction
         (b) Copper salts alter the endometrium and cervical mucus
      (2) Two hormone-containing IUDs:
         (a) Progesterone-releasing device
         - Releases to diffuse into the endometrial cavity, and cause decidualization and atrophy of the endometrium (approved for 1 year)
         (b) Levonorgestrel-releasing device
         - Releases levonorgestrel gradually at a rate of 20 micrograms/day (approved for 5 years)

> Progesterone-releasing IUDs preferred over copper containing IUDs.

      (3) Do *not* leave any one system in place for more than 5 years.
         - Pelvic actinomycosis may occur in 20% of cases.
      (4) Progestin contraceptive mechanisms
         (a) Thickening of cervical mucus
         (b) Inhibition of ovulation (but *not* always)
         (c) Inhibition of implantation
         (d) *Not* effective once the implantation process has occurred
      (5) Contraindication of IUDs
         (a) Patients with multiple sex partners
         - If in place with sexually transmitted diseases (STDs) there is increased risk of pelvic inflammatory disease (PID)

> IUDs should *not* be used in women with multiple sex partners.

B. **Mechanism of action of hormonal contraceptives**
1. Combination contraceptives
   a. Selectively inhibit pituitary function
      (1) LH and FSH release
      (2) Blocks ovulation
         • Blocks the positive feedback of estrogen on LH producing the LH surge, which is normally responsible for ovulation
   b. Pituitary most important site
2. Progestin-only contraceptives
   a. Affect ovarian function
   b. Cervical mucus

C. **Uses**
1. Contraception
2. Emergency contraception
   a. Higher dose of oral combination contraceptives
   b. Higher doses of oral progestin contraceptives
   c. Endometriosis
   d. Treatment of acne vulgaris
      (1) Norgestimate and ethinyl estradiol
      (2) Increase in SHBG, decreases free testosterone, which is important in development of acne (androgen receptors located on sebaceous glands)
   e. Treatment of dysfunctional uterine bleeding (ovulatory and anovulatory types)

D. **Adverse effects**
1. Venous thrombotic disease
2. Myocardial infarction
3. Cerebrovascular disease
4. Intrahepatic cholestasis with jaundice
5. Hepatic adenomas
   • Commonly rupture and produce intraperitoneal hemorrhage
6. Increased incidence of migraine headache
7. Mood changes
   • Norgestimate, a third-generation progestin, has high progestational, slight estrogenic, and low androgenic activity; it has little effect on serum lipoproteins and has very little negative effect on carbohydrate metabolism.
8. Lipid effects of combination hormonal contraceptives
   a. Estrogen compounds associated with lipid effects
      (1) Increased high-density lipoprotein (HDL)-cholesterol
      (2) Decreased low-density lipoprotein (LDL)-cholesterol
      (3) Triglycerides may increase
   b. Use with caution in patients with familial defects of lipoprotein metabolism.

E. **Beneficial effects of low dose oral contraceptives (OCs) compared with women *not* taking OCs**
1. Lower risks of:
   a. Ovarian cysts
   b. Ovarian (only surface-derived ovarian cancers) and endometrial cancer
   c. Benign breast disease
2. Lower incidence of:
   a. Ectopic pregnancy
   b. Iron deficiency
   c. Rheumatoid arthritis
3. Ameliorates:
   a. Premenstrual symptoms
   b. Dysmenorrhea
   c. Endometriosis
4. Adverse effect
   • Break through ovulation with pregnancy

F. **Therapeutic summary of selected estrogen-related drugs** (Table 26-2)

IV. **Androgens and Inhibitors** (see Box 26-2; Fig. 26-3)
   • Testosterone is the most important androgen in humans.
   A. **Androgens**
   1. Synthesis and secretion
      • Stimulated by LH

The pituitary is the most important site of action for estrogen/progestin combination contraceptives; they decrease LH and FSH secretion leading to decreased ovulation.

Norgestimate and ethinyl estradiol is used to treat acne vulgaris.

Oral contraceptives have a beneficial effect on the lipid profile.

Women on contraceptives are less likely to have an ectopic pregnancy.

Table 26-2. **Therapeutic Summary of Selected Estrogen-Related Drugs**

DRUGS	CLINICAL APPLICATIONS	ADVERSE EFFECTS	CONTRAINDICATIONS
Mechanism: *Stimulation of estrogen receptors*			

Estradiol
Estrogens (conjugated A/synthetic)
Estrogens (conjugated B/synthetic)
Estrogens (Conjugated/equine)
Estrogens (esterified)
Estropipate
	Oral contraception
	Estrogen replacement therapy (ERT)
	Treatment of vulvar and vaginal atrophy
	Treatment of postmenopausal urogenital symptoms
	Suppression of ovulation
		Postmenopausal bleeding during ERT
		Nausea
		Breast tenderness
		Increased incidence of:
		  Migraine headaches
		  Intrahepatic cholestasis
		  Hypertension
		  Cholesterol gallstones
		  Thrombophlebitis
		  Thromboembolism
		  Causes blood clots
		  Heart attack
		  Stroke
		  Markedly increased in smokers
		  Increased in family history of blood clots
		  Increased platelet aggregation
		  Accelerated blood clotting
			Estrogen-dependent
			Known or suspected carcinoma of the breast
			Liver disease
			History of thromboembolic disorders
			Smoking

Mechanism: *Selective estrogen receptor modulators; agonist in some tissues; antagonist at other tissues*			
Clomiphene Raloxifene Tamoxifen Toremifene	Treatment of infertility (clomiphene) Prevention or treatment of breast cancer (tamoxifen; toremifene) Prevention and treatment of osteoporosis (raloxifene)	Ovarian enlargement Multiple pregnancies (clomiphene) Hot flashes Flushing Hypertension Peripheral edema Fluid retention Vaginal bleeding Endometrial hyperplasia and cancer	Hypersensitivity Liver disease Abnormal uterine bleeding Uncontrolled thyroid or adrenal dysfunction Pregnancy History of deep vein thrombosis or pulmonary embolism
Mechanism: *Stimulation of progesterone receptors*			
Etonogestrel Levonorgestrel Medroxyprogesterone Megestrol Norethindrone Progesterone	Hormonal contraception Down-regulate endometrial lining to treat endometrial hyperplasia or cancer (non-surgical candidates) Dysmenorrhea, endometriosis, uterine bleeding disorders Hirsutism Hormonal replacement therapy (estrogens and progestins) Acne vulgaris	Increased risk of breast cancer Bone mineral density loss Risk of dementia in postmenopausal women Weight gain; stimulates appetite	Hypersensitivity History of or current thrombophlebitis Cerebral vascular disease Severe hepatic disease Carcinoma of the breast or genital organs Undiagnosed vaginal bleeding Missed abortion Pregnancy
Mechanism: *Antagonize the actions of progestins*			

Mifepristone
Danazol
	Mifepristone
	  Medical termination of intrauterine pregnancy
	Danazol
	  Endometriosis
	  Fibrocystic change
	  Hereditary angioedema
		Androgenic effects
		Weight gain
		Seborrhea
		Hirsutism
		Edema
		Alopecia (male pattern baldness)
			Hypersensitivity
			Undiagnosed genital bleeding
			Pregnancy
			Breast-feeding
			Porphyria
			Markedly impaired hepatic, renal, or cardiac function

Mechanism: *Stimulates both estrogen and progesterone receptors*			
Combinations of estrogens and progestins (see Box 26-20)	Hormonal replacement therapy Contraception	Venous thrombotic disease Myocardial infarction Cerebrovascular disease Intrahepatic cholestasis Hepatic adenomas (intraperitoneal hemorrhage) Increased incidence of migraine headache Increased risk of stroke Mood changes	Hypersensitivity Pregnancy Thrombophlebitis or venous thromboembolic disorders Heavy smoking Hormonal-dependent cancers Cardiovascular disease Undiagnosed vaginal bleeding

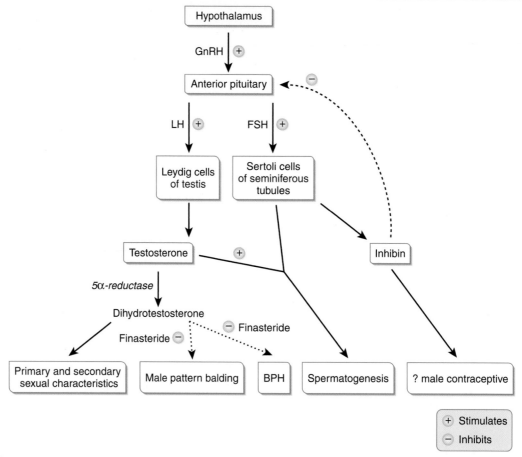

26-3: Male axis. BPH, benign prostatic hyperplasia; FSH, follicle-stimulating hormone; GnRH, gonadotropin-releasing hormone; LH, luteinizing hormone. *(From Brown TA: Rapid Review Physiology. Philadelphia, Mosby, 2007, Figure 3-13.)*

   a. Sites of production
      (1) Testes (Leydig cells) in males
      (2) Ovaries and adrenal cortex in females
   b. In males, testosterone is converted to 5α-dihydrotestosterone (DHT) by the enzyme 5α-reductase in peripheral tissues (e.g., prostate, skin).
   c. In females, testosterone is converted to estrogens by the enzyme aromatase.
2. Physiologic actions
   a. Stimulates libido (increased sex drive) in both males and females
   b. Accounts for the major changes that occur in males at puberty
   c. Has anabolic activity
3. Uses
   a. Replacement therapy in hypogonadism or hypopituitarism
   b. Acceleration of growth in childhood
   c. Anabolic agent (especially in debilitating diseases such as acquired immunodeficiency syndrome [AIDS]-associated wasting syndrome and breast cancer and in geriatric patients)
4. Adverse effects
   a. Masculinization (in women)
   b. Azoospermia
   c. Decrease in testicular size
5. Abuse potential
   • Because androgens stimulate muscle growth, some athletes misuse these agents in attempts to improve athletic performance.
B. **Androgen suppression and antiandrogens**
   1. Gonadotropin-releasing hormone (GnRH) analogues
      a. Examples
         (1) Leuprolide
         (2) Goserelin

Androgens are widely abused by athletes.

  b. Mechanism of action
   • Produce gonadal suppression when blood levels are continuous rather than pulsatile.

Continuous exposure to a long-acting GnRH analogue is useful in treating prostate cancer.

  c. Uses
   (1) Palliative treatment of advanced prostate cancer
   (2) Management of endometriosis
   (3) Treatment of anemia caused by uterine leiomyomata (fibroids)
   (4) Central precocious puberty
   (5) Down-regulation of ovaries prior to ovarian stimulation in infertility treatment
 2. 5α-Reductase inhibitors
  a. Examples
   (1) Dutasteride
   (2) Finasteride
  b. Mechanism of action
   (1) Inhibits the androgen-metabolizing enzyme 5α-reductase
   (2) Inhibits the formation of DHT
   (3) Androgen necessary for prostate growth and function
  c. Uses
   (1) Benign prostatic hyperplasia (BPH)
   (2) Male pattern baldness (finasteride)

5α-Reductase inhibitors are useful in treating BPH and male pattern baldness.

  d. Adverse effects
   (1) Teratogenic properties
    • Pregnant women are cautioned about working with finasteride or dutasteride because breathing the dust could result in teratogenesis.

Finasteride and dutasteride are extremely teratogenic.

   (2) Impotence
   (3) Decreased libido
 3. Receptor antagonists
  a. Examples
   (1) Flutamide
   (2) Bicalutamide
   (3) Nilutamide

Note common ending -lutamide for androgen receptor blockers

  b. Uses
   • Treatment of metastatic prostatic carcinoma in combination therapy with GnRH agonist analogues
 4. Ketoconazole (see Chapter 28; antifungal drug)
  a. Mechanism of action
   • Decreases testosterone synthesis (males)
  b. Use
   • Treatment of prostate cancer (experimental)
C. **Therapeutic summary of selected androgen-related drugs**: (Table 26-3)

Table 26-3. **Therapeutic Summary of Selected Androgen-Related Drugs**

DRUGS	CLINICAL APPLICATIONS	ADVERSE EFFECTS	CONTRAINDICATIONS
Mechanism: *Stimulate androgen receptors*			
Danazol Fluoxymesterone Methyltestosterone Nandrolone Oxandrolone Testolactone Testosterone	Replacement therapy in hypogonadism or hypopituitarism Acceleration of growth in childhood Anabolic agent	Masculinization (in women) Azoospermia, decrease in testicular size	Hypersensitivity Pregnancy Breast-feeding Carcinoma of the breast or prostate (men) Serious hepatic, renal, or cardiac disease
Mechanism: *Androgen receptor blockers*			
Bicalutamide Flutamide Nilutamide	Treatment of metastatic prostatic carcinoma in combination therapy with GnRH agonist analogues	Breast tenderness Galactorrhea Gynecomastia Hot flashes Impotence Tumor flare Edema Anemia	Hypersensitivity Pregnancy Liver disease

(Continued)

Table 26-3. **Therapeutic Summary of Selected Androgen-Related Drugs—Cont'd**

DRUGS	CLINICAL APPLICATIONS	ADVERSE EFFECTS	CONTRAINDICATIONS
Mechanism: *5α-Reductase inhibitors; inhibits the conversion of testosterone to dihydroxytestosterone*			
Dutasteride Finasteride	Benign prostatic hyperplasia (BPH) Male pattern baldness (finasteride)	Impotence Decreased libido Ejaculation disturbance Teratogenic	Hypersensitivity Pregnancy Use in children
Mechanism: *Inhibit gonadotropin release with continuous administration of longer-lasting synthetic analogues*			

Goserelin
Leuprolide
	Palliative treatment of advanced prostate cancer
	Management of endometriosis
	Treatment of anemia caused by uterine
	  leiomyomata (fibroids)
	Central precocious puberty
	Down-regulation of ovaries prior to ovarian
	  stimulation in infertility treatment
		Vaginal bleeding
		Headache
		Hot flashes
		GI distress
		Vaginitis
		Testicular atrophy
			Hypersensitivity
			Abnormal vaginal
			  bleeding
			Pregnancy
			Breast-feeding

GI, gastrointestinal; GnRH, gonadotropin releasing hormone.

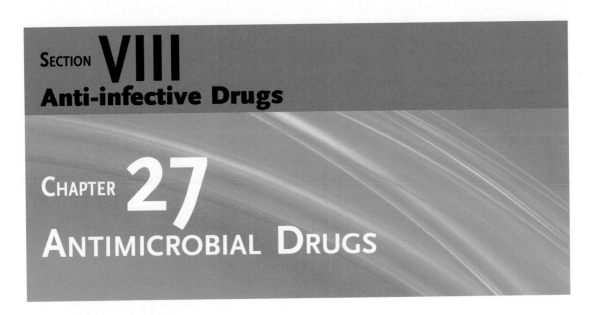

SECTION VIII
Anti-infective Drugs

CHAPTER 27
ANTIMICROBIAL DRUGS

I. General Considerations
A. Keys to successful antimicrobial therapy
1. Selective toxicity
   - Destroy pathogenic microorganisms with minimal adverse effects to host
2. Adequate blood levels
   - Sufficient levels to destroy microorganisms in order to prevent development of microbial resistance

B. Mechanism of action
1. Sites of action antimicrobial drugs (Fig. 27-1)
2. Molecular targets of antimicrobial drugs (see Fig. 27-1)
   a. Cell wall synthesis
   b. Cell membrane
   c. Folic acid metabolism
   d. DNA replication
   e. RNA synthesis
   f. Protein synthesis

C. Mechanisms of microbial resistance
1. Resistance often correlates with:
   a. Frequency of antimicrobial use
   b. Total quantity of drug dispensed
   c. Location of the patient when receiving the medication
   d. Immune status of the patient
2. Processes that contribute to resistance (see Table 27-1 for examples)
   a. Drug resistance due to altered targets
   b. Drug resistance due to decreased accumulation
      (1) Decreased uptake
      (2) Increased efflux
   c. Drug resistance due to enzymatic inactivation
3. Multidrug resistance is often transmitted by plasmids.
4. To minimize the emergence of resistance:
   a. Only use chemotherapeutic agents when they are clearly indicated
   b. Use a narrow-spectrum drug known to be effective against the pathogen.
   c. Use an effective dose of the chemotherapeutic agent.
   d. Ensure that the duration of chemotherapy is adequate.
   e. Use older chemotherapeutic drugs whenever possible.
   f. Use multiple drugs in combination chemotherapy when the pathogen is noted to develop resistance to an individual drug rapidly.

D. Functions
1. Antibacterial selection (Table 27-2)
   a. Bactericidal agents (Table 27-3)
      - Kill microorganisms

Antimicrobial therapy is an exercise in selective toxicity.

Inadequate blood levels of antimicrobials leads to drug resistance.

Know molecular target of individual drugs.

Overuse of antimicrobials markedly contributes to antimicrobial resistance.

Know modes of resistance for individual drugs.

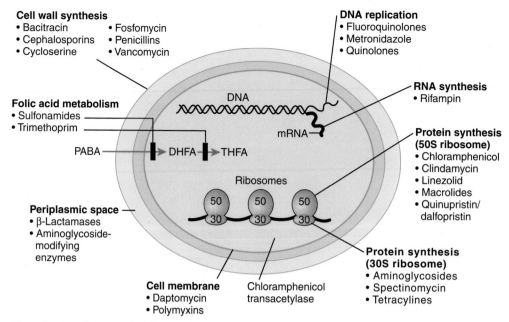

Cell wall synthesis
- Bacitracin
- Cephalosporins
- Cycloserine
- Fosfomycin
- Penicillins
- Vancomycin

DNA replication
- Fluoroquinolones
- Metronidazole
- Quinolones

Folic acid metabolism
- Sulfonamides
- Trimethoprim

RNA synthesis
- Rifampin

DNA

mRNA

PABA → DHFA → THFA

Protein synthesis (50S ribosome)
- Chloramphenicol
- Clindamycin
- Linezolid
- Macrolides
- Quinupristin/dalfopristin

Ribosomes

Periplasmic space
- β-Lactamases
- Aminoglycoside-modifying enzymes

Protein synthesis (30S ribosome)
- Aminoglycosides
- Spectinomycin
- Tetracylines

Cell membrane
- Daptomycin
- Polymyxins

Chloramphenicol transacetylase

27-1: Sites of action of antimicrobial drugs and enzymes that inactivate these drugs. DHFA, dihydrofolic acid; PABA, p-aminobenzoic acid; THFA, tetrahydrofolic acid.

TABLE 27-1. Mechanism of Microbial Resistance

DRUG RESISTANCE DUE TO ALTERED TARGETS	DRUG RESISTANCE DUE TO DECREASED ACCUMULATION		DRUG RESISTANCE DUE TO ENZYMATIC INACTIVATION
β-Lactams	**Decreased permeability**	**Increased efflux**	β-Lactams
Vancomycin	β-Lactams	Macrolides	Aminoglycosides
Aminoglycosides	Tetracyclines	Tetracyclines	Macrolides
Chloramphenicol	Fluoroquinolones	Fluoroquinolones	Tetracyclines
Clindamycin			Chloramphenicol
Macrolides			
Tetracyclines			
Rifampin			
Sulfonamides			
Trimethoprim			
Fluoroquinolones			

TABLE 27-2. Microbial Organisms with Sites of Infection and Drugs of Choice for Treatment

MICROORGANISM	INFECTION	DRUGS OF CHOICE	ALTERNATIVES*
Gram-positive			
Staphylococcus aureus	Abscess, Cellulitis, Bacteremia, Pneumonia, Endocarditis	Methicillin susceptible: Nafcillin, Oxacillin; Methicillin resistant: Vancomycin	Linezolid, Quinupristin/dalfopristin, TMP/SMX, Teicoplanin
Streptococcus pyogenes (group A)	Pharyngitis, Cellulitis	Penicillin G, Penicillin V	Other β-lactams, Macrolides
Streptococcus (group B)	Meningitis, Cellulitis, Sepsis	Penicillin G (+/– aminoglycoside), Clindamycin	Other β-lactams, Macrolides
Enterococcus	Bacteremia	Penicillin G (+/– aminoglycoside), Ampicillin	Vancomycin/gentamicin
Enterococcus	Endocarditis	Penicillin G (+/– aminoglycoside), Ampicillin	Vancomycin, Dalfopristin/quinupristin, Linezolid
Enterococcus	Urinary tract	Ampicillin	Fluoroquinolone, Nitrofurantoin
Streptococcus (viridans group)	Endocarditis	Penicillin G (+/– aminoglycoside), Ceftriaxone	Cephalosporin, Vancomycin
Streptococcus pneumoniae	Pneumonia	Penicillin G, Vancomycin (+/– rifampin)	Levofloxacin
Streptococcus pneumoniae	Otitis, Sinusitis	Amoxicillin (+/– clavulanic acid)	Azithromycin, TMP/SMX, Oral cephalosporin
Streptococcus pneumoniae	Meningitis	Ceftriaxone, Cefotaxime	Penicillin G

(Continued)

TABLE 27-2. Microbial Organisms with Sites of Infection and Drugs of Choice for Treatment—Cont'd

MICROORGANISM	INFECTION	DRUGS OF CHOICE	ALTERNATIVES
Listeria monocytogenes	Bacteremia Meningitis Endocarditis	Ampicillin	TMP/SMX
Gram-negative			
Escherichia coli	Urinary tract	TMP/SMX Ciprofloxacin	Nitrofurantoin Fosfomycin
Escherichia coli	Bacteremia	Third-generation cephalosporin	TMP/SMX Ciprofloxacin
Klebsiella pneumoniae	Urinary tract	Ciprofloxacin	TMP/SMX Oral cephalosporin
Klebsiella pneumoniae	Pneumonia Bacteremia	Third generation Cephalosporin	Fluoroquinolone TMP/SMX Imipenem Aztreonam
Proteus mirabilis	Urinary tract	Ampicillin	TMP/SMX
Haemophilus influenzae	Otitis Sinusitis Bronchitis	Cefotaxime Ceftriaxone	Fluoroquinolone TMP/SMX
Moraxella catarrhalis	Otitis Sinusitis	Amoxicillin/Clavulanic acid	TMP/SMX Macrolide
Neisseria gonorrhoeae	Genital	Ceftriaxone Cefixime	Sulfonamide Chloramphenicol
Pseudomonas aeruginosa	Urinary tract	Ciprofloxacin	TMP/SMX Imipenem Aztreonam Third generation cephalosporin
Pseudomonas aeruginosa	Pneumonia Bacteremia	Antipseudomonal penicillin + aminoglycoside Ceftazidime	Aztreonam Carbapenems Cefepime
Vibrio cholerae	Cholera	Doxycycline Fluoroquinolone	TMP/SMX

Helicobacter pylori	Peptic ulcer
	    (use multiple drugs)
		Amoxicillin
		Clarithromycin
		Tinidazole
		    (Rabeprazole, proton pump inhibitor)
			Tetracycline
			Bismuth
			Metronidazole

Anaerobes			
Bacteroides spp.	Abdominal infections Abscesses	Metronidazole	Clindamycin Carbapenems Cefoxitin Ticarcillin/clavulanic acid
Clostridium perfringens	Abscesses Gangrene	Penicillin G + clindamycin	Doxycycline
Clostridium difficile	Pseudomembranous colitis	Metronidazole	Vancomycin (oral)
Other			
Legionella spp.	Pulmonary	Azithromycin Levofloxacin	Clarithromycin
Mycoplasma pneumoniae	Pulmonary	Azithromycin Clarithromycin Erythromycin Levofloxacin	Doxycycline
Chlamydia pneumoniae	Pulmonary	Doxycycline	Erythromycin Fluoroquinolone
Chlamydia trachomatis	Genital	Doxycycline Azithromycin	Erythromycin
Rickettsia	Rocky Mountain spotted fever	Doxycycline	Chloramphenicol
Ehrlichia spp.	Ehrlichiosis	Doxycycline	Chloramphenicol
Borrelia burgdorferi	Lyme disease	Ceftriaxone Cefuroxime axetil Doxycycline Amoxicillin	Penicillin G (high dose) Cefotaxime

Mycobacterium tuberculosis	Tuberculosis
	    (Always use multiple
	    drugs)
		Isoniazid
		Rifampin
		Ethambutol
		Pyrazinamide
			Streptomycin
			Rifabutin

Treponema pallidum	Syphilis	Benzathine penicillin G	Doxycycline

*Only a few common alternative drugs are listed. TMP/SMX, trimethoprim/sulfamethoxazole

TABLE 27-3. **Bactericidal and bacteriostatic antibacterial agents**

BACTERICIDAL AGENTS	BACTERIOSTATIC AGENTS
β-lactam antibiotics	Tetracyclines
Bacitracin	Chloramphenicol
Fosfomycin	Macrolides
Vancomycin	Clindamycin
Isoniazid	Ethambutol
Aminoglycosides	Linezolid
Quinupristin/dalfopristin	Sulfonamides
Metronidazole	Trimethoprim
Polymyxins	Nitrofurantoin
Fluoroquinolones	
Tigecycline	
Rifampin	
Pyrazinamide	

Know which drugs are bacteriostatic versus bactericidal.

Drugs that cause hepatotoxicity: tetracyclines, isoniazid, erythromycin, clindamycin, sulfonamides, amphotericin B

Drugs that cause renal toxicity: cephalosporins, vancomycin, aminoglycosides, sulfonamides, amphotericin B

Candidiasis is most common superinfection caused by antimicrobial therapy.

Treat pseudomembranous colitis with metronidazole.

(1) Concentration-dependent killing
    (a) Aminoglycosides
    (b) Fluoroquinolones
(2) Time-dependent killing
    (a) β-Lactam antibiotics
    (b) Vancomycin
  b. Bacteriostatic agents (see Table 27-3)
    • Suppress bacterial growth and multiplication
2. Prophylactic use of anti-infective agents (Table 27-4)
E. **Adverse effects of antimicrobial drugs** (Table 27-5)
  1. Organ-directed toxicity
    a. Ototoxicity
    b. Hematopoietic toxicity
    c. Hepatotoxicity
    d. Renal toxicity
  2. Idiosyncrasies (unexpected individual reactions)
    a. Hemolytic anemias (e.g., in glucose-6-phosphate dehydrogenase [G6PD]-deficient people)
    b. Photosensitivity reactions (e.g., tetracycline)
  3. Hypersensitivity reactions
    • These reactions are most notable with penicillins and sulfonamides but can occur with most antimicrobial drugs.
  4. Superinfections
    a. Candidiasis
      • Treatment with oral nystatin (local effects), miconazole (local vaginal effects), fluconazole (oral medication for vaginal candidiasis)
    b. Pseudomembranous colitis caused by *Clostridium difficile*
      • Treatment with oral metronidazole or vancomycin
    c. Staphylococcal enterocolitis
      • Treatment with oral vancomycin

TABLE 27-4. **Prophylactic Use of Anti-infective Drugs**

DRUG	USE
Cefazolin	Surgical procedures
Cefoxitin, cefotetan	Surgical procedures in which anaerobic infections are common
Ampicillin or penicillin	Group B streptococcal infections
Trimethoprim-sulfamethoxazole	*Pneumocystis jiroveci* pneumonia UTIs
Rifampin	*Haemophilus influenzae* type B Meningococcal infection
Chloroquine, mefloquine	Malaria
Isoniazid, rifampin	Tuberculosis
Azithromycin	*Mycobacterium avium* complex in patients with AIDS
Ciprofloxacin	*Bacillus anthracis* (anthrax)
Ampicillin or azithromycin	Dental procedures in patients with valve abnormalities

AIDS, acquired immunodeficiency syndrome; UTI, urinary tract infection.

TABLE 27-5. **Adverse reactions to antimicrobials**

ORGAN-DIRECTED TOXICITY	IDIOSYNCRATIC RESPONSES	HYPERSENSITIVITY REACTIONS	SUPERINFECTIONS

Ototoxicity
  Aminoglycosides
  Vancomycin
  Minocycline
	Hemolytic anemia
	  (in G6PD deficiency)
	  Primaquine
	  Sulfonamides
	  Nitrofurantoin
		β-Lactams
		  Penicillins
		  Cephalosporins
		  Carbapenems
			Candidiasis
			Broad spectrum antibiotics
			Treatment
			  Nystatin
			  Fluconazole
			  Miconazole

Hematopoietic toxicity
Chloramphenicol
  Sulfonamides
	Photosensitivity
	  Tetracyclines
	  Sulfonamides
	  Fluoroquinolones
		Sulfonamides
		Stevens-Johnson
		  syndrome most serious
			Staphylococcal enterocolitis
			Treatment
			  Vancomycin

Hepatotoxicity
  Tetracyclines
  Macrolides
  Isoniazid
  Sulfonamides
  Amphotericin B
		Lower incidence with
		  other antimicrobials
			Pseudomembranous colitis
			  (Clostridium difficile)
			  Clindamycin
			Treatment
			  Metronidazole
			  Vancomycin

Renal toxicity
  Aminoglycosides
  Vancomycin
  Amphotericin B
  Cephalosporins
  Sulfonamides			

G6PD, Glucose-6-phosphate dehydrogenase

    5. Synergism
        a. Aminoglycosides plus penicillins
        b. Sulfamethoxazole plus trimethoprim
        c. Amphotericin B plus flucytosine
        d. Fosfomycin plus β-lactams
        e. Fosfomycin plus aminoglycosides
        f. Fosfomycin plus fluoroquinolones
    6. Potentiation
        a. Imipenem plus cilastatin
        b. Ampicillin plus sulbactam
        c. Amoxicillin plus clavulanic acid
        d. Piperacillin plus tazobactam
        e. Ticarcillin plus clavulanic acid
    7. Antagonism
        a. Penicillin G plus chloramphenicol
        b. Penicillin G plus tetracycline

> Be able to distinguish drug combinations that lead to synergism, potentiation, or antagonism.

II. Cell Wall Synthesis Inhibitors (Box 27-1)
  A. General information
    1. Intracellular or extracellular steps in the synthesis of the cell wall (Fig. 27-1 and Fig. 27-2)
    2. β-Lactam antibiotics are most often used
    3. Structural relationships of β-lactam antibiotics (Fig. 27-3)
  B. Penicillins
    1. Key characteristics of penicillin G (see Fig. 27-3)
        a. β-lactam ring
        b. Penicillinase sensitivity
        c. Acid labile
        d. Tubular secretion (organic anion)
        e. Inhibition of cell wall synthesis
        f. Hypersensitivity
    2. Pharmacokinetics
        a. Absorption
            (1) May be destroyed by gastric acid
            (2) Acid-resistant preparations for oral administration
                (a) Amoxicillin
                (b) Carbenicillin indanyl
                (c) Dicloxacillin
                (d) Oxacillin
                (e) Penicillin V

> β-Lactam antimicrobials include: penicillins, cephalosporins, carbapenems, monobactams.

> Learn how other β-lactams differ from penicillin G.

> Acid resistant (orally effective) penicillins include: penicillin V, amoxicillin, carbenicillin indanyl, oxacillin, and dicloxacillin.

BOX 27-1 β-LACTAM DRUGS AND OTHER CELL WALL SYNTHESIS INHIBITORS

Penicillins
Amoxicillin (O)
Ampicillin
Carbenicillin indanyl (O)
Dicloxacillin (O)
Nafcillin
Oxacillin (O)
Penicillin G
Penicillin V (O)
Piperacillin
Ticarcillin

Cephalosporins
First-Generation Drugs
Cefadroxil (O)
Cefazolin
Cephalexin (O)
Cephalothin (prototype; no longer available in the United States)
Second-Generation Drugs
Cefaclor (O)
Cefotetan
Cefoxitin
Cefoprozil (O)
Cefuroxime (O)
Loracarbef (O)

Third-Generation Drugs
Cefdinir (O)
Cefditoren (O)
Cefixime (O)
Cefoperazone
Cefotaxime
Cefpodoxime (O)
Ceftazidime
Ceftibuten (O)
Ceftizoxime
Ceftriaxone
Fourth-Generation Drugs
Cefepime

Other β-Lactam Drugs
Aztreonam
Doripenem
Ertapenem
Imipenem-cilastatin
Meropenem

Other Cell Wall Synthesis Inhibitors
Bacitracin (topical)
Fosfomycin (O)
Vancomycin

O, often given orally

27-2: Sites of action of cell wall synthesis inhibitors. The peptidoglycan substrate for Step 2 is inhibited by fosfomycin and cycloserine; the transport of the peptidoglycan across the cell membrane is inhibited by bacitracin (Step 1); the linkage of peptidoglycan monomers via transglycosylation is inhibited by vancomycin (Step 6); the cross-linking of strands by transpeptidation is inhibited by β-lactams (Site 6). *(From Brenner G and Stevens C: Pharmacology, 3rd ed. Philadelphia, Saunders, 2010, Figure 38-2.)*

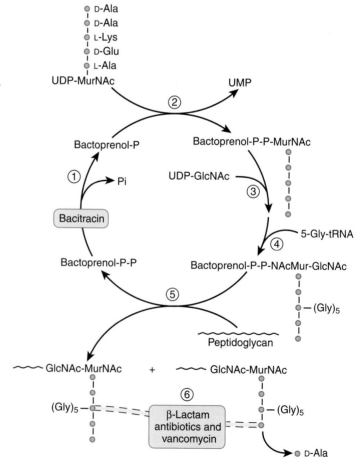

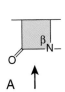

β-Lactam nucleus

A

Acyl side chain   Thiazolidine ring

R_1—C—N—C—C

Penicillins

Monobactams

B   Cephalosporins

Acyl side chain   Dihydrothiazine ring

R_1—C—N—C—C

Carbapenems

27-3: Structures of β-lactam drugs. *(From Wecker L, et al.: Brody's Human Pharmacology, 5th ed. Philadelphia, Mosby, 2010, Figure 46-1.)*

b. Distribution
  (1) Good to most tissues and fluids, including:
    (a) Pleural fluid
    (b) Pericardial fluid
    (c) Synovial fluid
  (2) Poor penetration
    (a) Eye
    (b) Prostate
    (c) Central nervous system (CNS) (except in meningitis)
c. Excretion
  (1) Unchanged in urine by tubular secretion
    • Exception; nafcillin is biliary excretion
  (2) Inhibited by probenecid
3. Pharmacodynamics
  a. Mechanism of action (see Fig. 27-2)
    (1) Bind to specific penicillin-binding proteins (PBPs)
      (a) Inhibit transpeptidase enzymes
        • Inhibits cross-linking of peptidoglycan chains
      (b) Activates autolytic enzymes
        • Causes holes in bacterial cell wall
    (2) Bactericidal
  b. Causes of resistance
    (1) Inactivation by β-lactamases (most common)
    (2) Alteration in target PBPs (methicillin-resistant species)
      • Methicillin-resistant *Staphylococcus aureus* (MRSA)
    (3) Permeability barrier, preventing drug penetration
      • Contributes to the resistance of many gram-negative bacteria
4. Uses
  a. Penicillin G
    (1) Pharyngitis (Group A *streptococcus*)
    (2) Syphilis *(Treponema pallidum)*
    (3) Pneumonia *(pneumococcus, streptococcus)*
    (4) Meningitis *(meningococcus, pneumococcus)*
  b. Benzathine penicillin G
    (1) Intramuscular injection gives low blood levels for up to 3 weeks.
    (2) Useful in situations in which organisms are very sensitive
      (a) *T. pallidum* in syphilis
      (b) β-Hemolytic streptococcal pharyngitis prophylaxis
        • Monthly injection prevents reinfection

Penicillins are poor for treating infections in the eye, prostate, or CNS (except in meningitis).

Exceptions: Nafcillin and, to a lesser extent, oxacillin and dicloxacillin depend on biliary secretion.

Inhibitors of cell wall synthesis cause osmotic rupture of the bacterial cell.

Alterations in PBPs: responsible for methicillin resistance in staphylococci (MRSA) and penicillin resistance in pneumococci.

Methicillin resistant strains are resistant to all β-lactam antibiotics.

Primary use of penicillin G: infections with gram-positive (+) bacteria.

Benzathine penicillin G is the drug of choice for syphilis.

c. Ampicillin and amoxicillin (extended spectrum penicillins)
  (1) Route of administration
      (a) Ampicillin is usually given by injection.
          • Often given with sulbactam
      (b) Amoxicillin is given orally.
          • Often given with clavulanic acid
  (2) Uses
      (a) Urinary tract infections (UTIs) *(Escherichia coli)*
      (b) Infectious diarrhea *(Salmonella)*
      (c) Otitis media or sinusitis *(Haemophilus)*
      (d) Meningitis *(Listeria)*
      (e) Endocarditis (prevention)
      (f) Bacteremia *(Enterococcus)* combined with an aminoglycoside

d. Ticarcillin (antipseudomonal penicillin) potent against nosocomial *(Pseudomonas)* infections
  (1) Usually combined with an aminoglycoside
  (2) Often given with clavulanic acid

e. Piperacillin (antipseudomonal penicillin)
  (1) More active against *Pseudomonas* than ticarcillin
  (2) Often given with tazobactam

f. Penicillinase-resistant β-lactam antibiotics
  (1) Examples
      (a) Nafcillin (parenteral)
          • Biliary excretion
      (b) Oxacillin (oral; parenteral)
          • Both biliary and renal excretion
      (c) Dicloxacillin (oral)
          • Both biliary and renal excretion
  (2) Used against penicillinase-producing microorganisms
      (a) Endocarditis (streptococci, staphylococci)
      (b) Osteomyelitis (staphylococci)

5. Adverse effects
  a. Allergic reactions (most serious)
  b. Seizures with high levels in brain

C. Cephalosporins
• Cephalothin, the prototype first-generation cephalosporin, is no longer available in the United States.
1. Key characteristics of cephalosporins
  a. β-Lactam ring (see Fig. 27-3)
  b. Increased resistance to penicillinases
  c. Inhibition of cell wall synthesis
  d. Acid resistance (some agents)
      • Some agents are orally effective (see Box 27-1)
  e. Nephrotoxicity
  f. Tubular secretion
      • Exception, ceftriaxone is eliminated by biliary excretion
2. Mechanism of action
  a. Similar to penicillins
  b. Bactericidal
  c. Penicillinase-resistant
  d. Many are cephalosporinase sensitive
3. Uses
  a. First-generation
      (1) Examples
          (a) Cefazolin (parenteral)
          (b) Cephalexin (oral)
          (c) Cefadroxil (oral)
      (2) Cefazolin has good activity against gram-positive bacteria and modest activity against gram-negative bacteria.
          (a) Cellulitis *(Staphylococcus, Streptococcus)*
          (b) Surgical prophylaxis
              • *Exception*, cefoxitin for abdominal surgery prophylaxis

---

Intravenous ampicillin is an excellent choice for treatment of following conditions: actinomycosis; cholangitis (acute); diverticulitis; endocarditis; group B strep prophylaxis (intrapartum); Listeria infections; sepsis/meningitis; urinary tract infections (enterococcus suspected).

Penicillins but not cephalosporins are active against Enterococcal infections in combination with aminoglycosides.

Antipseudomonal penicillins and cephalosporins are combined with aminoglycosides to prevent resistance.

Antistaphylococcal penicillins (e.g., nafcillin): ineffective against infections with MRSA

Ampicillin rash: nonallergic rash; high incidence in patients with Epstein-Barr virus infection (mononucleosis).

Exceptions: Cefoperazone and ceftriaxone are mostly eliminated by biliary secretion.

First-generation cephalosporins have good activity against gram-positive bacteria and modest activity against gram-negative bacteria.

b. Second-generation
   (1) Examples
       (a) Cefaclor (oral)
       (b) Cefotetan
       (c) Cefoxitin
       (d) Cefoprozil (oral)
       (e) Cefuroxime (parenteral, oral)
       (f) Loracarbef (oral)
   (2) Increased activity against gram-negative bacteria *(E. coli, Klebsiella, Proteus, Haemophilus influenzae, Moraxella catarrhalis)*
       (a) Pelvic inflammatory disease
       (b) Diverticulitis
       (c) Abdominal surgical prophylaxis
       (d) Pneumonia
       (e) Bronchitis *(H. influenzae)*
c. Third-generation
   (1) Examples
       (a) Cefdinir (oral)
       (b) Cefditoren (oral)
       (c) Cefixime (oral)
       (d) Cefotaxime (parenteral)
       (e) Cefpodoxime (oral)
       (f) Ceftazidime (parenteral)
       (g) Ceftibuten (oral)
       (h) Ceftizoxime (parenteral)
       (i) Ceftriaxone (parenteral)
   (2) Decreased activity against gram-positive bacteria but increased activity against gram-negative bacteria *(Enterobacter, Serratia)*
   (3) Activity against *Pseudomonas aeruginosa* in a subset
       (a) Ceftazidime
       (b) Cefoperazone
   (4) Specific uses
       (a) Meningitis *(Neisseria gonorrhoeae)*
           • Third-generation good penetration of blood-brain barrier
       (b) Community-acquired pneumonia
       (c) Lyme disease
       (d) Osteomyelitis (ceftazidime)
       (e) Gonorrhea
           • Ceftriaxone (parenteral) or cefixime (oral) are drugs of choice
d. Fourth-generation (cefepime)
   (1) Extensive gram-positive and gram-negative activity
   (2) Increased resistance to β-lactamases
   (3) Use
       (a) Neutropenic fever (parenteral)
       (b) Use when other drugs fail
           • The U.S. Food and Drug Administration (FDA) is monitoring concerns of increased mortality in cefepime-treated patients.
4. Adverse effects
   a. Disulfiram-like effect with alcohol
      • Some second- and third-generation cephalosporins (e.g., cefotetan, cefoperazone)
   b. Dose-dependent nephrotoxicity, especially when used with other nephrotoxic drugs (e.g., aminoglycosides, amphotericin B)
   c. Drug hypersensitivity
D. Other β-lactam drugs
   1. Aztreonam
      a. Monobactam (see Fig. 27-3)
      b. Given intravenously
      c. *No* activity against gram-positive or anaerobic bacteria
      d. *No* cross allergenicity with other β-lactams
      e. Use in life threatening infections with gram-negative rods

---

Second-generation cephalosporins have increased activity against gram-negative bacteria *(E. coli, Klebsiella, Proteus, Haemophilus influenzae, Moraxella catarrhalis).*

First or second generation cephalosporins are drugs of choice against *E. coli, Klebsiella* and *Proteus.*

Third-generation cephalosporins have decreased activity against gram-positive bacteria but increased activity against gram-negative bacteria *(Enterobacter, Serratia).*

Many third-generation cephalosporins that penetrate into the CNS are useful in treatment of meningitis.

Cephalosporins are *not* active against *Listeria,* Enterococci, MRSA and Atypicals.

Cephalosporins with a methylthiotetrazole group (e.g., cefamandole, cefmetazole, cefotetan, cefoperazone) may cause hypoprothrombinemia and bleeding disorders and cause severe disulfiram-like reactions when taken with alcohol.

Cross-sensitivity to cephalosporins: less than 5% of patients with penicillin allergy

Aztreonam has *no* cross-allergenicity with other β-lactams.

(1) *Serratia*
(2) *Klebsiella*
(3) *Pseudomonas*
f. Adverse effects
(1) Pseudomembranous colitis
(2) Candidiasis
2. Carbapenems (see Fig. 27-3)
a. Examples
(1) Imipenem
• Must be given with cilastatin, a dehydropeptidase inhibitor
(2) Meropenem
(3) Ertapenem
(4) Doripenem
b. Uses
• Broad-spectrum activity, including anaerobes
(1) Mixed aerobic anaerobic infections
(2) *P. aeruginosa* infection resistant to other drugs
• All carbapenems except ertapenem
(3) Febrile neutropenic patients
• Often with aminoglycoside
(4) *Enterobacter* infections
c. Adverse effects
(1) Nausea and vomiting
(2) Pseudomembranous colitis
(3) Confusion
(4) Myoclonia
(5) Seizures (imipenem)
3. β-Lactamase inhibitors
a. Used with extended spectrum β-lactams to protect from β-lactamase
(1) Clavulanic acid with
(a) Amoxicillin
(b) Ticarcillin
(2) Sulbactam with ampicillin
(3) Tazobactam with piperacillin
b. *Not* active against MRSA
E. Other cell wall synthesis inhibitors
1. Vancomycin
a. Mechanism of action (see Fig. 27-2)
(1) Binds to the D-ala-D-ala terminus of peptidoglycan monomer
(2) Inhibits transglycosylation
(3) Addition of monomer to growing chain via a sugar linkage
(4) Bactericidal
(5) Active against only gram-positive bacteria (aerobes and anaerobes)
b. Uses
(1) Infections caused by gram-positive, penicillin-resistant organisms
(a) *Staphylococcus aureus*
(b) Hospital-acquired MRSA
(c) Enterococci species (in combination with aminoglycosides)
(d) Other gram-positive bacteria in penicillin-allergic patients
(2) *C. difficile*-caused diarrhea; alternate treatment
(a) Oral vancomycin results in poor gastrointestinal (GI) absorption and local treatment
(b) Metronidazole is first choice, because oral vancomycin may result in the development of resistant strains of *C. difficile*.
c. Adverse effects
(1) Ototoxicity
(2) Nephrotoxicity
(3) "Red man syndrome"
• Flushing from histamine release when given too quickly
2. Fosfomycin (see Box 27-1)
a. Mechanism of action (see Fig. 27-2)
(1) Inhibits cell wall synthesis by inhibiting the first step of peptidoglycan formation
(2) Bactericidal

Aztreonam only effective against gram-negative organisms.

Imipenem must be given with cilastatin to prevent inactivation by renal tubule dehydropeptidases.

Note the common ending -penem for all carbapenems

Drugs always active against anaerobes: penicillin + penicillinase inhibitor, metronidazole, imipenem, chloramphenicol.

The resistance of MRSA is *not* based upon penicillinase; it is based upon the mutation of the PBPs.

Vancomycin inhibits a transglycosylation step; linking of monomers via sugar residues.

Vancomycin *only* effective against gram-positive organisms.

Drugs that often cause histamine release ("red man syndrome"): d-tubocurarine, morphine, vancomycin.

    b. Uses
      (1) Uncomplicated lower UTIs in women
      (2) Infections caused by gram-positive (enterococci) and gram-negative bacteria
    c. Adverse effects
      (1) Asthenia
      (2) Diarrhea
      (3) Dizziness
  3. Bacitracin (see Box 27-1)
    • Given in combination with polymyxin and/or neomycin ointments for prophylaxis of superficial infections
    a. Mechanism of action (see Fig. 27-2)
      (1) Inhibits the transmembrane transport of peptidoglycan units
      (2) Bactericidal
      (3) Active only against gram-positive organisms
      (4) *No* cross resistance with other antimicrobials
    b. Uses
      (1) Topical applications only (nephrotoxic when given systemically)
      (2) Skin and ocular infections (gram-positive cocci)
  F. Therapeutic summary of selected cell wall synthesis inhibitors (Table 27-6)
III. Drugs That Affect the Cell Membrane (Box 27-2)
  A. Daptomycin
    1. Mechanism of action
      a. Binds to components of the cell membrane
      b. Causes rapid depolarization
      c. Inhibits intracellular synthesis of DNA, RNA, and proteins
      d. Bactericidal in a concentration-dependent manner
      e. Similar antibacterial spectrum as vancomycin

> Fosfomycin is used to treat UTIs in women.

> Bacitracin is bactericidal: *only* used for gram-positive infections.

> Bacitracin is *only* used topically.

> Daptomycin and polymyxin target bacterial cell membranes.

TABLE 27-6. **Therapeutic Summary of Selected Cell Wall Synthesis Inhibitors**

DRUGS	CLINICAL APPLICATIONS	ADVERSE EFFECTS	CONTRAINDICATIONS
Mechanism: *Inhibits transpeptidase; cross-linking; mainly gram positive bacteria*			
Penicillin G Penicillin V (O)	Pharyngitis (hemolytic streptococcus) Syphilis (*Treponema pallidum*) Pneumonia (pneumococcus, streptococcus) Meningitis (meningococcus, pneumococcus)	Seizures (high CNS levels) Anaphylaxis, Urticaria, Rash Pruritus Pseudomembranous colitis	Hypersensitivity
Mechanism: *Inhibits transpeptidase; cross-linking; penicillinase resistant*			
Antistaphylococcal Dicloxacillin (O) Nafcillin Oxacillin (O)	Endocarditis Osteomyelitis (staphylococci)	Seizures (high CNS levels) Anaphylaxis Urticaria Rash Pruritus Pseudomembranous colitis	Hypersensitivity
Mechanism: *Inhibits transpeptidase; cross-linking; more effective against gram-negative bacteria*			
Extended spectrum Amoxicillin (O) Ampicillin	Urinary tract infections (UTIs) (*Escherichia coli*) Infectious diarrhea (*Salmonella*) Otitis media or sinusitis (*Haemophilus*) Meningitis (*Listeria*) Endocarditis (prevention)	Seizures (high CNS levels) Ampicillin rash Anaphylaxis Urticaria Rash Pruritus Pseudomembranous colitis	Hypersensitivity
Mechanism: *Inhibits transpeptidase; cross-linking; effective against pseudomonas*			
Antipseudomonal Carbenicillin indanyl (O) Piperacillin Ticarcillin	*Proteus* *Pseudomonas*	Seizures (high CNS levels) Anaphylaxis Urticaria Rash Pruritus Pseudomembranous colitis	Hypersensitivity

(Continued)

TABLE 27-6. **Therapeutic Summary of Selected Cell Wall Synthesis Inhibitors—Cont'd**

DRUGS	CLINICAL APPLICATIONS	ADVERSE EFFECTS	CONTRAINDICATIONS
Mechanism: *Inhibits transpeptidase; cross-linking; somewhat broader spectrum than penicillin G*			
First-Generation Drugs Cefadroxil (O) Cefazolin Cephalexin (O)	Cellulitis (*Staphylococcus, Streptococcus*) Surgical prophylaxis (cefazolin)	Seizures (high CNS levels) GI distress Added nephrotoxicity Anaphylaxis, Urticaria Rash Pruritus Pseudomembranous colitis	Hypersensitivity
Mechanism: *Inhibits transpeptidase; cross-linking; Increased activity against gram-negative bacteria (E. coli, Klebsiella, Proteus, Haemophilus influenzae, Moraxella catarrhalis)*			
Second-Generation Drugs Cefaclor (O) Cefotetan Cefoxitin Cefoprozil (O) Cefuroxime (O) Loracarbef (O)	Pelvic inflammatory disease Diverticulitis Abdominal surgical prophylaxis (cefoxitin) Pneumonia Bronchitis (*H. influenzae*)	Seizures (high CNS levels) GI distress Added nephrotoxicity Anaphylaxis Urticaria Rash Pruritus Pseudomembranous colitis	Hypersensitivity
Mechanism: *Inhibits transpeptidase; cross-linking; Decreased activity against gram-positive bacteria but increased activity against gram-negative bacteria (Enterobacter, Serratia)*			
Third-Generation Drugs Cefdinir (O) Cefditoren (O) Cefixime (O) Cefoperazone Cefotaxime Cefpodoxime (O) Ceftazidime Ceftibuten (O) Ceftizoxime Ceftriaxone	Meningitis (*Neisseria gonorrhoeae*) Community-acquired pneumonia Lyme disease Osteomyelitis (ceftazidime) Gonorrhea (ceftriaxone, cefixime) *Pseudomonas aeruginosa* in a subset (ceftazidime)	Seizures (high CNS levels) GI distress Added nephrotoxicity Anaphylaxis Urticaria Rash Pruritus Pseudomembranous colitis Platelet dysfunction Disulfiram like effect (cefoperazone)	Hypersensitivity
Mechanism: *Inhibits transpeptidase; cross-linking; Extensive gram-positive and gram-negative activity; increased resistance to β-lactamases*			
Fourth-Generation Drugs Cefepime	Neutropenic fever (parenteral) Use when other drugs fail	Same as other cephalosporins May be increased mortality in cefepime treated patients	Hypersensitivity
Mechanism: *Inhibits transpeptidase; cross-linking; No activity against gram-positive or anaerobic bacteria*			
Aztreonam	Gram-negative rods *Serratia* *Klebsiella* *Pseudomonas*	GI distress Added nephrotoxicity Anaphylaxis Urticaria Rash Pruritus Pseudomembranous colitis	Hypersensitivity No cross allergenicity with other β-lactams
Mechanism: *Inhibits transpeptidase; cross-linking; Broad-spectrum activity, including anaerobes*			
Doripenem Ertapenem Imipenem-cilastatin Meropenem	Mixed aerobic anaerobic infection *Pseudomonas aeruginosa* infection resistant to other drugs, but not ertapenem Febrile neutropenic patients Often with aminoglycoside *Enterobacter* infections	Nausea and vomiting Pseudomembranous colitis Confusion Myoclonic seizures (Imipenem) Anaphylaxis	Hypersensitivity
Mechanism: *Inhibits the synthesis of peptidoglycan monomers*			
Fosfomycin (O)	UTIs in women due to susceptible strains of *E. coli* and *Enterococcus faecalis*	Headache GI distress Vaginitis Rhinitis	Hypersensitivity
Mechanism: *Inhibits transglycosylation; linking of monomers*			
Vancomycin	*Staphylococcus aureus* Methicillin-resistant *S. aureus* (MRSA) Enterococci species Other gram-positive bacteria in penicillin-allergic patients	Ototoxicity Nephrotoxicity "Red man syndrome" (histamine release)	Hypersensitivity

CNS, central nervous system; GI, gastrointestinal; O, effective orally.

BOX 27-2 DRUGS THAT AFFECT THE CELL MEMBRANE

Daptomycin
Polymyxin

    2. Uses
        a. Treatment of complicated skin infections caused by susceptible aerobic gram-positive organisms
        b. *S. aureus* bacteremia
        c. Right-sided infective endocarditis caused by methicillin-sensitive *Staphylococcus aureus* (MSSA) or MRSA
        d. Treatment of severe infections caused by MRSA or vancomycin-resistant *Enterococcus faecium* (VRE)
    3. Adverse effects
        a. Diarrhea
        b. Anemia
        c. Peripheral edema
        d. Electrolyte disturbances
        e. Renal failure
B. Polymyxin B
    1. Mechanism of action
        a. Interacts with specific lipopolysaccharide component of the outer cell membrane
        b. Increases permeability to polar molecules
        c. Bactericidal
        d. Active *only* against gram-negative bacteria
    2. Use
        a. Topical treatment of gram-negative bacteria infections (main use)
        b. Systemic use limited
           • Reserved for life-threatening infections caused by organisms resistant to the preferred drugs (e.g., pseudomonal meningitis—intrathecal administration)
IV. Protein Synthesis Inhibitors (Box 27-3)
    • These drugs reversibly bind to the 30S or 50S ribosomal subunit (Fig. 27-4; also see Fig. 27-1).
    A. Aminoglycosides
        1. Examples
           a. Amikacin
           b. Gentamicin
           c. Streptomycin
           d. Tobramycin
        2. Key characteristics
           a. Bind to the 30S ribosomal subunit
           b. Bactericidal
           c. Multiple mechanisms of resistance
           d. Adverse effects

> Polymyxin is effective against gram-negative; daptomycin is effective against gram-positive organisms.

> Polymyxin B is mainly used topically.

> Gentamicin is the most widely used aminoglycoside.

> Aminoglycosides are bactericidal.

BOX 27-3 PROTEIN SYNTHESIS INHIBITORS

Inhibitors of the 30S Ribosomal Subunit
Aminoglycosides
  Amikacin
  Gentamicin
  Kanamycin
  Neomycin
  Streptomycin
  Tobramycin
Tetracyclines
  Demeclocycline
  Doxycycline
  Minocycline
  Tetracycline

Inhibitors of the 50S Ribosomal Subunit
Macrolides
  Azithromycin
  Clarithromycin
  Erythromycin
Other Antibiotics
  Chloramphenicol
  Clindamycin
  Linezolid
  Quinupristin-dalfopristin
  Telithromycin
  Mupirocin

27-4: Bacterial protein synthesis and sites of drug action. *(From Brenner G and Stevens C: Pharmacology, 3rd ed. Philadelphia, Saunders, 2010, Figure 39-1.)*

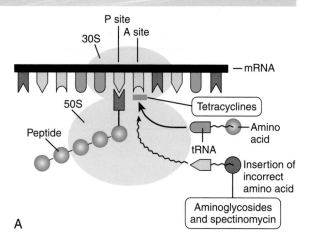

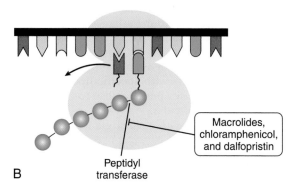

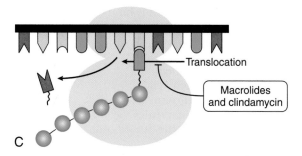

Dose adjustment required for aminoglycosides in the elderly to reduce nephrotoxicity.

Aminoglycosides are effective in single daily dosing because of their long post-antibiotic effect and concentration dependent killing.

Aminoglycosides are taken up by bacteria via an oxygen-dependent process; not effective against anaerobes.

Aminoglycosides: bactericidal inhibitors of protein synthesis.

(1) Nephrotoxicity
  • Commonly occurs in elderly because physicians do *not* dose-adjust the drug to the patient's reduced glomerular filtration rate that normally occurs in the aging process.
(2) Ototoxicity
(3) Neuromuscular junction blockade
3. Pharmacokinetics
  a. Usually given by intramuscular or intravenous injection
    • Poorly absorbed from the GI tract
  b. Dosage monitoring using plasma levels
  c. Often used for once-a-day dosing
  d. Eliminated by glomerular filtration
4. Pharmacodynamics
  a. Mechanism of action
    (1) Undergo active transport across cell membrane via an oxygen-dependent process after crossing the outer membrane via a porin channel
      • *Not* effective against anaerobes
    (2) Bactericidal inhibitor of protein synthesis
    (3) Bactericidal

(4) Once bound to specific 30S ribosome proteins

    (a) Interfere with the "initiation complex" of peptide formation

    (b) Misread mRNA, causing the incorporation of incorrect amino acids into the peptide

    (c) Synergy with β-lactam antibiotics

  b. Causes of resistance

    (1) Adenylation, acetylation, or phosphorylation (occurs via plasmids) as the result of the production of an enzyme by the inactivating microorganism

    (2) Alteration in porin channels or proteins involved in the oxygen-dependent transport of aminoglycosides

    (3) Deletion or alteration of the receptor on the 30S ribosomal subunit that binds the aminoglycosides

5. General uses

  a. Infections with aerobic gram-negative bacteria

    (1) *E. coli*

    (2) *Proteus*

    (3) *Klebsiella*

    (4) *Serratia*

    (5) *Enterobacter*

  b. Infection with *P. aeruginosa* in combination with:

    (1) Antipseudomonal penicillins

      (a) Piperacillin

      (b) Ticarcillin

    (2) Third- or fourth-generation cephalosporins

      (a) Ceftazidime (third)

      (b) Cefepime (fourth)

    (3) Fluoroquinolone (ciprofloxacin)

    (4) Carbapenem

      (a) Imipenem

      (b) Meropenem

      (c) Doripenem

    (5) Monobactam (aztreonam)

6. Specific uses of agents

  a. Streptomycin

    (1) Tuberculosis

    (2) Streptococcal or enterococcal endocarditis

      • Streptomycin has better gram-positive activity than gentamicin.

    (3) Mycobacterial infections

    (4) Plague

    (5) Tularemia

    (6) Brucellosis

  b. Amikacin, gentamicin, tobramycin

    (1) Gram-negative coverage

    (2) Often in combination with penicillins or cephalosporins

  c. Neomycin

    (1) Skin and eye infections (topical)

    (2) Preparation for colon surgery (oral; *not* absorbed))

7. Adverse effects

  a. Ototoxicity

  b. Nephrotoxicity (acute tubular necrosis)

  c. Neuromuscular junction blockade (high doses; see Chapter 6)

B. Tetracyclines

1. Examples

  a. Demeclocycline

  b. Doxycycline

  c. Minocycline

  d. Tetracycline

2. Key characteristics

  a. Chelation with multivalent metals

  b. Bacteriostatic action

  c. Reversible inhibition of protein synthesis (30S inhibitor)

  d. Broad spectrum of action

Margin notes:

Aminoglycosides bind to 30S ribosome.

Aminoglycosides: treatment of gram-negative infections

Aminoglycosides plus antipseudomonal penicillins are used for *P. aeruginosa*.

Streptomycin is used for: Tuberculosis; streptococcal or enterococcal endocarditis; mycobacterial infections; plague; tularemia.

Tetracyclines have the broadest spectrum of action of antibacterial protein synthesis inhibitors.

e. Multiple drug resistance
f. Adverse effects
   (1) GI toxicity
   (2) Bone growth retardation
   (3) Tooth discoloration
   (4) Photosensitivity
3. Pharmacokinetics
  a. Absorption
   (1) Decreased by chelation with divalent and trivalent cations
   (2) Do *not* give with foods or medicines that contain calcium
   (3) Do *not* give with antacid or iron-containing medicinals
  b. Distribution:
   (1) High concentration
    (a) Bones
    (b) Teeth
    (c) Kidneys
    (d) Liver
   (2) Low concentration
    (a) CNS
    (b) Adipose tissues
   (3) Crosses placenta and is excreted in milk
  c. Excretion
   (1) Tetracycline
    • Cleared mostly by the kidney
   (2) Minocycline, doxycycline
    • Cleared mostly by biliary excretion
4. Pharmacodynamics
  a. Mechanism of action (see Fig. 27-4)
   (1) Reversible inhibitor of protein synthesis
   (2) Bind to the 30S subunit of the ribosome
   (3) Blocks binding of aminoacyl-tRNA to the acceptor site (A site) on the mRNA-ribosome complex
   (4) Bacteriostatic
   (5) Broad spectrum of action
  b. Causes of resistance
   (1) Decreased intracellular accumulation caused by impaired influx or increased efflux via an active transport protein pump (encoded on a plasmid)
   (2) Ribosomal protection by synthesis of proteins that interfere with the binding of tetracyclines to the ribosome
   (3) Enzymatic inactivation of tetracyclines
    • The practice of using tetracycline in food for animals has contributed to resistance of tetracyclines globally.
5. Uses
  a. Infections with gram-positive and gram-negative bacteria, including
   (1) *Mycoplasma pneumoniae*
   (2) *Chlamydia*
   (3) *Vibrio cholerae*
   (4) Rocky Mountain spotted fever *(Rickettsia)*
   (5) Lyme disease *(Borrelia burgdorferi)* (doxycycline)
  b. Syndrome of inappropriate antidiuretic hormone (SIADH) (demeclocycline)
  c. Syphilis and gonorrhea (alternative treatment)
  d. Plague *(Yersinia pestis)* (doxycycline)
  e. Alternative to mefloquine for malaria prophylaxis (doxycycline)
  f. Treatment of inflammatory lesions associated with rosacea
  g. As part of a multidrug regimen for *Helicobacter pylori* eradication (tetracycline)
6. Adverse effects
  a. Nausea
  b. Diarrhea *(C. difficile)*
  c. Inhibition of bone growth (fetuses, infants, and children)
  d. Discoloration of teeth
  e. Superinfections (e.g., candidiasis)
  f. Photosensitivity

Margin notes:

Tetracyclines bind to divalent and trivalent cations.

Tetracyclines concentrate in tissues high in calcium or DNA.

Tetracyclines bind to the 30S ribosome.

Tetracyclines are bacteriostatic.

Tetracyclines: antibiotic of choice for chlamydial infection, brucellosis, mycoplasma pneumonia, rickettsial infections, some spirochetes (Lyme disease, alternative for syphilis)

Tetracyclines are category D in pregnancy and contraindicated in children younger than 8 years of age.

C. Macrolides
1. Examples
   a. Erythromycin
   b. Clarithromycin
   c. Azithromycin
2. Key characteristics
   a. Bacteriostatic but bactericidal for some bacteria
   b. Reversible inhibitors of protein synthesis (50S inhibitors)
   c. Elimination by biliary secretion
3. Pharmacokinetics
   a. Absorbed from GI tract, but acid-labile (erythromycin)
   b. Erythromycin esters or enteric coated erythromycin base provides sufficient oral absorption
   c. Also administered IV
   d. Excellent distribution, except to CNS
   e. Crosses placenta
   f. Excreted in bile (levels 50 times higher than in plasma)
   g. Half-life 2-5 hours except for azithromycin (60 or more hours)
4. Mechanism of action (see Fig. 27-4)
   a. Binds reversibly to the 50S ribosomal subunit
   b. Blocks peptidyl transferase and prevents translocation from the aminoacyl site to the peptidyl site
5. Causes of resistance
   a. Plasma-encoded reduced permeability
   b. Intracellular metabolism of the drug
   c. Modification of the ribosomal binding site (methyltransferases)
6. General uses
   a. Gram positive bacteria, some gram negative
   b. Backup for penicillins in penicillin-sensitive patient
   c. Azithromycin and clarithromycin have a broader spectrum
   d. Good for:
      (1) *Mycoplasma* pneumonia
      (2) Legionnaires' disease
      (3) Chlamydia
7. Use of specific drugs
   a. Erythromycin
      (1) Legionnaires' disease
      (2) *M. pneumoniae*
      (3) Neonatal genital or ocular infections
      (4) Chlamydial infections
   b. Azithromycin
      (1) *Mycobacterium avium* complex prophylaxis in patients with advanced human immunodeficiency virus (HIV)
      (2) Sinusitis and otitis media (*H. influenzae, M. catarrhalis*)
      (3) Chlamydial infections
   c. Clarithromycin
      (1) Infection caused by *H. pylori*
      (2) Also, for infections treated with azithromycin
      (3) Treatment of *M. avium*-intracellulare
8. Adverse effects
   a. Erythromycin (cytochrome P450 system inhibitor) increases the effects of:
      (1) Carbamazepine
      (2) Clozapine
      (3) Cyclosporine
      (4) Digoxin
      (5) Midazolam
      (6) Quinidine
      (7) Protease inhibitors
   b. GI effects
      (1) Anorexia
      (2) Nausea
      (3) Vomiting
      (4) Diarrhea

Note common ending of -thromycin for all macrolides.

Azithromycin does not inhibit cytochrome P450.

Azithromycin only has to be administered 3 to 5 days for treatment of most infections.

Macrolides bind to 50S ribosome.

Erythromycin has similar antibacterial coverage as Penicillin G.

Macrolides are good for respiratory infections.

Single-dose azithromycin is the drug of choice for the treatment of chlamydial infections concomitant with gonorrhea.

Erythromycin inhibits cytochrome P450; causes many drug-drug interactions.

c. Hepatotoxicity
  - Intrahepatic cholestasis (erythromycin estolate)
  d. Pseudomembranous colitis

D. Other protein synthesis inhibitors
  1. Chloramphenicol
    a. Pharmacokinetics
      (1) Well absorbed from all routes
      (2) CNS levels equal serum levels
      (3) Glucuronidation in liver is rate-limiting step for inactivation/clearance.
      (4) 100% excreted in urine
        (a) 10% filtration of parent
        (b) 90% tubular secretion of glucuronide
    b. Mechanism of action (see Fig. 27-4)
      (1) Inhibits protein synthesis at the 50S ribosome
      (2) Inhibits peptidyl transferase
      (3) Bacteriostatic
    c. Uses
      (1) Therapy should be limited to infections for which the benefits outweigh the risks.
      (2) Ampicillin-resistant *H. influenzae* meningitis
      (3) Alternative drug for infections caused by:
        (a) *Bacteroides*
        (b) *Neisseria meningitidis*
        (c) *Rickettsia*
        (d) *Salmonella*
    d. Adverse effects
      (1) Aplastic anemia (idiosyncratic with oral administration)
      (2) Dose dependent inhibition of erythropoiesis
      (3) Gray baby syndrome
        - Deficiency of glucuronyl transferase at birth
      (4) Inhibits cytochrome P-450s
  2. Clindamycin (oral, IV, topical)
    a. Mechanism of action (see Fig. 27-4)
      (1) Inhibits protein synthesis at the 50S ribosome
      (2) Bacteriostatic
    b. Uses
      (1) Severe gram-positive anaerobic infections (*Bacteroides* and others)
      (2) Aspiration pneumonia
      (3) Bacterial (*Gardnerella, Mycoplasma, Prevotella)* vaginosis (vaginal cream, vaginal suppository)
      (4) Pelvic inflammatory disease (IV)
      (5) Topically in treatment of severe acne
    c. Adverse effects
      (1) Severe diarrhea
      (2) Pseudomembranous colitis *(C. difficile)*
  3. Linezolid (oral, IV)
    a. Mechanism of action
      (1) Binds to the 50S ribosome
      (2) Interferes with protein synthesis
      (3) Bacteriostatic against enterococci and staphylococci
      (4) Bactericidal against most strains of streptococci.
    b. Uses
      (1) Treatment of VRE infections
      (2) Nosocomial pneumonia caused by *S. aureus* including MRSA or *Streptococcus pneumoniae*
      (3) Skin infections (including diabetic foot infections without concomitant osteomyelitis)
      (4) Community-acquired pneumonia caused by susceptible gram-positive organisms
    c. Adverse effects
      (1) Diarrhea, nausea and vomiting
      (2) Headache
      (3) Thrombocytopenia and neutropenia

Erythromycin and clarithromycin similarly inhibit the P-450 system, azithromycin is much less inhibitory.

Erythromycin causes the most frequent GI adverse effects, clarithromycin and azithromycin produce much fewer.

Chloramphenicol binds to 50S ribosome.

Chloramphenicol is active against gram positive and negative anaerobes.

Chloramphenicol: potential to cause lethal aplastic anemia; gray baby syndrome in newborns

Chloramphenicol: inhibitor of microsomal oxidation that increases blood levels of phenytoin, tolbutamide, and warfarin

Clindamycin binds to 50S ribosome.

Clindamycin is effective against anaerobes.

Linezolid used to treat vancomycin-resistant organisms.

(4) Inhibits monoamine oxidase (MAO)
- Patients should avoid consuming tyramine-containing foods (e.g., aged cheese, red wine)

Linezolid inhibits MAO.

4. Quinupristin-dalfopristin (IV)
   a. Mechanism of action (see Fig. 27-4)
      (1) Binds to multiple sites on 50S ribosome
      (2) Interferes with protein synthesis
      (3) Bactericidal
   b. Uses
      (1) Treatment of serious or life-threatening infections associated with VRE bacteremia
      (2) Treatment of complicated skin infections caused by MRSA or *Streptococcus pyogenes*
   c. Adverse effects
      (1) Nausea and vomiting
      (2) Diarrhea
   d. Drug interactions
      (1) Potent inhibitors of CYP3A4
      (2) Increase plasma levels of:
         (a) Cyclosporine
         (b) Diazepam
         (c) Nucleoside reverse transcriptase inhibitors
         (d) Warfarin

Quinupristin-dalfopristin used to treat vancomycin-resistant organisms.

Quinupristin-dalfopristin potent inhibitor of CYP3A4; causes many drug-drug interactions.

5. Telithromycin
   a. Broad-spectrum antibiotic
   b. Binds to the 50S ribosomal subunit
   c. Similar to macrolides
   d. Used for upper and lower respiratory tract infections
   e. May cause severe hepatotoxicity

Telithromycin similar to macrolides.

6. Mupirocin
   a. Mechanism of action
      (1) Binds to bacterial isoleucyl transfer-RNA synthetase
      (2) Inhibits ribosomal protein synthesis
   b. Uses
      (1) Intranasal
         - Eradication of nasal colonization with MRSA
      (2) Topical
         - Treatment of impetigo or secondary infected traumatic skin lesions due to *S. aureus* and *S. pyogenes*
   c. Adverse effects
      (1) Nasal irritation
      (2) Pharyngitis
   E. **Therapeutic summary of selected protein synthesis inhibitors:** (Table 27-7)
V. **Antimetabolites Used for Microorganisms** (Box 27-4)
   A. **General**
      - These antimicrobials interfere with the metabolism of folic acid (see Fig. 27-1 and Fig. 27-5).
   B. **Sulfonamides**
      1. Key characteristics
         a. Competitive inhibition of *p*-aminobenzoic acid (PABA) incorporation
         b. Synergistic action with trimethoprim
         c. Primary use is for UTIs
         d. Adverse effects
            (1) Acute hemolytic anemia
            (2) Crystalluria (crystals in the urine)
      2. Pharmacodynamics
         a. Mechanism of action
            - Bacteriostatic
               (1) Competitive inhibitor of dihydropteroate synthase (see Fig. 27-5)
               (2) Have a synergistic action when given with trimethoprim
               (3) Combination causes a sequential blockade of the formation of tetrahydrofolate.
               (4) Trimethoprim inhibits dihydrofolate reductase in folate metabolism.
         b. Causes of resistance
            - Mutations cause excess production of PABA.

Primary use for sulfonamides: UTIs

Force fluids with sulfonamide therapy to prevent crystalluria.

TABLE 27-7. **Therapeutic Summary of Selected Protein Synthesis Inhibitors**

Drugs	Clinical Applications	Adverse Effects	Contraindications
Mechanism: *Bactericidal inhibitor of 30S ribosomes; bactericidal*			
Aminoglycosides Amikacin Gentamicin Kanamycin Neomycin Streptomycin Tobramycin	Infections with aerobic gram-negative bacteria *Escherichia coli* *Proteus* *Klebsiella* *Serratia* *Enterobacter* *Pseudomonas*	Ototoxicity Nephrotoxicity (acute tubular necrosis) Neuromuscular junction blockade	Hypersensitivity Severe renal dysfunction
Mechanism: *Reversible inhibitor of 30S ribosomes; bacteriostatic*			
Tetracyclines Demeclocycline Doxycycline Minocycline Tetracycline	*Mycoplasma pneumoniae* *Chlamydia* *Vibrio cholerae* Rocky Mountain spotted fever *(Rickettsia)* Lyme disease (doxycycline) Syndrome of inappropriate antidiuretic hormone (SIADH) (demeclocycline) Syphilis and gonorrhea (alternative treatment) Plague *(Yersinia pestis)* (doxycycline) Alternative to mefloquine for malaria prophylaxis (doxycycline) Treatment of inflammatory lesions associated with rosacea As part of a multidrug regimen for *Helicobacter pylori* eradication (tetracycline)	Nausea Diarrhea *(Clostridium difficile)* Inhibition of bone growth (fetuses, infants, and children) Discoloration of teeth Superinfections (e.g., candidiasis) Photosensitivity	Hypersensitivity Children ≤8 years of age Severe hepatic dysfunction Pregnancy
Mechanism: *Reversible inhibitor of 50S ribosomes; bacteriostatic*			
Macrolides Azithromycin Clarithromycin Erythromycin	*Erythromycin* Legionnaires' disease Mycoplasma pneumonia Neonatal genital or ocular infections Chlamydial infections *Azithromycin* *Mycobacterium avium* complex prophylaxis in patients with advanced HIV Sinusitis and otitis media *(Haemophilus influenzae, Moraxella catarrhalis)* Chlamydial infections *Clarithromycin* Infection caused by *H. pylori* Also, for infections treated with azithromycin	Inhibition of drug metabolism (erythromycin and clarithromycin) GI effects (erythromycin) Anorexia Nausea Vomiting Diarrhea Hepatotoxicity Cholestatic hepatitis (erythromycin estolate) Pseudomembranous colitis	Hypersensitivity
Mechanism: *Reversible inhibitor of 50S ribosomes; bacteriostatic*			
Clindamycin	Aspiration pneumonia Bacterial vaginosis (vaginal cream, vaginal suppository) Osteomyelitis Pelvic inflammatory disease (IV) Severe gram-positive anaerobic infections (Bacteroides and others) Topically in treatment of severe acne	Severe diarrhea Pseudomembranous colitis *(C. difficile)*	Hypersensitivity

---

BOX 27-4 ANTIMETABOLITES

Sulfonamides
Silver sulfadiazine
Sulfacetamide
Sulfadiazine
Sulfisoxazole

Dihydrofolate Reductase Inhibitors
Trimethoprim/sulfamethoxazole (TMP/SMX)
Trimethoprim

---

3. Uses
    a. Sulfisoxazole
        (1) UTIs
        (2) Otitis media
        (3) Chlamydia
        (4) Nocardiosis
    b. Sulfadiazine
        (1) Urinary tract infections
        (2) Nocardiosis
        (3) Adjunctive treatment in toxoplasmosis
        (4) Uncomplicated attack of malaria

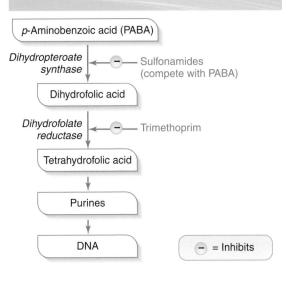

27-5: Sequential inhibition of tetrahydrofolic acid synthesis. Dihydropteroate is inhibited by sulfonamides and sulfones (dapsone). Dihydrofolate reductase is inhibited by trimethoprim (bacteria, protozoa); pyrimethamine (protozoa); and methotrexate (mammals). Trimethoprim is used in the treatment of certain infections; pyrimethamine is used in the treatment of malaria; and methotrexate is used as an anticancer and immunosuppressive agent. PABA, p-aminobenzoic acid.

   c. Sulfacetamide
     (1) Ophthalmic
       • Treatment and prophylaxis of conjunctivitis
     (2) Dermatologic
       (a) Scaling dermatosis (seborrheic)
       (b) Bacterial infections of the skin
       (c) Acne vulgaris
   c. Silver sulfadiazine
     (1) Applied topically
     (2) Prevention and treatment of infection in second- and third-degree burns
  4. Adverse effects
   a. Blood dyscrasias
     (1) Agranulocytosis
     (2) Leukemia
     (3) Aplastic anemia (rare)
     (4) Methemoglobinemia and hemolysis in G6PD deficient patients
     (5) Folate deficiency with macrocytic anemia
   b. Crystalluria and hematuria
   c. Hypersensitivity reactions
     • Stevens-Johnson syndrome most severe form
   d. Kernicterus in infants
  5. Contraindications
   a. Relative contraindications
     (1) Preexisting bone marrow suppression
     (2) Blood dyscrasias
     (3) Megaloblastic anemia secondary to folate deficiency
   b. Absolute contraindications
     (1) G6PD deficiency
     (2) Megaloblastic anemia
     (3) Porphyria
     (4) Neonatal period
   c. Sulfonamide hypersensitivity
C. Trimethoprim
  1. Mechanism of action (see Fig. 27-5)
   a. Inhibits dihydrofolate reductase
   b. Bacteriostatic
  2. Uses
   a. Prostatitis
   b. Vaginitis
   c. Otitis media and bronchitis (in combination with sulfonamide)
  3. Adverse effects
   • Similar to those of sulfonamides

Sulfacetamide used for eye infections; neutral pH so not irritating.

Silver sulfadiazine used to treat and prevent infections in burn patients.

Sulfonamides may cause Stevens-Johnson syndrome (severe skin rashes)

Sulfonamides may produce kernicterus in newborns.

Don't use sulfonamides in patients with G6PD deficiency.

Many drugs are contraindicated in patients with sulfonamide allergies: Sulfonamide antimicrobials; sulfonylurea oral hypoglycemics; All thiazide and loop (except ethacrynic acid) diuretics; celecoxib.

D. **Trimethoprim/sulfamethoxazole (TMP/SMX) combination** (see Fig. 27-5)
   1. These two selected because of similar pharmacokinetics
   2. Given both orally and intravenously
   3. Use
      a. Oral treatment
         (1) Urinary tract infections due to *E. coli*, *Klebsiella* and *Enterobacter* spp., *Morganella morganii*, *Proteus mirabilis* and *Proteus vulgaris*
         (2) Acute otitis media in children
         (3) Acute exacerbations of chronic bronchitis in adults due to susceptible strains of *H. influenzae* or *S. pneumoniae*
         (4) Treatment and prophylaxis of *Pneumocystis jiroveci* pneumonitis (PCP)
         (5) Traveler's diarrhea due to enterotoxigenic *E. coli*
         (6) Treatment of enteritis caused by *Shigella flexneri* or *Shigella sonnei*
      b. IV treatment for severe or complicated infections
         (1) Documented PCP
         (2) Empiric treatment of PCP in immune compromised patients
         (3) Treatment of documented or suspected shigellosis
         (4) Typhoid fever
         (5) *Nocardia asteroides* infection
E. **Therapeutic summary of selected antimetabolites and fluoroquinolones used as antimicrobials** (Table 27-8)
VI. **Inhibitors of DNA gyrase: fluoroquinolones** (Box 27-5)
   A. **General information**
      1. Fluoroquinolones interfere with bacteria DNA synthesis (see Fig. 27-1).
      2. Classified by "generation"
         a. First-generation
            (1) Norfloxacin
            (2) Activity against common pathogens that cause UTIs
            (3) Similar to nalidixic acid
               (a) Quinolone used to treat UTIs
               (b) Predecessor to the fluoroquinolones
         b. Second-generation
            (1) Ciprofloxacin
            (2) Ofloxacin
            (3) Excellent activity against:
               (a) Gram-negative bacteria including gonococcus
               (b) Many gram-positive cocci
               (c) *Mycobacteria*
               (d) *M. pneumoniae*
         c. Third-generation
            (1) Levofloxacin
            (2) Gatifloxacin
            (3) Less activity against gram-negative bacteria but greater activity against some gram-positive cocci
               (a) *S. pneumoniae*
               (b) Enterococci
               (c) MRSA
         d. Fourth-generation
            (1) Gemifloxacin
            (2) Moxifloxacin
            (3) Broadest spectrum fluoroquinolones
            (4) Good activity against anaerobes and pneumococci
            (5) Good CNS penetration
   B. **Pharmacokinetics**
      1. Good oral bioavailability
         • Absorption is affected by antacids containing divalent and trivalent cations
      2. Excretion of most fluoroquinolones is by tubular secretion
         • Blocked by probenecid
   C. **Mechanism of action**
      1. Inhibits DNA-gyrase (topoisomerase II)
      2. Also, inhibits topoisomerase IV
      3. Inhibits the relaxation of supercoiled DNA
      4. Promotes breakage of double-stranded DNA
      5. Bactericidal

Trimethoprim and sulfamethoxazole are used to together because of similar pharmacokinetics; they inhibit sequential steps in folate utilization.

TMP/SMX preferred drug for treatment and prophylaxis of *Pneumocystis jiroveci* pneumonitis (PCP).

Ciprofloxacin and ofloxacin good for gram-negative organisms.

Levofloxacin and gatifloxacin good for gram-positive organisms.

Gemifloxacin and moxifloxacin good for anaerobes and pneumococci.

Note the common ending of -floxacin for most fluoroquinolones.

TABLE 27-8. **Therapeutic Summary of Selected Antimetabolites and Fluoroquinolones**

Drugs	Clinical Applications	Adverse Effects	Contraindications
Mechanism: *Competitive inhibitor of dihydropteroate synthase; bacteriostatic*			

Sulfacetamide
Sulfadiazine
Sulfisoxazole
Silver sulfadiazine
	Sulfisoxazole
	  Urinary tract infections
	  Otitis media
	  Chlamydia
	  Nocardiosis
	Sulfadiazine
	  Urinary tract infections
	  Nocardiosis
	  Adjunctive treatment in toxoplasmosis
	  Uncomplicated attack of malaria
	Sulfacetamide
	  Ophthalmic: Treatment and prophylaxis of conjunctivitis
	  Dermatologic:
	    Scaling dermatosis (seborrheic)
	    Bacterial infections of the skin
	    Acne vulgaris
	Silver sulfadiazine
	  Prevention and treatment of infection in second- and
	    third-degree burns
		Blood dyscrasias
		Agranulocytosis
		Leukemia
		Aplastic anemia
		  (rare)
		Crystalluria and
		  hematuria
		Hypersensitivity
		  reactions
		Stevens-Johnson
		  syndrome most
		  severe form
			Relative contraindications
			Preexisting bone marrow
			  suppression
			Blood dyscrasias
			Megaloblastic anemia
			  secondary to folate
			  deficiency
			Absolute contraindications
			Glucose-6-phosphate
			  dehydrogenase (G6PD)
			  deficiency
			Megaloblastic anemia
			Porphyria
			Neonatal period
			Sulfonamide
			  hypersensitivity

Mechanism: *Competitive inhibitor of dihydrofolate reductase; bacteriostatic*			
Trimethoprim	Prostatitis Vaginitis Otitis media and bronchitis	Similar to sulfonamides	
Mechanism: *Sequential inhibition of tetrahydrofolate; bacteriostatic*			

Trimethoprim/
  sulfamethoxazole
  (TMP/SMX)
	Oral treatment
	  Urinary tract infections due to *Escherichia coli, Klebsiella*
	    and Enterobacter spp., *Morganella morganii, Proteus mirabilis*
	    and *Proteus vulgaris*
	  Acute otitis media in children
	  Acute exacerbations of chronic bronchitis in adults due to
	    susceptible strains of *Haemophilus influenzae* or *Streptococcus*
	    pneumoniae
	  Treatment and prophylaxis of *Pneumocystis jiroveci*
	    pneumonitis (PCP)
	  Traveler's diarrhea due to enterotoxigenic *E. coli*
	  Treatment of enteritis caused by *Shigella flexneri* or *Shigella*
	    sonnei
	IV treatment for severe or complicated infections
	  Documented PCP
	  Empiric treatment of PCP in immune compromised patients
	  Treatment of documented or suspected shigellosis
	  Typhoid fever
	  Nocardia asteroides infection
		See sulfonamides	See sulfonamides

Mechanism: *DNA gyrase inhibitors; bactericidal*			

Ciprofloxacin
Gatifloxacin
Gemifloxacin
Levofloxacin
Moxifloxacin
Norfloxacin
Ofloxacin
Trovafloxacin
	Infections with aerobic gram-negative rods
	  Enterobacteriaceae
	  Pseudomonas
	  Neisseria
	Infections caused by:
	  Campylobacter jejuni
	  Salmonella
	  Shigella
	  Mycobacterium avium complex
	Types of infections:
	  Sinusitis
	  Bronchitis
	  Pneumonia
	  UTIs
	  Neutropenic fever (ciprofloxacin)
	  Anthrax prophylaxis (ciprofloxacin)
		Nausea
		Interactions with
		  other drugs
		Avoid:
		Calcium containing
		  medications
		Theophylline
		Caffeine.
		Interference with
		  collagen synthesis
		Causes tendon
		  rupture
			Hypersensitivity
			Pregnancy
			Children

BOX 27-5   DNA GYRASE INHIBITORS: FLUOROQUINOLONES

Ciprofloxacin	Moxifloxacin
Gatifloxacin	Norfloxacin
Gemifloxacin	Ofloxacin
Levofloxacin	Trovafloxacin

Overuse of fluoroquinolones is leading to increased resistance to this class of antimicrobials.

D. **Resistance**
   1. Due to a change in the gyrase enzyme
   2. Decreased permeability
E. **Uses**
   1. Infections with aerobic gram-negative rods
      a. Enterobacteriaceae
      b. *Pseudomonas*
   2. Infections caused by:
      a. *Campylobacter jejuni*
      b. *Salmonella*
      c. *Shigella*
      d. *M. avium* complex
      e. *N. gonorrhoeae*
   3. Types of infections
      a. Sinusitis
      b. Bronchitis
      c. Pneumonia
      d. UTIs
      e. Neutropenic fever (ciprofloxacin)
      f. Anthrax prophylaxis (ciprofloxacin)
F. **Adverse effects**
   1. Nausea
   2. Interactions with other drugs
      a. Patients taking fluoroquinolones should avoid:
         (1) Calcium-containing medications
         (2) Theophylline
         (3) Caffeine
      b. Divalent, trivalent cations decrease the absorption of fluoroquinolones
   3. Interference with collagen synthesis
      a. Causes tendon rupture
         • The U.S. Food and Drug Administration (FDA) boxed warning; Increased risk of tendonitis and tendon rupture associated with the use of fluoroquinolones.
      b. Should be avoided during pregnancy
   4. Abnormal liver function tests
      • Trovafloxacin use is limited because of hepatotoxicity
   5. Seizures
   6. All quinolones prolong QT interval
G. **Therapeutic summary of selected antimetabolites and fluoroquinolones used as antimicrobials** (see Table 27-8)

Fluoroquinolones are good for UTIs and respiratory infections.

Ciprofloxacin recommended for bioengineered anthrax used in bioterrorism.

Divalent, trivalent cations decrease the bioavailability of fluoroquinolones.

Ciprofloxacin may cause rupture of the Achilles tendon.

Trovafloxacin use is limited to life- and limb-threatening infections.

Fluoroquinolones prolong QT interval in electrocardiogram (ECG).

CHAPTER 28
OTHER ANTI-INFECTIVE DRUGS

I. Antimycobacterial Drugs (Box 28-1)
- The management of tuberculosis is summarized in Table 28-1.
  A. Isoniazid (INH)
  1. Pharmacokinetics
     a. Metabolism occurs by acetylation (*N*-acetyltransferase; NAT)
        - This enzyme is under genetic control
     b. Individuals are either *fast* or *slow* acetylators.
  2. Mechanism of action
     a. Inhibits synthesis of mycolic acids
     b. Thus, inhibits mycobacterial cell wall synthesis
     c. Bactericidal
     d. Resistance
        (1) Mutations in catalase-peroxidase *(katg)* preventing conversion of the prodrug isoniazid to its active metabolite
        (2) Mutation in the mycobacterial *inhA* and *KasA* genes involved in mycolic acid biosynthesis
        (3) Mutations in nicotinamide-adenine dinucleotide (NADH) dehydrogenase *(ndh)*
  3. Use
     - Tuberculosis (Mycobacterium tuberculosis)
        a. Prophylaxis in tuberculin converters (positive skin test)
        b. Treatment along with rifampin, ethambutol, pyrazinamide, or streptomycin (see Table 28-1)
  4. Adverse effects
     a. Hepatic damage (especially in individual's >50 years of age); boxed warning
        (1) Severe and sometimes fatal hepatitis may occur
        (2) Usually occurs within the first 3 months of treatment, although may develop even after many months of treatment
     b. Peripheral neuritis
        (1) Reversed by pyridoxine
        (2) More prominent in "slow" acetylators
     c. Sideroblastic anemia due to pyridoxine deficiency
  B. Rifampin
  1. Pharmacokinetics
     a. Well absorbed orally
     b. Hepatic metabolism
     c. Undergoes enterohepatic recirculation
     d. Marked inducer of cytochrome P-450s
     e. Penetrates well into tissues and phagocytic cells
  2. Mechanism of action
     a. Binds to the β-subunit of bacterial DNA-dependent RNA polymerase
     b. Inhibits binding of the enzyme to DNA
        - Blocks RNA transcription
     c. Resistance
        - Mutations reduce binding of the drug to the polymerase

To prevent resistance anti-TB drugs are often administered under direct observed therapy (DOT).

Isoniazid is metabolized by acetylation; *fast* or *slow* acetylators.

Isoniazid inhibits mycolic acid cell wall synthesis.

Use rifampin for prophylactic treatment in those older than 50 years of age.

Isoniazid is hepatotoxic.

Pyridoxine protects against isoniazid peripheral neurotoxicity.

Rifampin inhibits DNA-dependent RNA synthesis.

BOX 28-1 ANTIMYCOBACTERIAL DRUGS

Dapsone (leprosy)
Ethambutol
Isoniazid
Pyrazinamide
Rifabutin
Rifampin
Streptomycin

Clofazimine
Levofloxacin
Ofloxacin
Ethionamide
Para-aminosalicylic acid (PAS)
Capreomycin
Cycloserine
Rifapentine

Alternative Drugs Used in Treatment of Tuberculosis
Amikacin
Ciprofloxacin

TABLE 28-1. **Management of Tuberculosis**

THERAPEUTIC GOAL AND DRUG-RELATED PATIENT FEATURES	INITIAL DRUG TREATMENT	SUBSEQUENT DRUG TREATMENT
Prevention of Tuberculosis		
Not resistant to isoniazid	Isoniazid (6mo)	None
HIV-negative; resistant to isoniazid; >50 years of age	Rifampin (6mo)	None
HIV-positive	Rifampin* or rifabutin (12 months)	None
Treatment of Tuberculosis		
Not resistant to isoniazid	Combination of isoniazid, rifampin, ethambutol, and pyrazinamide for 2 months	Combination of isoniazid and rifampin (4 more months if HIV-negative or 7 more months if HIV-positive)
Possibly resistant to isoniazid	Combination of isoniazid, rifampin, pyrazinamide, and either ethambutol or streptomycin (6 months)	Individualized therapy based on microbial susceptibility testing
Resistant to multiple drugs†	Combination of at least four drugs believed to be active in patient population (6 months)	Individualized therapy based on microbial susceptibility testing

*In HIV-infected patients, substitution of rifabutin for rifampin minimizes drug interactions with protease inhibitors and nucleoside reverse transcriptase inhibitors.
†Patients suspected of having multidrug resistance include those from certain demographic populations, those who have failed to respond to previous treatment, and those who have experienced a relapse of tuberculosis.
HIV, human immunodeficiency virus.

3. Uses
   a. Tuberculosis *(M. tuberculosis)*
      (1) Prophylaxis in cases of isoniazid resistance or in individuals who are older than 50 years of age
      (2) Treatment in combination with other drugs (see Table 28-1)
   b. Prophylaxis in contacts of:
      (1) *Neisseria meningitidis*
      (2) *Haemophilus influenzae* type B
   c. Legionnaires' disease (in combination with azithromycin)
   d. Leprosy *(Mycobacterium leprae)* (combination therapy)
4. Adverse effects
   a. Red-orange discoloration of urine, tears, saliva
   b. Hepatotoxicity
   c. Drug interactions
      (1) Rifampin, a potent inducer of the cytochrome P450 hepatic enzyme systems, can reduce the plasma concentrations of many drugs, including:
         (a) Anticonvulsants
         (b) Contraceptive steroids
         (c) Cyclosporine
         (d) Ketoconazole
         (e) Methadone
         (f) Terbinafine
         (g) Warfarin

Treatment with rifampin often results in permanent discoloration of soft contact lenses.

Rifampin: potent inducer of cytochrome P450 hepatic enzymes

Rifampin decrease the effectiveness if contraceptive steroids.

(2) Rifabutin is a less potent inducer of the cytochrome P450 hepatic enzyme system.
   (a) Thus, it causes less robust drug-drug interactions
   (b) It is preferred for patients on human immunodeficiency virus (HIV) medications

Drug-drug interactions are less with rifabutin than rifampin.

C. Ethambutol
1. Pharmacokinetics
   a. Well absorbed orally
   b. Elimination
      (1) Urine (50% unchanged drug)
      (2) Feces (20% unchanged drug)
      (3) Hepatic metabolism (20%)
2. Mechanism of action
   a. Inhibits glycan synthesis (component of the mycobacterial cell wall)
   b. Inhibits RNA synthesis
   c. Bacteriostatic
3. Use
   • Tuberculosis (combination therapy; see Table 28-1)
4. Adverse effects
   a. Optic neuritis
   b. Reduction in red-green visual acuity
      • Annual eye examination required
   c. Hepatic toxicity
      • Likely due to combination therapy

Ethambutol use requires regular eye examinations.

D. Pyrazinamide
1. Pharmacokinetics
   a. Well absorbed orally
   b. Hepatic metabolism
2. Mechanism of action
   a. Requires metabolic conversion to pyrazinoic acid
   b. Bacteriostatic or bactericidal depending on drug's concentration at infection site
   c. Exact mechanism unknown
      • May relate to lowered pH
3. Use
   • Tuberculosis (combination therapy; see Table 28-1)
4. Adverse effects
   a. Hyperuricemia
   b. Hepatotoxicity
   c. Photosensitivity
   d. Use with caution in following patients:
      (1) Diabetes mellitus
      (2) Porphyria
      (3) History of alcoholism

Pyrazinamide is converted to pyrazinoic acid (active agent).

Pyrazinamide produces hepatotoxicity.

E. Rifabutin
1. General information
   a. Like rifampin
   b. *But* a less potent inducer of cytochrome P450 hepatic enzymes
2. Uses
   a. Substitute for rifampin in the treatment of tuberculosis in HIV-infected patients
   b. Prevention and treatment of *Mycobacterium avium* complex

F. Streptomycin (see aminoglycosides in Chapter 27)
1. This aminoglycoside is used more frequently today because of increased incidence of drug-resistant *M. tuberculosis* strains
2. Other uses include:
   a. Tularemia *(Francisella tularensis)*
   b. Plague *(Yersinia pestis)*
   c. In combination with a penicillin for the treatment of endocarditis.

Rifabutin preferred to use with HIV highly active antiretroviral therapy (HAART) cocktails since it is a less potent inducer of drug metabolisms than rifampin.

Streptomycin *only* used in initial therapy because it has to be injected and other agents are orally administered.

G. Alternative drugs used in treatment of tuberculosis (Box 28-1)
1. Use increasing because of drug resistance
2. Referred to as second line drugs and include:
   a. Amikacin
   b. Clofazimine

Because of resistance to first line drugs, second line drugs have to be used frequently.

c. Levofloxacin
d. Ofloxacin
e. Ethionamide
f. Para-aminosalicylic acid (PAS)
g. Capreomycin
h. Cycloserine
i. Rifapentine

H. Dapsone
1. Mechanism of action
   a. Inhibitor of folic acid synthesis
      • Like sulfonamides
   b. Bacteriostatic
2. Use
   • Treatment of leprosy *(M. leprae)*
3. Adverse effects
   a. Optic neuritis
   b. Neuropathy
   c. Contraindicated with glucose-6-phosphate dehydrogenase (G6PD) deficiency
      • Leads to hemolytic anemia

II. Therapeutic Summary of Selected Drugs used in Treatment of Tuberculosis: Table 28-2

III. Antiviral Drugs (Box 28-2)
   • The mechanism of viral replication and the effects of antiviral drugs are shown in Fig. 28-1.
A. Drugs used in the prevention and treatment of influenza
   1. Amantadine and rimantadine
      a. Mechanism of action
         (1) Blocks viral uncoating by blocking M2 proton channel
         (2) Prevents release of viral nucleic acid into the host cell
      b. Uses
         (1) Influenza A (prophylaxis)
         (2) Parkinson's disease (see Chapter 11)

> Dapsone used to treat leprosy.

> Amantadine blocks viral uncoating.

Table 28-2. **Therapeutic Summary of Selected Drugs used in Treatment of Tuberculosis**

DRUGS	CLINICAL APPLICATIONS	ADVERSE EFFECTS	CONTRAINDICATIONS
Mechanism: *Inhibits synthesis of mycolic acids*			
Isoniazid	TB prophylaxis TB treatment in combination with other drugs	Hepatic damage Peripheral neuritis	Hypersensitivity Liver disease
Mechanism: *Inhibits DNA-dependant RNA synthesis*			

Rifampin
Rifabutin
	TB treatment in combination with other drugs
	TB Prophylaxis (alternative)
	Prophylaxis in contacts of:
	  (1) *Neisseria meningitides*
	  (2) *Haemophilus influenzae* type B
	Legionnaires' disease (in combination with azithromycin)
	Leprosy *(Mycobacterium leprae)* (combination therapy)
		Red orange color of tissue fluids
		Hepatotoxicity
		Drug-drug interactions
			Hypersensitivity
			Concurrent use of amprenavir, saquinavir/ritonavir

Mechanism: *Inhibits glycan and RNA synthesis*			
Ethambutol	TB treatment in combination with other drugs	Optic neuritis Reduction in red-green visual acuity Hepatotoxicity	Hypersensitivity Optic neuritis Unconscious patients
Mechanism: *Requires metabolic conversion to pyrazinoic acid (low pH)*			
Pyrazinamide	TB treatment in combination with other drugs	Hyperuricemia Hepatotoxicity Photosensitivity	Hypersensitivity Acute gout Severe hepatic damage
Mechanism: *Bactericidal 30S ribosomal inhibitor of protein synthesis*			
Streptomycin	TB treatment in combination with other drugs Treatment of: Streptococcal or enterococcal endocarditis Plague Tularemia Brucellosis	Ototoxicity Nephrotoxicity (acute tubular necrosis) Neuromuscular junction blockade	Hypersensitivity Pregnancy

BOX 28-2   ANTIVIRAL DRUGS

Drugs Used in the Treatment and Prophylaxis of Influenza
Amantadine
Oseltamivir
Rimantadine
Zanamivir

Antiherpes Drugs
Acyclovir
Acyclovir congeners: famciclovir, penciclovir, valacyclovir
Cidofovir
Foscarnet
Ganciclovir
Valganciclovir

Interferons
Interferon alfa-2a
Interferon alfa-2b
Interferon alfacon-1
Interferon alfa-n3
Interferon beta-1a
Interferon beta-1b
Interferon gamma-1b
Peginterferon alfa-2a
Peginterferon alfa-2b

Antiretroviral Drugs
Nucleoside Reverse Transcriptase Inhibitors (NRTIs)
Abacavir
Adefovir
Didanosine (ddI)
Emtricitabine
Entecavir

Lamivudine (3TC)
Stavudine (d4T)
Telbivudine
Zalcitabine (ddC)
Zidovudine (AZT)
Nucleotide Reverse Transcriptase Inhibitor
Tenofovir
Nonnucleoside Reverse Transcriptase Inhibitors (NNRTIs)
Delavirdine
Efavirenz
Etavirine
Nevirapine
Protease Inhibitors (PIs)
Amprenavir
Atazanavir
Indinavir
Lopinavir
Nelfinavir
Ritonavir
Saquinavir
Tipranavir
Fusion Inhibitor
Enfuvirtide
Integrase Inhibitor
Raltegravir
CCR5 antagonist
Maraviroc

Other Antiviral Drugs
Docosanol
Fomivirsen
Ribavirin
Trifluridine

    c. Adverse effects
       (1) Dizziness
       (2) Anxiety
       (3) Impaired coordination
       (4) Livedo reticularis
    d. Amantadine or rimantadine: Advisory Committee on Immunization Practices (ACIP) 2008-2009 Influenza Guidelines (July 2008)
       (1) Do *not* recommend the use for the treatment or chemoprophylaxis of influenza A infection for residents of the United States.

> Influenza A highly resistant to amantadine.

       (2) Based on current patterns of resistance to these medications.
  2. Oseltamivir and zanamivir
    a. Administration
       (1) Oseltamivir: a prodrug given orally

> Oseltamivir taken orally.

       (2) Zanamivir given by inhalation

> Zanamivir taken by inhalation.

    b. Mechanism of action
       (1) Inhibit viral neuraminidase
       (2) Prevents extrusion from host cell

> -amivir drugs inhibit viral neuraminidase.

       (3) Prevents infection of new cells
    c. Uses
       (1) Treatment of influenza virus A and B in patients who have been symptomatic for *no* more than 2 days
       (2) Prophylaxis against influenza virus A and B
    d. Adverse effects
       (1) Headache
       (2) Throat/tonsil discomfort/pain

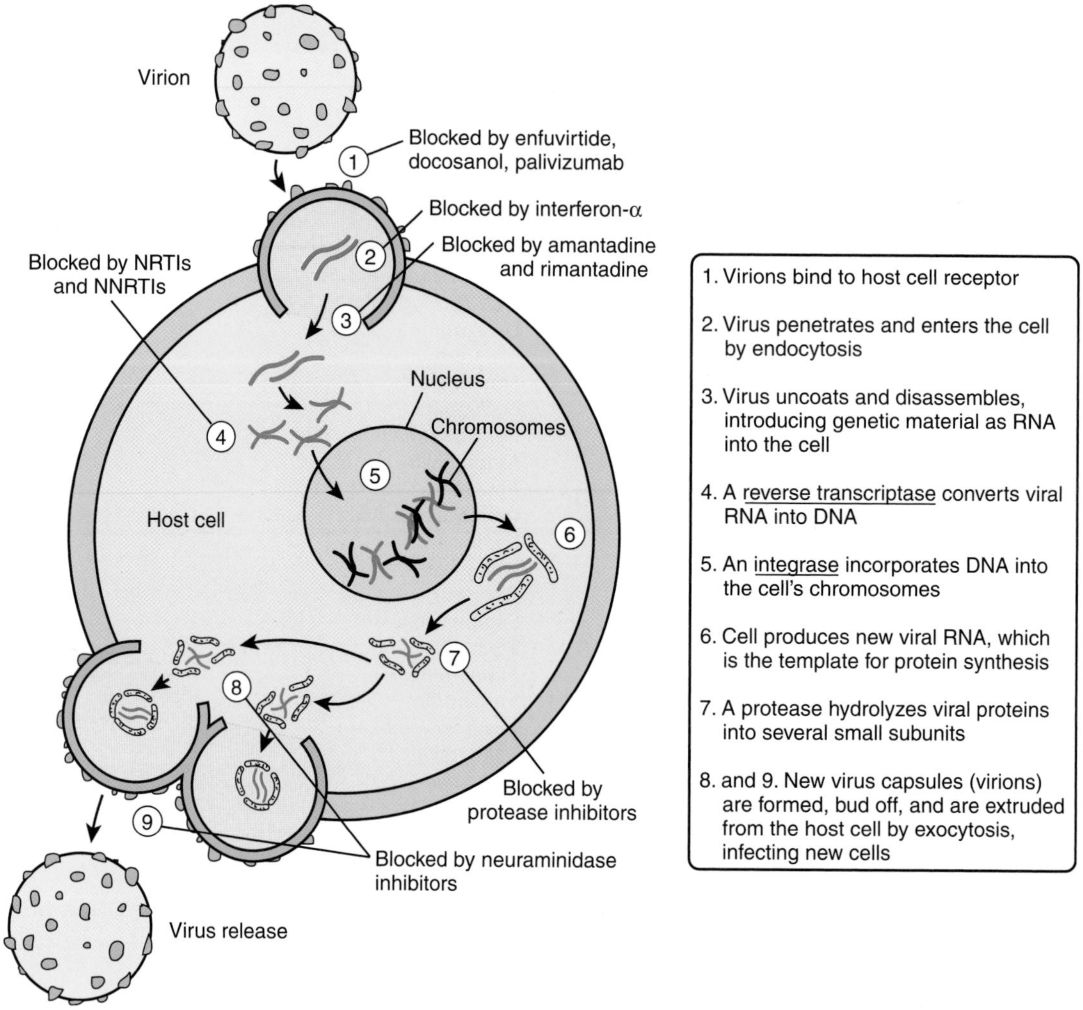
Virion
Blocked by enfuvirtide, docosanol, palivizumab
Blocked by interferon-α
Blocked by amantadine and rimantadine
Blocked by NRTIs and NNRTIs
Nucleus
Chromosomes
Host cell
Blocked by protease inhibitors
Blocked by neuraminidase inhibitors
Virus release
1. Virions bind to host cell receptor
2. Virus penetrates and enters the cell by endocytosis
3. Virus uncoats and disassembles, introducing genetic material as RNA into the cell
4. A reverse transcriptase converts viral RNA into DNA
5. An integrase incorporates DNA into the cell's chromosomes
6. Cell produces new viral RNA, which is the template for protein synthesis
7. A protease hydrolyzes viral proteins into several small subunits
8. and 9. New virus capsules (virions) are formed, bud off, and are extruded from the host cell by exocytosis, infecting new cells

28-1: Mechanism of viral replication and the site of action of antiviral drugs. NRTI, nucleoside reverse transcriptase inhibitors; NNRTI, nonnucleoside reverse transcriptase inhibitors. *(From Wecker L, et al.: Brody's Human Pharmacology, 5th ed. Philadelphia, Mosby, 2010, Figure 51-2.)*

(3) Nasal signs and symptoms
(4) Cough
(5) Bronchospasm in asthmatics (zanamivir)

B. Interferons

1. Mechanism of action
   a. Inhibit viral penetration
   b. Inhibit viral uncoating
   c. Inhibit peptide elongation
2. Uses
   a. Interferon alfa (see Box 28-2)
      (1) Hairy-cell leukemia
      (2) Acquired immunodeficiency syndrome (AIDS)-related Kaposi's sarcoma
      (3) Condyloma acuminatum (venereal wart)
      (4) Chronic hepatitis B
      (5) Chronic hepatitis C
   b. Interferon beta (see Box 28-2)
      • Multiple sclerosis (MS)
   c. Interferon gamma-1b (see Box 28-2)
      (1) Reduce frequency and severity of serious infections associated with chronic granulomatous disease
      (2) Delay time to disease progression in patients with severe, malignant osteopetrosis

Interferon alfa for tumors and viral infections

Interferon beta for MS

Interferon gamma-1b for chronic granulomatous disease

3. Adverse effects
   a. Neutropenia
   b. Anemia
   c. Influenza symptoms
C. Antiherpes drugs
   1. Acyclovir and congeners
      a. Examples
         (1) Famciclovir (prodrug to penciclovir)
         (2) Penciclovir (topically)
         (3) Valacyclovir (prodrug to acyclovir)
      b. Bioavailability
         (1) Acyclovir poor; has to be given 5 times a day
         (2) Prodrugs excellent; given 2 to 3 times a day
      c. Mechanism of action
         (1) Converted to monophosphates by virus-specific thymidine kinase
         (2) Then converted to triphosphate by cellular enzymes
         (3) Triphosphates inhibit DNA synthesis and viral replication
         (4) Compete with deoxyguanosine triphosphate for viral DNA polymerase
      d. Resistance
         • Involves loss of thymidine kinase activity
      e. Uses
         (1) Herpes simplex (cold sores)
         (2) Herpes genitalis
         (3) Herpes zoster (shingles)
         (4) Varicella zoster (chickenpox)
         (5) Acyclovir given IV in immunocompromised patients
      f. Adverse effects
         (1) Malaise
         (2) Headache
         (3) Gastrointestinal (GI) distress
         (4) Nephrotoxicity (IV administration)
   2. Ganciclovir and valganciclovir
      a. General
         (1) Given IV for severe CMV retinitis
         (2) Available as ocular implant
         (3) Valganciclovir a prodrug to ganciclovir
            • Better oral bioavailability
      b. Mechanism of action
         (1) Phosphorylated first to a monophosphate by viral specific thymidine kinase (in herpes simplex virus [HSV]) or phosphotransferase (in CMV)
         (2) It is further phosphorylated into a triphosphate
         (3) Triphosphate competitively inhibits DNA polymerase
         (4) This inhibits viral DNA synthesis
      c. Uses
         (1) Treatment of CMV retinitis
         (2) Prophylaxis of CMV infection in transplantation patients
         (3) Prophylaxis of CMV infection in patients with advanced HIV infections
      d. Adverse effects
         (1) Fever
         (2) Rash
         (3) GI distress
         (4) Anemia
         (5) Avoid during pregnancy
   3. Foscarnet
      a. Mechanism of action
         (1) Pyrophosphate analogue
         (2) *No* dependence on thymidine kinase for bioactivation
         (3) Selective inhibition of the viral-specific DNA polymerases
      b. Uses
         • Treats drug-resistant viral infections
            (1) CMV
            (2) HSV
            (3) Varicella zoster virus

Prodrugs actively transported from gastrointestinal (GI) tract with marked improvement of bioavailability requiring less frequent dosing.

Bioactivation by viral kinases provide selective toxicity to virus but mutations in kinases contribute to resistance.

Drugs must be converted to the triphosphate to inhibit viral polymerases.

Cytomegalovirus (CMV) has *no* thymidine kinase, acyclovir is not effective.

Ganciclovir for CMV.

In AIDS patients with CMV and pneumocystosis, combine ganciclovir (bone marrow toxicity) with pentamidine (nephrotoxicity)

Ganciclovir analogues much more toxic to host than acyclovir analogues.

Foscarnet already phosphorylated so effective in resistant strains with mutated vial kinases.

c. Adverse effects
   (1) Fever and headache
   (2) Renal impairment
   (3) Hypokalemia
   (4) Hypocalcemia
   (5) Hypomagnesemia
   (6) Hypophosphatemia
   (7) Seizures
4. Cidofovir
   a. Acyclic phosphonate nucleotide analogue
   b. Does *not* require intracellular activation for antiviral activity
   c. Used for the treatment of CMV retinitis in patients with AIDS
   d. Needs to be administered with probenecid
   e. Nephrotoxicity is a major dose-limiting toxicity

D. Antiretroviral drugs (see Box 28-2)
1. Nucleoside reverse transcriptase inhibitors (NRTIs)
   a. Examples
      (1) Abacavir
      (2) Adefovir
      (3) Didanosine (ddI)
      (4) Emtricitabine
      (5) Entecavir
      (6) Lamivudine (3TC)
      (7) Stavudine (d4T)
      (8) Telbivudine
      (9) Zalcitabine (ddC)
      (10) Zidovudine (AZT)
   b. Mechanism of action
      (1) Converted to triphosphate
      (2) Triphosphates inhibit viral RNA-directed DNA polymerase
         (reverse transcriptase)
   c. Uses
      (1) Treatment of HIV infection in combination with at least two other
         antiretroviral agents
      (2) Prevention of maternal/fetal HIV transmission as monotherapy (zidovudine)
2. Nucleotide reverse transcriptase inhibitors
   a. Tenofovir
   b. Uses
      (1) Management of HIV infections in combination with at least two other
         antiretroviral agents
      (2) Treatment of chronic HBV
3. Nonnucleoside reverse transcriptase inhibitors (NNRTIs)
   a. Examples
      (1) Delavirdine
      (2) Efavirenz
      (3) Etravirine
      (4) Nevirapine
   b. Mechanism of action
      (1) NNRTIs
      (2) Do *not* require intracellular phosphorylation
      (3) Directly block RNA-dependent and DNA-dependent DNA polymerase
         activities including HIV-1 replication
   c. Uses
      (1) Treatment of HIV-1 infections in combination with at least two other
         antiretroviral agents
      (2) Prevention of maternal-fetal HIV transmission in women with *no* prior
         antiretroviral therapy (nevirapine)
4. Protease inhibitors (PIs)
   a. Examples
      (1) Amprenavir
      (2) Atazanavir
      (3) Indinavir
      (4) Lopinavir

In AIDS patients with CMV and pneumocystosis, combine foscarnet (nephrotoxicity) with sulfonamides (bone marrow toxicity)

Cidofovir already phosphorylated so effective in resistant strains with mutated viral kinases.

Zidovudine is the prototypic reverse transcriptase inhibitor.

Nucleosides must be converted to the triphosphate to inhibit viral reverse transcriptase.

Zidovudine used to prevent vertical transmission of HIV from mother to fetus.

Tenofovir is a nucleotide reverse transcriptase inhibitor used to treat HIV and hepatitis B virus (HBV).

NNRTIs have no cross resistance to NRTIs.

Nevirapine is used to prevent vertical transmission of HIV from mother to fetus.

(5) Nelfinavir

(6) Ritonavir

(7) Saquinavir

(8) Tipranavir

b. Pharmacokinetic considerations

(1) Produce many drug-drug interactions

(2) Indinavir and ritonavir inhibit the cytochrome P450 system

(3) Ritonavir used as a pharmacokinetic "booster" for other protease inhibitors

(4) Saquinavir metabolized by the cytochrome P450 system but does *not* inhibit the enzyme

c. Mechanism of action

(1) Inhibit HIV protease

(2) Thus, the enzyme is incapable of processing the gag-pol polyprotein precursor.

(3) This leads to production of noninfectious immature HIV particles.

d. Uses

(1) Treatment of HIV-1 infections in combination with at least two other antiretroviral agents

(2) Ritonavir used as a pharmacokinetic "booster" for other protease inhibitors

e. Adverse effects

(1) Effects on carbohydrate and lipid metabolism including:

(a) Hyperglycemia

(b) Insulin resistance

(c) Hyperlipidemia

(d) Altered body fat distribution (buffalo hump, facial wasting, gynecomastia, and truncal obesity)

(2) GI distress

(3) Altered hepatic and renal function

5. Fusion inhibitor

• Enfuvirtide

a. It interferes with the entry of HIV-1 into host cells by inhibiting the fusion of the virus and cell membranes.

b. Reserved for individuals who have advanced disease or show resistance to current HIV treatments

6. Integrase inhibitor

• Raltegavir

a. Inhibits the catalytic activity of integrase

b. Prevents integration of the proviral gene into human DNA

c. Used with other agents in treatment-experienced patients with virus that shows multidrug resistance and active replication

7. CCR5 antagonist

• Maraviroc

a. Selectively and reversibly binds to the chemokine (C-C motif receptor 5 [CCR5]) coreceptors located on human CD4 cells

b. Inhibits gp120 conformational change required for CCR5-tropic HIV-1 fusion with the CD4 cell and subsequent cell entry

c. Used in combination with other antiretroviral agents in treatment-experienced patients with evidence of viral replication and HIV-1 strains resistant to multiple antiretroviral therapy

8. Highly active antiretroviral therapy (HAART)

a. Typically use a combination of 3 to 4 drugs

b. Preferred NNRTI-based regimen combines efavirenz with lamivudine or emtricitabine and zidovudine or tenofovir

c. Preferred PI-based regimen combines lopinavir; ritonavir with zidovudine and lamivudine or emtricitabine

d. Patients are prone to opportunistic infections (Table 28-3)

e. Numerous drug-drug interactions amongst the numerous drugs needed in treating HIV patients

f. Some selected adverse effects of HIV drugs (see Table 28-5)

E. Other antiviral drugs

1. Docosanol

a. Prevents viral entry and replication at the cellular level

b. Topical treatment of herpes simplex of the face or lips

Note common ending -navir for protease inhibitors, whereas many antivirals have the ending: -vir.

HIV protease inhibitors inhibit the processing of gag-pol polyprotein precursor required for production of HIV infectious particles.

Adverse effects of protease inhibitors are very similar to Cushing's syndrome except facial wasting instead of "moon face."

Enfuvirtide inhibits the entry of HIV-1 into host cells.

Raltegavir prevents the integration of the HIV proviral gene into human DNA.

Maraviroc inhibits HIV-1 fusion with CD4 cells.

The preferred NNRTI-based regimen combines efavirenz with lamivudine or emtricitabine and zidovudine or tenofovir; the preferred PI-based regimen combines lopinavir, ritonavir with zidovudine, and lamivudine or emtricitabine (available on the Internet at www.aidsinfo.nih.gov).

Docosanol used to treat cold sores.

TABLE 28-3. **Treatment of opportunistic infections in AIDS patients**

OPPORTUNISTIC INFECTION	TREATMENT
Pneumocystis jiroveci infection	Trimethoprim/sulfamethoxazole
Mycobacterium avium complex infection	Clarithromycin plus ethambutol; or azithromycin (less drug interactions)
Toxoplasmosis	Pyrimethamine/sulfadiazine plus folinic acid
Cryptococcal meningitis	Amphotericin B/flucytosine Fluconazole
Cytomegalovirus infection	Valganciclovir (orally) Ganciclovir (IV) Foscarnet (resistant strains)
Esophageal candidiasis or recurrent vaginal candidiasis	Fluconazole
Herpes simplex infection	Acyclovir Famciclovir Valacyclovir Foscarnet (resistant strains)
Herpes zoster	Acyclovir Famciclovir Valacyclovir Foscarnet (resistant strains)

2. Fomivirsen
   a. Antisense inhibitor viral protein of viral protein synthesis
   b. Local treatment of CMV retinitis in HIV patients
   c. Used when other treatments are contraindicated
3. Ribavirin
   a. General information
      (1) Synthetic nucleoside
      (2) Antiviral action requires intracellular phosphorylation
   b. Mechanism of action
      (1) Inhibits replication of RNA and DNA viruses
      (2) Inhibits influenza virus RNA polymerase activity
      (3) Inhibits the initiation and elongation of RNA fragments
      (4) Thus, inhibits viral protein synthesis
   c. Uses
      (1) Inhalation therapy in respiratory syncytial virus (RSV) infections and influenza
      (2) Orally for hepatitis C with alpha interferons
   d. Adverse effects
      (1) Fatigue
      (2) Nausea and anorexia
      (3) Anemia
      (4) Dyspnea
      (5) Teratogenic (pregnancy category X)
4. Trifluridine
   a. Interferes with viral replication by incorporating into viral DNA in place of thymidine
   b. Used topically to treat primary keratoconjunctivitis and recurrent epithelial keratitis caused by herpes simplex virus types I and II
   F. **Therapeutic Summary of Selected Drugs used in Treatment of Viral Infections:** Table 28-4
   G. **Adverse Effects of some Antiretroviral Agents:** Table 28-5
IV. **Antiparasitic Drugs** (Box 28-3)
   A. **Antimalaria drugs**
      1. Chloroquine
         a. Pharmacokinetics
            (1) Rapid oral absorption
            (2) Extensive tissue binding, with a very large volume of distribution (13,000 L)
            (3) Slow release from the tissues
            (4) Liver metabolism
            (5) Renal excretion
            (6) Long half-life (once a week dosing)

Ribavirin is given by inhalations to treat RSV; palivizumab, a monoclonal antibody, is given to prevent RSV in high risk infants.

Patients exposed to ribavirin should not conceive children for at least 6 months following the exposure.

Trifluridine treats primary keratoconjunctivitis and recurrent epithelial keratitis.

TABLE 28-4. **Therapeutic Summary of Selected Drugs used in Treatment of Viral Infections**

DRUGS	CLINICAL APPLICATIONS	ADVERSE EFFECTS	CONTRAINDICATIONS
Mechanism: *Converted to monophosphates by virus-specific thymidine kinase; then converted to triphosphate by cellular enzymes; triphosphates inhibits DNA synthesis and viral replication*			

Antiherpes Drugs
Acyclovir
Acyclovir congeners:
  Famciclovir
  Penciclovir
  Valacyclovir
	Herpes simplex (cold sores)
	Herpes genitalis
	Herpes zoster (shingles)
	Varicella zoster (chickenpox)
		Malaise
		Headache
		GI distress
		Nephrotoxicity (IV
		  administration)
			Hypersensitivity

Mechanism: *Converted to monophosphates by virus-specific thymidine kinase (except phosphorylated analogues); then converted to triphosphate by cellular enzymes; triphosphates inhibits DNA synthesis and viral replication*			

Cidofovir
Foscarnet
Ganciclovir
Valganciclovir
	Treatment and prophylaxis of cytomegalovirus (CMV)
	Foscarnet for resistant
	  Herpes simplex virus
	  Varicella zoster virus
		Fever
		Rash
		GI distress
		Anemia
		Avoid during pregnancy
		Foscarnet
		  Renal impairment
		    (also cidofovir)
		  Hypokalemia
		  Hypocalcemia
		  Hypomagnesemia
		  Hypophosphatemia
		  Seizures
			Hypersensitivity

Mechanism: *Blocks viral uncoating by blocking M2 proton channel*			
Amantadine Rimantadine	Influenza A (prophylaxis) High resistance Parkinson's disease (amantadine)	Dizziness Anxiety Impaired coordination Livedo reticularis	Hypersensitivity
Mechanism: *Inhibits viral neuraminidase*			

Oseltamivir (oral
  prodrug)
Zanamivir
  (inhalation)
	Treatment of influenza virus A and B
	Prophylaxis against influenza virus A and B
		Headache
		Throat/tonsil discomfort/pain
		Nasal signs and symptoms
		Cough
		Bronchospasm in asthmatics
		  (zanamivir)
			Hypersensitivity

Mechanism: *Inhibit viral penetration, uncoating, and peptide elongation*			

Interferons
Interferon alfa-2a
Interferon alfa-2b
Interferon alfacon-1
Interferon alfa-n3
Interferon beta-1a
Interferon beta-1b
Interferon
  gamma-1b
Peginterferon alfa-2a
Peginterferon alfa-2b
	Interferon alfa:
	  Hairy-cell leukemia
	  AIDS-related Kaposi's sarcoma
	  Condyloma acuminatum
	  Chronic hepatitis B
	  Chronic Hepatitis C
	  Interferon beta:
	  Multiple sclerosis
	Interferon Gamma-1b:
	  Chronic granulomatous disease
	  Delay time to disease progression in patients with severe,
	    malignant osteopetrosis
		Neutropenia
		Anemia
		Influenza symptoms
			Hypersensitivity

Mechanism: *Converted to triphosphate which inhibits viral RNA–directed DNA polymerase (reverse transcriptase)*			

*Nucleoside Reverse
  Transcriptase
  Inhibitors*
Abacavir
Adefovir
Didanosine (ddI)
Emtricitabine
Entecavir
Lamivudine (3TC)
Stavudine (d4T)
Telbivudine
Zalcitabine (ddC)
Zidovudine (AZT)
	Treatment of HIV infection in combination with at least two
	  other antiretroviral agents
	Prevention of maternal/fetal HIV transmission as monotherapy
	  (zidovudine)
		See Table 28-5	Hypersensitivity

Mechanism: *Nucleotide reverse transcriptase inhibitor; inhibits replication of HBV by inhibiting HBV polymerase*			

*Nucleotide Reverse
  Transcriptase
  Inhibitor*
Tenofovir
	Management of HIV infections in combination with at least two
	  other antiretroviral agents
	Treatment of chronic hepatitis B virus (HBV)
		Chest pain
		Neurological pain
		GI distress
		Neuromuscular weakness	

(Continued)

TABLE 28-4. **Therapeutic Summary of Selected Drugs used in Treatment of Viral Infections—Cont'd**

DRUGS	CLINICAL APPLICATIONS	ADVERSE EFFECTS	CONTRAINDICATIONS
Mechanism: *Non-nucleoside reverse transcriptase inhibitors; do not require phosphorylation*			
Nonnucleoside Reverse Transcriptase Inhibitors Delavirdine Efavirenz Etavirine Nevirapine	Treatment of HIV-1 infections in combination with at least two other antiretroviral agents Prevention of maternal-fetal HIV transmission in women with no prior antiretroviral therapy (nevirapine)	See Table 28-5	Hypersensitivity Severe hepatic disease
Mechanism: *Inhibit HIV protease; thus, the enzyme is incapable of processing the gag-pol polyprotein precursor*			
Protease Inhibitors Amprenavir Atazanavir Indinavir Lopinavir Nelfinavir Ritonavir Saquinavir Tipranavir	Treatment of HIV-1 infections in combination with at least two other antiretroviral agents Ritonavir used as a pharmacokinetic "booster" for other protease inhibitors	Hyperglycemia Insulin resistance Hyperlipidemia Altered body fat distribution (buffalo hump, gynecomastia, and truncal obesity)	Hypersensitivity Pregnancy Renal or hepatic failure Beware of drug-drug interactions
Mechanism: *Interferes with the entry of HIV-1 into host cells by inhibiting the fusion of the virus and cell membranes*			
Fusion Inhibitor Enfuvirtide	Advanced disease or show resistance to current HIV treatments	Fatigue Insomnia Eosinophilia Injection site reactions	Hypersensitivity
Mechanism: *Prevents integration of the proviral gene into human DNA*			
Integrase Inhibitor Raltegravir	Treatment of experienced HIV patients with virus that shows multidrug resistance and active replication	Hypercholesterolemia Hypertension Fatigue GI distress Anemias	Hypersensitivity
Mechanism: *Inhibits gp120 conformational change required for CCR5-tropic HIV-1 fusion with the CD4 cell and subsequent cell entry*			
CCR5 antagonist Maraviroc	Used in combination with other antiretroviral agents in treatment-experienced patients with evidence of viral replication and HIV-1 strains resistant to multiple antiretroviral therapy	Fever Upper respiratory tract infections Rash GI disturbance	

TABLE 28-5. **Adverse Effects of some Individual Antiretroviral Agents**

DRUG	ADVERSE EFFECT(S)
Nucleoside Reverse Transcriptase Inhibitors	
Abacavir	Rash, hypersensitivity
Didanosine (ddI)	Peripheral neuropathy, pancreatitis (dose-dependent)
Emtricitabine	Hyperpigmentation, rash, GI distress, cough
Lamivudine (3TC)	Headache, ↑ liver enzymes, hyperbilirubinemia (dose-reduction is necessary in renal disease)
Stavudine (d4T)	Peripheral sensory neuropathy, myelosuppression
Zalcitabine (ddC)	Peripheral sensory neuropathy, esophageal ulcers, pancreatitis
Zidovudine (AZT)	Bone marrow suppression, anemia, neuropathy
Nonnucleoside Reverse Transcriptase Inhibitors	
Delavirdine	Rash, pruritus, ↑ liver enzymes
Efavirenz	Rash, pruritus, diarrhea, hypercholesterolemia, ↑ liver enzymes
Nevirapine	Rash, ↑ liver enzymes, hepatitis
Protease Inhibitors (all produce cushingoid-like effects)	
Indinavir	Hyperbilirubinemia, nephrolithiasis, hyperbilirubinemia
Nelfinavir	Diarrhea, anaphylactoid reactions, inhibition of metabolism of many drugs
Ritonavir	Multiple drug interactions, hepatitis
Saquinavir	Gastrointestinal disturbance, rhinitis

b. Mechanism of action
(1) Binds to and inhibits DNA and RNA polymerase
(2) Interferes with metabolism and hemoglobin utilization by parasites
(3) Concentrates within parasite acid vesicles and raises internal pH resulting in inhibition of parasite growth

BOX 28-3   ANTIPARASITIC DRUGS

Antimalarial Drugs
Atovaquone plus proguanil
Chloroquine
Mefloquine
Primaquine
Pyrimethamine
Quinine; quinidine
Sulfadoxine plus pyrimethamine

Other Antiprotozoal Drugs
Iodoquinol
Metronidazole
Paromomycin

Pentamidine
Tinidazole

Antihelmintic Drugs
Albendazole
Ivermectin
Mebendazole
Piperazine
Praziquantel
Pyrantel pamoate
Thiabendazole

    c. Mechanism of resistance
      • Membrane P-glycoprotein pump expels chloroquine from the parasite
    d. Uses
      (1) Clinical cure and prophylaxis (all species of *Plasmodium*)
      (2) Treatment of infections caused by *Plasmodium vivax* and *Plasmodium ovale* requires use of chloroquine in combination with primaquine
      (3) Extraintestinal amebiasis
    e. Adverse effects
      (1) Visual impairment
      (2) Hearing loss
      (3) Tinnitus
      (4) Aplastic anemia
  2. Mefloquine
    a. Destroys asexual form of malarial pathogens
    b. Used for prophylaxis and treatment
      (1) Chloroquine-resistant falciparum malaria
      (2) Multidrug-resistant falciparum malaria
    c. Long half-life (once a week dosing)
    d. Adverse effects
      (1) Central nervous system CNS effects
        (a) Dizziness
        (b) Loss of balance
        (c) Seizures
      (2) Psychiatric effects
        (a) Anxiety
        (b) Paranoia
        (c) Depression
        (d) Hallucinations
        (e) Psychosis
  3. Primaquine
    a. Mechanism of action
      (1) Disrupts mitochondria and binds to DNA
      (2) Active against late hepatic stages (hypnozoites and schizonts) of:
        (a) *P. vivax*
        (b) *P. ovale*
    b. Uses
      (1) Malaria (in combination with chloroquine)
      (2) *Pneumocystis jiroveci* pneumonia (alternative therapy; in combination with clindamycin)
    c. Adverse effects
      (1) Anorexia
      (2) Weakness
      (3) Hemolytic anemia
        (a) Use with caution in patients with known G6PD deficiency
        (b) Use with caution in patients with NADH methemoglobin reductase deficiency
      (4) Leucopenia

Membrane P-glycoprotein pump responsible for resistance of malaria to chloroquine.

Chloroquine should be avoided or used cautiously in patients with ocular, hematologic, neurologic, or hepatic diseases.

Mefloquine for chloroquine- and multidrug-resistant falciparum malaria.

Mefloquine associated with psychiatric disturbances.

Primaquine only drug available for hepatic stages of P. vivax or P. ovale.

Pneumocystis jiroveci pneumonia was previously referred to as Pneumocystis carinii pneumonia (PCP); PCP is still used to refer to this infection

Individuals with G6PD deficiency who take primaquine are susceptible to hemolytic anemia.

4. Atovaquone plus proguanil
   a. Mechanism of action
      (1) Atovaquone selectively inhibits parasite mitochondrial electron transport
      (2) Proguanil's metabolite cycloguanil, inhibits dihydrofolate reductase
   b. Used to prevent or treat acute, uncomplicated *Plasmodium falciparum* malaria
   c. Adverse effects
      (1) GI distress
      (2) Increased hepatic transaminase
      (3) Headache
      (4) Dizziness
5. Quinine and quinidine
   a. Still used to treat uncomplicated chloroquine-resistant *P. falciparum* malaria
   b. Cinchonism
      (1) Overdose of quinine or its natural source, cinchona bark
      (2) Symptoms
         (a) Flushed and sweaty skin
         (b) Ringing of the ears (tinnitus)
         (c) Blurred vision
         (d) Impaired hearing
         (e) Confusion
6. Pyrimethamine
   a. High affinity for protozoan dihydrofolate reductase
   b. Uses
      (1) Prophylaxis of malaria
      (2) With quinine and sulfadiazine for the treatment of uncomplicated attacks of chloroquine-resistant *P. falciparum* malaria
      (3) Synergistic in combination with sulfonamide in treatment of toxoplasmosis
      (4) Often used with sulfadoxine for presumptive treatment or chloroquine-resistant malaria
   c. Adverse effects
      (1) Megaloblastic anemia
      (2) Leukopenia
      (3) Thrombocytopenia
      (4) Pancytopenia
7. Artemether and lumefantrine
   a. A co-formulation with activity against *P. falciparum*
   b. Used for acute, uncomplicated malaria from *P. falciparum*

B. Therapeutic Summary of Selected Drugs used in Treatment of Malaria: Table 28-6
C. Other antiprotozoal drugs
1. Metronidazole and tinidazole
   a. Mechanism of action
      (1) Disrupts helical DNA structure
      (2) Causes DNA strand breaks
      (3) Results in protein synthesis inhibition
   b. Uses
      (1) Urogenital trichomoniasis *(Trichomonas vaginalis)*
      (2) Giardiasis *(Giardia)*
      (3) Amebiasis *(Entamoeba histolytica)*
      (4) Aspiration pneumonia
      (5) Anaerobic infections (including *Clostridium difficile, Bacteroides fragilis*)
      (6) *Helicobacter pylori*
   c. Adverse effects
      (1) Metallic taste
      (2) Disulfiram-like effect with alcohol
      (3) GI distress
2. Iodoquinol
   a. Used for the local treatment of acute and chronic intestinal amebiasis
   b. Used for asymptomatic cyst passers
3. Paromomycin
   a. Acts locally on ameba
   b. Used to treat acute and chronic intestinal amebiasis

Both quinine and its dextro isomer quinidine are still used some to treat chloroquine-resistant *P. falciparum* malaria.

Cinchonism is a term used to describe adverse symptoms of quinine and quinidine.

Quinidine and doxycycline is used IV to treat complicated malaria in unconscious patients.

Pyrimethamine has a high affinity for protozoan dihydrofolate reductase.

Artemether is derived from the herb, artemisinin, used in Chinese traditional medicine to treat multi-drug resistant strains of falciparum malaria.

Metronidazole used to treat protozoan and anaerobic bacterial infections.

Metronidazole is *not* effective against aerobic bacterial infections.

Metronidazole: Patients who are taking this drug should *not* consume alcohol.

Table 28-6. **Therapeutic Summary of Selected Drugs used in Treatment of Malaria**

DRUGS	CLINICAL APPLICATIONS	ADVERSE EFFECTS	CONTRAINDICATIONS
Mechanism: *Binds to and inhibits DNA and RNA polymerase; interferes with metabolism and hemoglobin utilization by parasites*			
Chloroquine	Clinical cure and prophylaxis (all species of *Plasmodium*) Treatment of infections caused by *Plasmodium vivax* and *Plasmodium ovale* requires use of chloroquine in combination with primaquine Extraintestinal amebiasis	Visual impairment Hearing loss Tinnitus Aplastic anemia	Hypersensitivity Retinal or visual field changes
Mechanism: *Destroys asexual form of malarial pathogens*			
Mefloquine	Used for prophylaxis and treatment: Chloroquine-resistant falciparum malaria Multidrug-resistant falciparum malaria	CNS effects: Dizziness Loss of balance Seizures Psychiatric effects Anxiety Paranoia Depression Hallucinations Psychosis	Hypersensitivity Seizures Severe psychiatric disorders
Mechanism: *Disrupts mitochondria and binds to DNA; Active against late hepatic stages (hypnozoites and schizonts) of P. vivax and P. ovale*			
Primaquine	Malaria (in combination with chloroquine) *Pneumocystis jiroveci* pneumonia (alternative therapy; in combination with clindamycin)	Anorexia Weakness Hemolytic anemia	In acutely-ill patients who have a tendency to develop granulocytopenia (e.g., rheumatoid arthritis, SLE) Concurrent use with other medications causing hemolytic anemia or myeloid bone marrow suppression
Mechanism: *Atovaquone selectively inhibits parasite mitochondrial electron transport; Proguanil's, metabolite cycloguanil, inhibits dihydrofolate reductase*			
Atovaquone plus proguanil	Prevents or treats acute, uncomplicated *P. falciparum* malaria	GI distress Increased hepatic transaminase Headache Dizziness	Hypersensitivity Severe renal impairment
Mechanism: *High affinity for protozoan dihydrofolate reductase*			
Pyrimethamine	Prophylaxis of malaria With quinine and sulfadiazine for the treatment of uncomplicated attacks of chloroquine-resistant *P. falciparum* malaria Synergistic in combination with sulfonamide in treatment of toxoplasmosis Often used with sulfadoxine for chloroquine-resistant malaria	Megaloblastic anemia Leukopenia Thrombocytopenia Pancytopenia	Hypersensitivity Resistant malaria Megaloblastic anemia secondary to folate deficiency

4. Pentamidine
   a. Mechanism of action
      (1) Interferes with DNA/RNA function
      (2) Inhibits oxidative phosphorylation
   b. Use
      (1) Treatment and prevention of pneumonia caused by *P. jiroveci* (PCP)
         • Given by inhalation
      (2) Treatment of *Trypanosoma gambiense*
      (3) Treatment of visceral leishmaniasis
   c. Adverse effects
      (1) Pancreatitis
      (2) Nephrotoxicity
      (3) Abnormal liver function tests

D. Antihelmintic drugs
   1. Praziquantel
      a. Mechanism of action
         (1) Increases calcium permeability
            • Depolarizing cells
         (2) Causes contraction and paralysis of worm musculature
      b. Uses
         (1) Schistosomiasis
         (2) Infections with flukes (trematodes)
         (3) Some infections with tapeworms (cestodes)

Given by inhalation for pneumonia by PCP as an alternative to trimethoprim/sulfamethoxazole

Praziquantel paralyzes worms by increasing calcium permeability.

Praziquantel is useful for flukes and tapeworms.

c. Adverse effects
  (1) Headache
  (2) Dizziness
  (3) Drowsiness
  (4) GI disturbances
2. Thiabendazole and mebendazole
  a. Mechanism of action
  b. Block microtubule formation
  c. Uses
    (1) Thiabendazole
      (a) Strongyloidiasis
      (b) Cutaneous larva migrans (alternative drug)
    (2) Mebendazole
      (a) Ascariasis
      (b) Trichuriasis
      (c) Hookworm
      (d) Pinworm *(Enterobius vermicularis)*
      (e) Cysticercosis *(Taenia solium)*
      (f) *Echinococcus* infestations
  d. Adverse effects
    (1) Abdominal pain
    (2) Diarrhea
3. Pyrantel pamoate
  a. Mechanism of action
    (1) Acts as a depolarizing neuromuscular blocking agent on the nicotinic receptor
    (2) Increases the effects of acetylcholine and inhibits cholinesterase in the worm
  b. Uses
    (1) Ascariasis
    (2) Pinworm *(E. vermicularis)*
    (3) Hookworm
    (4) Whipworm *(Trichuris trichiura)*
    (5) *Trichostrongylus*
  c. Adverse effects
    (1) Nausea
    (2) Vomiting
    (3) Diarrhea
    (4) Anorexia
4. Piperazine
  a. Blocks the effects of acetylcholine at the worm neuromuscular junction
  b. Used as an alternative to treat pinworm and roundworm infections
5. Ivermectin
  a. Mechanism of action
    (1) Increases chloride permeability
    (2) Polarizes cells leading to paralysis
  b. Uses
    (1) Strongyloidiasis
    (2) Onchocerciasis
  c. Adverse effects
    (1) Pruritus
    (2) Fever
    (3) Arthralgia
    (4) Lymph node enlargement
E. Therapeutic Summary of Selected Drugs used in Treatment of Worms:
  Table 28-7:
V. Antifungal Drugs (Box 28-4)
  A. General information
    1. Antifungal agents are commonly used in debilitated and immunosuppressed patients with conditions such as:
      a. Leukemia
      b. Lymphoma
      c. Immunodeficiencies
      d. Diabetes
    2. The mechanisms of action of some antifungal agents are shown in Fig. 28-2.

Thiabendazole and mebendazole inhibit microtubule function in worms.

Pyrantel pamoate paralyzes worms via depolarizing neuromuscular junctions in worm musculature.

Thiabendazole, mebendazole, pyrantel pamoate, and piperazine are used to treat various roundworms.

Ivermectin paralyzes worms by increasing chloride permeability.

Increased fungal infections in immunosuppressed patients.

Table 28-7. **Therapeutic Summary of Selected Drugs used in Treatment of Worms**

DRUGS	CLINICAL APPLICATIONS	ADVERSE EFFECTS	CONTRAINDICATIONS
Mechanism: *Increases calcium permeability → depolarizing cells leading to contraction and paralysis of worm musculature*			
Praziquantel	Schistosomiasis Infections with flukes (trematodes) Some infections with tapeworms (cestodes)	Headaches Dizziness Drowsiness GI disturbances	Hypersensitivity
Mechanism: *Block microtubule formation*			

Thiabendazole
Mebendazole
	Thiabendazole
	  Strongyloidiasis
	  Cutaneous larva migrans (alternative drug)
	Mebendazole
	  Ascariasis
	  Trichuriasis
	  Hookworm
	  Pinworm *(Enterobius vermicularis)*
	  Cysticercosis *(Taenia solium)*
	  Echinococcus infestations
		Abdominal pain
		Diarrhea
			Hypersensitivity

Mechanism: *Acts as a depolarizing neuromuscular blocking agent on the nicotinic receptors of the worm musculature*			
Pyrantel pamoate	Ascariasis Pinworm *(Enterobius vermicularis)* Hookworm Whipworm *(Trichuris trichiura)* Trichostrongylus	Nausea Vomiting Diarrhea Anorexia	Hypersensitivity
Mechanism: *Increases chloride permeability polarizing cells leading to paralysis*			
Ivermectin	Strongyloidiasis Onchocerciasis	Pruritus Fever Arthralgia Lymph node enlargement	Hypersensitivity

BOX 28-4 ANTIFUNGAL DRUGS

Azole Antifungal Derivatives
Clotrimazole (topical)
Econazole (topical)
Fluconazole (oral; IV)
Itraconazole (oral; IV)
Ketoconazole (oral)
Miconazole (topical)
Oxiconazole (topical)
Posconazole (oral)
Sertaconazole (topical)
Sulconazole (topical)
Voriconazole (oral; IV)

Polyene Antifungal Drugs
Amphotericin B
Liposomal amphotericin B
Nystatin (topical)

Echinocandin Antifungal Drugs
Anidulafungin (IV)
Caspofungin (IV)
Micafungin (IV)

Other Antifungal Drugs
Butenafine (topical)
Flucytosine (oral)
Griseofulvin (oral)
Naftifine (topical)
Terbinafine (oral; topical)
Tolnaftate (topical)

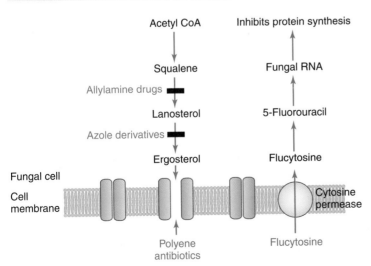

28-2: Mechanism of action of some antifungal drugs. Amphotericin B and nystatin are polyenes; terbinafine is an allylamine; and ketoconazole, fluconazole, and itraconazole are azoles. CoA, coenzyme A.

B. Azole antifungal drugs
1. Examples
   a. Clotrimazole (topical)
   b. Econazole (topical)
   c. Fluconazole (oral; IV)
   d. Itraconazole (oral; IV)
   e. Ketoconazole (oral)
   f. Miconazole (topical)
   g. Oxiconazole (topical)
   h. Posaconazole (oral)
   i. Sertaconazole (topical)
   j. Sulconazole (topical)
   k. Voriconazole (oral; IV)
2. Pharmacokinetics
   a. Systemic drugs are well absorbed orally
   b. Fluconazole
      • Good CNS penetration
   c. Renal clearance
      • Fluconazole
   d. Hepatic clearance
      (1) Ketoconazole
      (2) Itraconazole
      (3) Posaconazole
      (4) Voriconazole
3. Mechanism of action (see Fig. 28-2)
   a. Inhibit ergosterol synthesis
   b. Prevents conversion of lanosterol to ergosterol
   c. Essential component of the fungal cell membrane
4. Use
   a. Topical treatments
      (1) *Tinea pedis* (athlete's foot)
      (2) *Tinea cruris* (jock itch)
      (3) *Tinea corporis* (ringworm)
      (4) *Tinea versicolor*
      (5) Cutaneous candidiasis
   b. Systemic treatment of susceptible fungal infections
      (1) Candidiasis
      (2) Oral thrush
      (3) Blastomycosis
      (4) Histoplasmosis
      (5) Paracoccidioidomycosis
      (6) Coccidioidomycosis
      (7) Chromomycosis
      (8) Candiduria
      (9) Chronic mucocutaneous candidiasis
      (10) Recalcitrant cutaneous dermatophytoses
   c. Cryptococcal meningitis (fluconazole)
   d. *Aspergillus*
      (1) Itraconazole
      (2) Voriconazole
5. Adverse effects
   a. Elevation of serum transaminase levels
   b. Gynecomastia (blocks adrenal steroid synthesis)
   c. Inhibition of cytochrome P450 enzymes (drug-drug interactions)
      • Especially ketoconazole

C. Amphotericin B (polyene antibiotic)
1. Pharmacokinetics
   a. Administered intravenously or intrathecally
   b. *Not* absorbed orally
   c. Liposomal amphotericin B
      (1) Active drug in a lipid delivery system
      (2) Increased efficacy
      (3) Decreased toxicity

Fluconazole is the azole antifungal that best penetrates blood-brain barrier (BBB).

Azole antifungals inhibit cytochrome P-450s that are involved in ergosterol synthesis in fungi, as well as host steroidogenesis, and drug metabolism.

Azole derivatives: inhibition of cytochrome P450 enzymes - fluconazole is the least inhibitory

2. Mechanism of action (See Fig. 28-2)
   a. Binds to ergosterol in fungal cell membranes
   b. Increases membrane permeability
3. Uses
   a. Drug of choice for severe systemic and CNS infections caused by susceptible fungi:
      (1) *Candida* species
      (2) *Histoplasma capsulatum*
      (3) *Cryptococcus neoformans* (combined with flucytosine)
      (4) *Aspergillus* species
      (5) *Blastomyces dermatitidis*
      (6) *Torulopsis glabrata*
      (7) *Coccidioides immitis*
   b. Fungal peritonitis
   c. Irrigant for bladder fungal infections
   d. Fungal infection in patients with bone marrow transplantation
   e. Chemoprophylaxis (low-dose IV)
4. Adverse effects
   a. Nephrotoxicity
   b. Pancytopenia, anemia
   c. Hepatotoxicity
   d. Fever and chills
      • U.S. boxed warning: Should be used primarily for treatment of progressive, potentially life-threatening fungal infections, *not* noninvasive forms of infection.

D. Flucytosine
1. Pharmacokinetics
   a. Good oral absorption
   b. Good CNS penetration
   c. Renal clearance
2. Mechanism of action (See Fig. 28-2)
   a. Converted to fluorouracil (an antimetabolite) only in fungal cells
   b. Competes with uracil by interfering with pyrimidine metabolism and disrupting both RNA and protein synthesis
3. Uses
   a. Systemic fungal infections due to *Candida* species
      (1) *C. glabrata*
      (2) *Cryptococcus neoformans*
   b. Always used in combination with amphotericin B
   c. Resistance occurs rapidly when used alone
4. Adverse effects
   a. Nausea and vomiting
   b. Diarrhea
   c. Bone marrow suppression

E. Echinocandin antifungal drugs
1. Examples
   a. Anidulafungin
   b. Caspofungin (prototype)
   c. Micafungin
2. Mechanism of action
   • Inhibits the synthesis of β (1,3)-D-glucan, which is an essential component of the fungal cell wall
3. Uses
   a. Treatment of invasive *Aspergillus* infections in patients who are refractory or intolerant of other therapy
   b. Treatment of candidemia and other *Candida* infections
      (1) Intra-abdominal abscesses
      (2) Esophageal candidiasi and peritonitis in pleural space
      (3) Empirical treatment for presumed fungal infections in febrile neutropenic patients
4. Adverse effects
   a. Hypotension and tachycardia
   b. Fever, chills and headache

Polyene antifungals bind to ergosterol in fungal cells (fungicidal) and cholesterol in host cells (toxicity) increasing membrane permeability.

Nephrotoxicity is dose limiting toxicity of amphotericin B.

Because of patient ill feeling, amphotericin B is known as Ampho-terrible.

Resistance develops to flucytosine rapidly when it is used alone.

Echinocandins, inhibitors of fungal β (1,3)-D-glucan, are a new class of drugs available to treat fungal infections refractory to conventional drugs.

c. Rash
d. Anemias
e. Hypokalemia

F. **Griseofulvin**

1. Pharmacokinetics
   a. Micronized formulations are adequately absorbed
   b. Absorption enhanced by fatty meals
   c. Concentrates in keratinized tissue
   d. Selectively localizes in the skin
   e. Higher affinity for diseased skin
   f. Extensive hepatic metabolism
2. Mechanism of action
   a. Decreases microtubule function
   b. Disrupts the mitotic spindle structure of the fungal cell
   c. Causes an arrest of the M phase of the cell cycle
3. Uses
   • Treatment of susceptible tinea infections of the skin, hair, and nails
4. Adverse effects
   a. Headache
   b. Dizziness
   c. GI distress
   d. Granulocytopenia
   e. Photosensitivity
   f. Rash
   g. Hepatotoxicity

G. **Allylamine antifungal drugs**

1. Examples
   a. Butenafine (topical)
   b. Naftifine (topical)
   c. Terbinafine (oral; topical)
2. Pharmacokinetics
   a. Terbinafine absorbed orally
   b. Concentrates in keratinized tissue (like griseofulvin)
3. Mechanism of action (see Fig. 28-2)
   a. Inhibits the fungal enzyme squalene epoxidase
   b. Interferes with ergosterol biosynthesis (like azoles)
4. Uses
   a. Dermatophytosis (topical)
   b. Onychomycosis (oral, replaces griseofulvin)
5. Adverse effects (rare)
   a. Headache
   b. GI upset

H. **Nystatin**

1. Polyene antifungal with mechanism similar to amphotericin B
2. Use
   a. Orally (not absorbed from the GI tract) for intestinal candidiasis
   b. Topically for candidiasis of the oral and vaginal cavity

I. **Tolnaftate**

1. Distorts the hyphae and stunts mycelial growth of fungi
2. Topical treatment
   a. *Tinea pedis* (athlete's foot)
   b. *Tinea cruris* (jock itch)
   c. *Tinea corporis* (ringworm)

J. **Therapeutic Summary of Selected Drugs used in Treatment of Fungal Infections:** Table 28-8

Griseofulvin is best absorbed when taken with a fatty meal.

Griseofulvin causes severe headaches.

Griseofulvin and terbinafine concentrate in keratinized tissues.

Allylamines, like terbinafine, inhibit the fungal enzyme squalene epoxidase.

Terbinafine is used to treat onychomycosis of finger and toe nails.

Nystatin swish is often used for the treatment of oral thrush.

Table 28-8. **Therapeutic Summary of Selected Drugs used in Treatment of Fungal Infections**

Drugs	Clinical Applications	Adverse Effects	Contraindications
Mechanism: *Inhibit ergosterol synthesis by preventing the conversion of lanosterol to ergosterol*			
Clotrimazole (topical) Econazole (topical) Fluconazole (oral; IV) Itraconazole (oral; IV) Ketoconazole (oral) Miconazole (topical) Oxiconazole (topical) Posconazole (oral) Sertaconazole (topical) Sulconazole (topical) Voriconazole (oral; IV)	*Topical treatments* *Tinea pedis* (athlete's foot) *Tinea cruris* (jock itch) *Tinea corporis* (ringworm) *Tinea versicolor* Cutaneous candidiasis *Systemic treatments* Candidiasis Oral thrush Blastomycosis Histoplasmosis Paracoccidioidomycosis Coccidioidomycosis Chromomycosis Candiduria Chronic mucocutaneous candidiasis Recalcitrant cutaneous dermatophytoses Cryptococcal meningitis (fluconazole) Aspergillus (itraconazole, voriconazole)	↑ serum transaminase levels Gynecomastia Inhibition of cytochrome P-450 enzymes (Fluconazole is the lowest)	Hypersensitivity Be aware of drug-drug interactions
Mechanism: *Binds to ergosterol in fungal cell membranes*			
Polyene Antifungal *Drugs* Amphotericin B Liposomal amphotericin B Nystatin (topical)	*Candida* species *Histoplasma capsulatum* *Cryptococcus neoformans* *Aspergillus* species *Blastomyces dermatitidis* *Torulopsis glabrata* *Coccidioides immitis* Fungal peritonitis Irrigant for bladder fungal infections Fungal infection in patients with bone marrow transplantation chemoprophylaxis (low-dose IV)	NephrotoxicityPancytopenia Anemia Hepatotoxicity Fever and chills	Hypersensitivity
Mechanism: *Selectively converted to fluorouracil (an antimetabolite) in fungal cells*			
Flucytosine (oral)	*Candida* species *C. glabrata* *Cryptococcus neoformans* Always used in combination with amphotericin B	Nausea and vomiting Diarrhea Bone marrow suppression	Hypersensitivity
Mechanism: *Inhibits synthesis of β (1,3)-D-glucan; essential component of the fungi cell wall*			
Echinocandins Anidulafungin (IV) Caspofungin (IV) Micafungin (IV)	Treatment of invasive *Aspergillus* infections in patients who are refractory or intolerant of other therapy Treatment of candidemia and other *Candida* infections Intra-abdominal abscesses Esophageal candidiasis and peritonitis Empirical treatment for presumed fungal infections in febrile neutropenic patients	Hypotension and tachycardia Fever, chills and headache Rash Anemias Hypokalemia	Hypersensitivity
Mechanism: *Inhibits final microtubules; concentrates in keratinized tissues*			
Griseofulvin (oral)	Treatment of susceptible tinea infections of the skin, hair, and nails	Headache Dizziness GI distress Granulocytopenia Photosensitivity Rash	Hypersensitivity Liver disease Pregnancy Porphyria
Mechanism: *Inhibits the fungal enzyme squalene epoxidase; concentrates in keratinized tissues*			
Allylamines Butenafine (topical) Naftifine (topical) Terbinafine (oral; topical)	Dermatophytosis (topical) Onychomycosis (oral, replaces griseofulvin)	Headache GI upset	Hypersensitivity

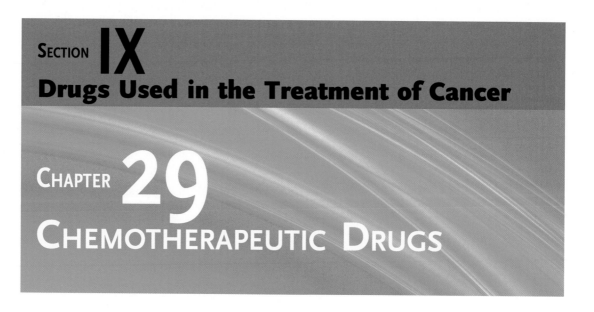

SECTION **IX**

Drugs Used in the Treatment of Cancer

CHAPTER **29**
CHEMOTHERAPEUTIC DRUGS

I. General Considerations
- Cancer is a disease in which the cellular control mechanisms that govern proliferation and differentiation are changed.

A. Pathology of cancers (See Rapid Review Pathology)

B. Drugs used in cancer chemotherapy

Know the molecular targets of antineoplastic drugs.

    1. Target important biosynthetic processes in proliferating cells (Fig. 29-1)
    2. Affect different stages of the cell cycle (Fig. 29-2)
       a. Cell cycle-specific (CCS) drugs
         (1) Antimetabolites
         (2) Bleomycin
         (3) Podophyllotoxins
         (4) Taxanes
         (5) Vinca alkaloids
       b. Cell cycle-nonspecific (CCNS) drugs

Know CCS and CCNS antineoplastic agents.

         (1) Alkylating agents
         (2) Anthracyclines
         (3) Dactinomycin
         (4) Mitomycin
         (5) Platinum analogues

C. Goals of cancer chemotherapy
    1. Selectively destroy cancer cells
    2. Minimize toxicity to normal cells

D. Adverse effects of chemotherapeutic drugs (Table 29-1)
    1. Individual drugs have "signature" adverse effects
    2. Common shared adverse effects

Learn the "shared" and "signature" adverse effects of antineoplastic agents.

       a. Bone marrow suppression
       b. Toxicity to mucosal cells of the gastrointestinal tract
         (1) Nausea and vomiting
         (2) Ulcers
         (3) Diarrhea
       c. Toxicity to skin
       d. Toxicity to hair follicles (hair loss)
       e. Teratogenic effects
       f. Sterility
       g. Immunosuppression (opportunistic infections)
    3. Acute effects

Antineoplastic drugs are toxic to rapidly proliferating cells: bone marrow, GI, skin, hair follicles, reproductive organs.

       a. Nausea and vomiting
         (1) Most prominent acute effect
         (2) Can cause dehydration, malnutrition, metabolic disorders

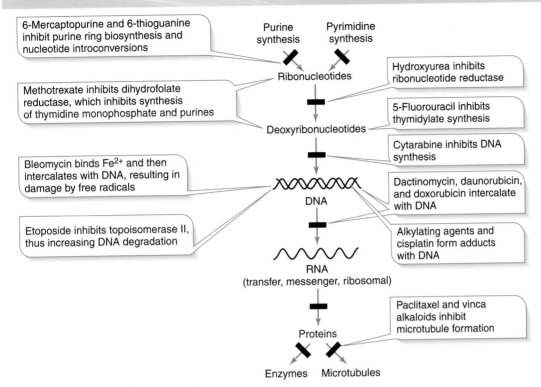

6-Mercaptopurine and 6-thioguanine inhibit purine ring biosynthesis and nucleotide introconversions

Methotrexate inhibits dihydrofolate reductase, which inhibits synthesis of thymidine monophosphate and purines

Bleomycin binds Fe^{2+} and then intercalates with DNA, resulting in damage by free radicals

Etoposide inhibits topoisomerase II, thus increasing DNA degradation

Purine synthesis   Pyrimidine synthesis

Hydroxyurea inhibits ribonucleotide reductase

5-Fluorouracil inhibits thymidylate synthesis

Cytarabine inhibits DNA synthesis

Dactinomycin, daunorubicin, and doxorubicin intercalate with DNA

Alkylating agents and cisplatin form adducts with DNA

Paclitaxel and vinca alkaloids inhibit microtubule formation

Ribonucleotides

Deoxyribonucleotides

DNA

RNA
(transfer, messenger, ribosomal)

Proteins

Enzymes   Microtubules

29-1: Sites of action of chemotherapeutic drugs.

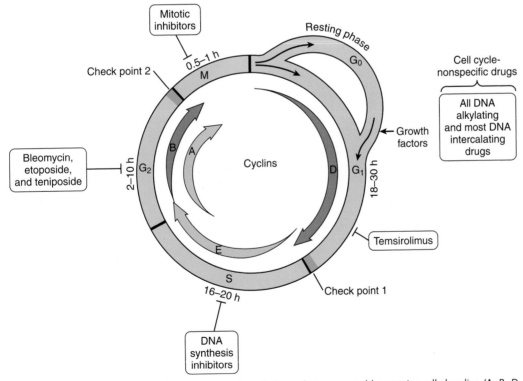

Mitotic inhibitors

Resting phase

Check point 2

Cell cycle-nonspecific drugs

All DNA alkylating and most DNA intercalating drugs

Bleomycin, etoposide, and teniposide

Cyclins

Growth factors

Temsirolimus

DNA synthesis inhibitors

Check point 1

29-2: Cell cycle activity of anticancer drugs. Progress through the cycle is promoted by proteins called cyclins (A, B, D, E), which are controlled by the cyclin-dependent kinases. *(From Brenner G and Stevens C: Pharmacology, 3rd ed. Philadelphia, Saunders, 2010, Figure 45-1.)*

    (3) Treat with antiemetics
        (a) 5-HT$_3$ antagonists (ondansetron)
        (b) Phenothiazines (prochlorperazine)
  4. Delayed effects
    a. Myelosuppression
      (1) Usually leukopenia (neutropenia) and thrombocytopenia
      (2) Risk of infection, bleeding

Ondansetron and other -setron drugs are used to treat the nausea and vomiting associated with anticancer drugs.

TABLE 29-1. **Therapeutic Uses and Adverse Effects of Selected Drugs Used in Cancer Chemotherapy**

DRUG	USE: TYPE(s) OF CANCER*	IMPORTANT ADVERSE EFFECT(s)
Aminoglutethimide	Breast, prostate	Adrenal suppression, dizziness, rash
Anastrozole	Breast	Hot flashes
Bleomycin	Testicular, ovarian, cervical, thyroid	Pulmonary fibrosis; very little bone marrow toxicity
Busulfan	CML, polycythemia vera	Interstitial pulmonary fibrosis
Carmustine/lomustine	Brain	Leukopenia, thrombocytopenia, hepatotoxicity
Cisplatin	Head and neck, lung, testicular, cervical, thyroid, ovarian	Ototoxicity, severe nephrotoxicity, mild bone marrow suppression
Cyclophosphamide	Leukemias/lymphomas	Hemorrhagic cystitis, alopecia
Cytarabine	Leukemias	Bone marrow suppression, CNS toxicity, immunosuppression
Dactinomycin	Wilms' tumor	Hepatotoxicity
Daunorubicin/doxorubicin	Acute leukemia, Hodgkin's disease, breast and lung	Cardiomyopathy (daunorubicin)
Etoposide	Lung, testicular	Bone marrow suppression
5-Fluorouracil	Colon, stomach, prostate, breast	Bone marrow suppression, GI toxicity
Imatinib	CML, gastrointestinal stromal tumors	Fluid retention
Irinotecan	Colon	Bone marrow suppression
Leuprolide	Prostate, breast	Hot flashes
Melphalan	Multiple myeloma	Bone marrow suppression
6-Mercaptopurine	Leukemias	Bone marrow suppression
Methotrexate	Wilms' tumor, choriocarcinoma, leukemias	Bone marrow suppression, oral and GI tract ulceration, diarrhea, hepatotoxicity[†]
Paclitaxel	Breast, ovarian	Bone marrow suppression
Procarbazine	Hodgkin's disease	Secondary malignancies, teratogenic
Tamoxifen	Breast	Hot flashes
Trastuzumab	Breast	Fever and chills
Vinblastine	Lymphomas	Bone marrow suppression
Vincristine	Acute lymphocytic leukemia	Neurotoxicity/peripheral neuropathy, low bone marrow suppression

*Not a complete list; for most cancers, drug combinations are used.
[†]Adverse effects, especially toxicity, may be reversed with folic acid ("leucovorin rescue").
CML, chronic myelogenous leukemia; CNS, central nervous system; GI, gastrointestinal.

Give growth factors to facilitate recovery of hematopoietic cells after dosing with antineoplastic drugs: Erythropoietin, GM-CSF, G-CSF, Oprelvekin.

Fluorouracil noted for causing hand-and foot syndrome.

    (3) Treat with:
       (a) Granulocytic/monocytic colony stimulating factor (GM-CSF)
       (b) Granulocytic colony stimulating factor (G-CSF)
       (c) Oprelvekin (IL-11)
         • Supports megakaryocytopoiesis
       (d) Platelet transfusions
       (e) Erythropoietin
         • Supports erythropoiesis
    (4) Gastrointestinal effects
       (a) Diarrhea
       (b) Mucositis
       (c) Stomatitis
    (5) Alopecia (e.g., cyclophosphamide)
    (6) Neuropathies (e.g., vicristine)
    (7) Hand and foot syndrome (ex. fluorouracil)
    (8) Know "signature" adverse effects of individual agents
  E. Drug Resistant Mechanisms
    1. Therapy selects for resistance
      a. Can't achieve total kill
      b. Combination chemotherapy is the rule, *not* the exception
    2. Primary resistance
      a. Tumor cells initially *not* sensitive to a given drug
      b. Test by *in vitro* sensitivity
    3. Secondary resistance
      a. Tumor cells develop resistance during therapy.
        (1) Changes in drug permeability
        (2) Amplification/alteration of targets

BOX 29-1   CHEMOTHERAPEUTIC DRUGS

Drugs That Alter DNA

Alkylating Drugs
  Bendamustine
  Busulfan
  Carboplatin
  Chlorambucil
  Carmustine
  Cisplatin
  Cyclophosphamide
  Dacarbazine
  Estramustine
  Ifosfamide
  Lomustine
  Mechlorethamine
  Melphalan
  Oxaliplatin

  Procarbazine
  Streptozocin
  Temozolomide
  Thiotepa
Antibiotics and related drugs
  Bleomycin
  Dactinomycin
  Daunorubicin
  Daunorubicin liposomal
  Doxorubicin
  Doxorubicin liposomal
  Epirubicin
  Idarubicin
  Mitoxantrone
  Valrubicin

    (3) Enhanced repair
    (4) P-glycoprotein (Pgp, mdr1) can export multiple classes of anti-cancer drugs (multidrug resistance)

> Extrusion of drugs from cancer cells by P-glycoprotein is one mechanism of multidrug resistance.

        (a) Antimetabolites
        (b) Antibiotics
        (c) Plant alkaloids
  b. Multi-drug resistance can be blocked by inhibition of transporters (ex. verapamil)

II. Drugs That Alter DNA (Box 29-1)

A. Alkylating drugs

1. Cyclophosphamide
  a. Mechanism of action
    (1) Prodrug that requires activation by the cytochrome P-450 system (Fig. 29-3)
        (a) Phosphoramide mustard (active)
        (b) Acrolein (bladder cystitis)
    (2) Cross-links DNA strands
    (3) Stops DNA processing

> Bifunctional alkylating agents cross-link DNA strands.

    (4) Cell cycle nonspecific (CCNS)
  b. Uses
    (1) Chronic lymphocytic leukemia (CLL)
    (2) Acute lymphocytic leukemia (ALL)
    (3) Non-Hodgkin's lymphoma
    (4) Multiple myeloma
    (5) Breast cancer
    (6) Ovarian cancer
    (7) Lung cancer

> Cyclophosphamide widely used as an anticancer and immunosuppressive drug.

    (8) Immunologic disorders such as
        (a) Lupus nephritis
        (b) Nephrotic syndrome
        (c) Wegener's granulomatosis
        (d) Rheumatoid arthritis
        (e) Graft-versus-host disease or graft rejection

> "Signature" adverse effect of cyclophosphamide: hemorrhagic cystitis treated with mesna

2. Ifosfamide
  a. Mechanism of action
    (1) Cross-links strands of DNA
    (2) Inhibits protein and DNA synthesis
  b. Uses
    (1) Testicular cancer
    (2) Used off label for several other cancers
3. Busulfan
  a. Mechanism of action
    (1) Cell cycle nonspecific (CCNS)
    (2) Bifunctional alkylating agent

29-3: Bioactivation of cyclophosphamide. *(From Wecker L, et al.: Brody's Human Pharmacology, 5th ed. Philadelphia, Mosby, 2010, Figure 54-6.)*

Cyclophosphamide

Cytochrome P-450 enzymes

Open ring aldehyde form of alcohol

Non-enzymatic

Phosphoramide mustard (active)

Acrolein (toxic)

(Reactive species)

  b. Use
    (1) Chronic granulocytic leukemia (drug of choice)
    (2) Conditioning regimens for bone marrow transplantation
 4. Mechlorethamine
  a. Mechanism of action
    (1) Nitrogen mustard alkylating agent
    (2) Cell cycle nonspecific (CCNS)
  b. Use
    (1) Hodgkin's disease
    (2) Non-Hodgkin's lymphoma (NHL)
    (3) Mycosis fungoides
 5. Chlorambucil
  a. Mechanism of action
    (1) Cross-links strands of DNA
    (2) Interferes with DNA replication and RNA transcription
  b. Uses
    (1) Chronic lymphocytic leukemia (CLL)
    (2) Hodgkin's lymphoma
    (3) Non-Hodgkin's lymphoma (NHL)
 6. Melphalan
  a. Mechanism of action
    (1) Cross-links strands of DNA
    (2) Acts on both resting and rapidly dividing tumor cells
  b. Uses
    (1) Palliative treatment of multiple myeloma
    (2) Nonresectable epithelial ovarian carcinoma
 7. Nitrosoureas
  a. Mechanism of action
    (1) Cross blood-brain barrier (BBB)
      (a) Carmustine
      (b) Lomustine
    (2) Cell cycle nonspecific (CCNS)
    (3) Cross-links strands of DNA and RNA

   b. Uses
     (1) Carmustine
       (a) Primary and metastatic brain tumors
       (b) Multiple myeloma
       (c) Hodgkin's disease (relapsed or refractory)
       (d) Non-Hodgkin's lymphomas (relapsed or refractory)
       (e) Melanoma (off-label)
     (2) Lomustine
       (a) Brain tumors
       (b) Hodgkin's disease
     (3) Streptozocin
       (a) Metastatic islet cell carcinoma of the pancreas
       (b) Carcinoid tumor and syndrome
       (c) Hodgkin's disease
       (d) Palliative treatment of colorectal cancer

> Carmustine and lomustine for brain tumors

> Streptozocin used experimentally to create animal models of diabetes mellitus

8. Platinum compounds
   a. Mechanism of action
     (1) Cross-links DNA stands or protein structures
     (2) Inhibits DNA replication
     (3) Inhibits RNA transcription
     (4) Inhibits protein synthesis
     (5) Cell cycle nonspecific (CCNS)
   b. Uses
     (1) Cisplatin
       (a) Testicular cancer (in combination with vinblastine and bleomycin)
       (b) Ovarian cancer
       (c) Urinary bladder cancer
       (d) Non-small cell lung cancer
     (2) Carboplatin
       (a) Ovarian cancer
       (b) Several other cancers (off-label)
     (3) Oxaliplatin
       (a) Stage III colon cancer and advanced colorectal cancer
       (b) Several other cancers (off-label)
   c. Dose-limiting toxicities
     (1) Cisplatin: Nephrotoxicity, ototoxicity
     (2) Carboplatin produces severe bone marrow suppression
     (3) Oxaliplatin produces neurotoxicity

> "Signature" adverse effects of cisplatin: nephrotoxicity (treated with amifostine), ototoxicity

> "Signature" adverse effect of carboplatin is bone marrow toxicity.

> "Signature" adverse effect of oxaliplatin is neurotoxicity.

9. Bendamustine
   a. Mechanism of action
     (1) Alkylating structure (nitrogen mustard) linked to a purine structure
     (2) Causes cell death via single and double strand DNA cross-linking
     (3) Active against quiescent and dividing cells
   b. Uses
     (1) CLL
     (2) Progressed indolent B-cell NHL

> Bendamustine is a nitrogen mustard alkylating structure linked to a purine structure.

10. Estramustine
   a. Mechanism of action
     (1) Nitrogen mustard linked to estradiol
     (2) Antitumor effect due to an estrogenic effect
     (3) Causes a marked decrease in plasma testosterone and increase in estrogen levels
   b. Uses
     • Palliative treatment of progressive or metastatic prostate cancer

> Estramustine is a nitrogen mustard alkylating structure linked to estradiol.

11. Thiotepa
   a. Mechanism of action
     (1) Alkylating agent that reacts with DNA phosphate groups
     (2) Cross-links DNA strands
     (3) Causes inhibition of DNA, RNA, and protein synthesis
   b. Uses
     (1) Superficial tumors of the bladder
     (2) Palliative treatment of adenocarcinoma of breast or ovary

(3) Lymphomas and sarcomas
(4) Central nervous system (CNS) leukemia/lymphoma; CNS metastases (intrathecal)
12. Drugs related to alkylating agents
a. Procarbazine
(1) Used in the treatment of Hodgkin's disease
(2) Highly teratogenic
(3) Causes secondary malignancy
b. Dacarbazine
(1) Cross-links strands of DNA
(2) Uses
(a) Metastatic malignant melanoma
(b) Osteogenic sarcoma
(c) Soft-tissue sarcoma
(d) Hodgkin's disease
c. Temozolomide
(1) A prodrug similar to dacarbazine that is converted to an active alkylating metabolite
(2) Uses
(a) Treatment of glioblastoma multiforme
(b) Treatment of refractory anaplastic astrocytoma

B. Antibiotics and related compounds that alter DNA
1. Dactinomycin (actinomycin D)
a. Mechanism of action
(1) Cell cycle-nonspecific (CCNS)
(2) Intercalates between base pairs of DNA
(3) Prevents DNA and RNA synthesis
b. Uses
(1) Trophoblastic tumors
(2) Wilms' tumor in combination with surgery and vincristine
(3) Ewing's sarcoma
2. Anthracyclines
a. Examples
(1) Daunorubicin
(2) Doxorubicin
(3) Epirubicin
(4) Idarubicin
b. Pharmacokinetic
(1) Administered intravenously
(2) Hepatic clearance
(3) Liposomal preparation of daunorubicin and doxorubicin
(a) Decrease the incidence of severe toxicity
(b) Increase efficacy
c. Mechanism of action
(1) Cell cycle-nonspecific (CCNS)
(2) Intercalates between base pairs of DNA
(3) Inhibits topoisomerase II, causing faulty DNA repairs
d. Uses
(1) Daunorubicin
(a) Acute granulocytic leukemia (AGL)
(b) Acute lymphocytic leukemia (ALL)
(2) Doxorubicin
(a) Breast cancer
(b) Endometrial cancer
(c) Ovarian cancer
(d) Testicular cancer
(e) Thyroid cancer
(f) Lung cancer
(g) Sarcomas
(3) Epirubicin
• Adjuvant therapy for primary breast cancer
(4) Idarubicin

MOPP (**M**echlorethamine, vincristine [**O**ncovin], **P**rocarbazine, and **P**rednisone) is used less today for Hodgkin's disease because both procarbazine and mechlorethamine are amongst the most carcinogenic antineoplastic agents.

Procarbazine is highly carcinogenic.

ABVD (doxorubicin [**A**driamycin], **B**leomycin, **V**inblastine, and **D**acarbazine) is preferred today over MOPP for treatment of Hodgkin's disease.

Dactinomycin (tumor cells) and rifampin (bacteria) inhibit DNA-dependent RNA synthesis.

Dactinomycin is used for treating pediatric tumors

Note the common ending of -rubicin for anthracycline anticancer drugs.

(a) Acute leukemias

(b) Accelerated phase or blast crisis of chronic myelogenous leukemia (CML)

(c) Breast cancer

(5) Valrubicin
- Intravesical therapy of Bacillus Calmette-Guerin (BCG)-refractory carcinoma *in situ* of the urinary bladder

e. Adverse effects

(1) Bone marrow toxicity

(2) Cardiotoxicity

(a) Free radicals require iron

(b) Dexrazoxane (iron chelator) is a chemoprotectant

(3) Idarubicin and epirubicin have lower cardiotoxicity

3. Mitoxantrone

a. Similar to the anthracyclines

b. Sometimes substituted for doxorubicin or daunorubicin

c. Has considerably less cardiotoxicity

4. Bleomycin

a. Mechanism of action

(1) Concentrates in skin and lungs

(2) Causes formation of free radicals, which affects DNA

(3) Cell cycle-specific (CCS)

(4) Most active during the G_2 and M phases

b. Uses

(1) Squamous cell carcinoma of the head, neck, and skin

(2) Lymphomas

(3) Testicular cancer

III. Antimetabolites (Box 29-2)

A. Folic acid antagonists

1. Methotrexate (MTX)

a. Mechanism of action

(1) Cell cycle-specific (CCS)
- S phase

(2) Dihydrofolate reductase inhibitor

(3) Inhibits conversion of folic acid to tetrahydrofolic acid

(4) Inhibits purine and thymidylic acid synthesis

(5) Inhibits aminoimidazolecarboxamide ribonucleotide (AICAR) formyltransferase (low doses)

b. Uses

(1) Choriocarcinoma (women)

(2) Acute lymphocytic leukemia (ALL)

(3) Non-Hodgkin's lymphoma

(4) Tumors of:

(a) Breast

(b) Testis

(c) Bladder

(d) Lung

(5) Systemic lupus erythematosus

(6) Rheumatic arthritis

Anthracyclines have strong bone marrow toxicity.

"Signature" adverse effect of daunorubicin and doxorubicin: cardiotoxicity (cardiomyopathy) treated with dexrazoxane

"Signature" adverse effect of bleomycin: pulmonary fibrosis

Antimetabolites are generally active in the S phase

Trimethoprim is a potent inhibitor of the bacterial dihydrofolate reductase, methotrexate inhibits the mammalian isoenzyme

Methotrexate is also a potent immunosuppressant drug.

BOX 29-2 CHEMOTHERAPEUTIC DRUGS

Antimetabolites
Folic Acid Antagonist
  Methotrexate
  Pemetrexed
  Trimetrexate
Purine Antagonists
  [Cladribine
  Fludarabine
  Mercaptopurine
  Pentostatin
  Nelarabine

  Thioguanine
Pyrimidine Antagonists
  Capecitabine
  Cytarabine
  Cytarabine liposomal
  5-Fluorouracil
  Gemcitabine

Ribonucleotide Reductase Inhibitor
  Hydroxyurea

(7) Crohn's disease

(8) Psoriasis

(9) With misoprostol to terminate early pregnancies

c. Leucovorin (folinic acid) "rescue" therapy

(1) High dose methotrexate to kill cancer cells

(2) Followed by leucovorin to reduce myelosuppression and mucositis

2. Pemetrexed

a. Mechanism of action

(1) Folic acid analogue antimetabolite

(2) Actions similar to methotrexate

b. Uses

(1) Treatment of malignant pleural mesothelioma

(2) Treatment of locally advanced or metastatic nonsquamous non-small cell lung cancer (NSCLC)

3. Trimetrexate

a. Mechanism of action

(1) Folate antimetabolite

(2) Decreases DNA synthesis by inhibiting dihydrofolate reductase

b. Uses

(1) Off label for following cancers

(a) Non-small cell lung cancer

(b) Metastatic colorectal cancer

(c) Metastatic head and neck cancer

(d) Pancreatic adenocarcinoma

(e) Cutaneous T-cell lymphoma

(2) Alternative therapy for the treatment of moderate-to-severe *Pneumocystis jiroveci* pneumonia (PCP)

B. Purine antagonist

1. Mercaptopurine (6-MP)

a. Pharmacokinetics

(1) Orally effective

(2) Bioactivated via purine salvage pathway

• Hypoxanthine/guanine phosphoribosyl transferase (HGPRT)

(3) Metabolism

(a) Hepatically via xanthine oxidase

• Allopurinol increases actions

(b) Methylated via thiopurine methyl transferase (TMPT)

• Determine TMPT genotype before dosing

b. Mechanism of action

(1) Cell cycle-specific (CCS)

(2) Inhibits purine synthesis

(3) Tumor resistance due to:

(a) Increase in alkaline phosphatase

(b) Decreases in HGPRT

c. Use

(1) Acute lymphoblastic leukemia (ALL)

(a) Induction

(b) Maintenance

(2) Steroid-sparing agent for corticosteroid-dependent

(a) Crohn's disease

(b) Ulcerative colitis

2. Thioguanine

a. Mechanism similar to 6-MP

b. Used to treat

(1) Acute myelogenous (nonlymphocytic) leukemia

(2) Chronic myelogenous leukemia

(3) Granulocytic leukemia

3. Fludarabine

a. Mechanism similar to 6-MP

b. Used to treat

(1) Progressive or refractory B-cell CLL

(2) Off label for several lymphocytic cancers

Leucovorin rescue (folinic acid) can be used to overcome the effects of high blood levels of methotrexate in non-cancerous cells.

"Signature" adverse effect of methotrexate: acute and chronic hepatotoxicity

Effects of purine antagonists are potentiated by allopurinol.

Mercaptopurine is very toxic in patients with TMPT deficiency.

Purine antimetabolites are used to treat cancer include: mercaptopurine, thioguanine, fludarabine, claridabine, and pentostatin.

4. Cladribine
   a. Mechanism of action
      (1) Phosphorylated to a 5′-triphosphate
      (2) Incorporates into DNA
      (3) Result in the breakage of DNA strands
      (4) Inhibits DNA synthesis
      (5) Cell-cycle specific (CCS)
   b. Uses
      (1) Treatment of hairy cell leukemia
      (2) Off label
         (a) Several lymphocytic cancers
         (b) Progressive multiple sclerosis
5. Pentostatin
   a. Mechanism of action
      (1) Purine antimetabolite
      (2) Inhibits adenosine deaminase
   b. Uses
      (1) Treatment of hairy cell leukemia
      (2) Off label for treatment of:
         (a) Cutaneous T-cell lymphoma
         (b) Chronic lymphocytic leukemia (CLL)
         (c) Acute and chronic graft-versus-host-disease (GVHD)
C. Pyrimidine antagonists
1. Fluorouracil (5-FU)
   a. Mechanism of action
      (1) Cell cycle-specific (CCS)
         • Most active during the S phase
      (2) Active metabolite inhibits
         (a) Thymidylate synthase
            • Leucovorin (folinic acid) enhances its binding to thymidylate synthase.
         (b) Interferes with DNA and RNA synthesis
   b. Uses
      (1) Treatment of carcinomas of:
         (a) Breast
         (b) Colon
         (c) Head and neck
         (d) Pancreas
         (e) Rectum
         (f) Stomach
      (2) Topically for the management of:
         (a) Actinic or solar keratoses
         (b) Superficial basal cell carcinomas
2. Cytarabine (Ara-C)
   a. Mechanism of action
      (1) Cell cycle-specific (CCS)
         • Active during the S phase
      (2) Active metabolite inhibits DNA polymerase
      (3) Thus interferes with DNA synthesis
   b. Uses
      (1) Treatment of:
         (a) Acute myeloid leukemia (AML)
         (b) Acute lymphocytic leukemia (ALL)
         (c) Chronic myelocytic leukemia (CML; blast phase)
         (d) Lymphomas
      (2) Prophylaxis and treatment of meningeal leukemia
      (3) Cytarabine Liposomal for treatment of lymphomatous meningitis
3. Capecitabine
   a. A prodrug of fluorouracil
   b. Uses
      (1) Treatment of metastatic colorectal cancer
      (2) Adjuvant therapy of Dukes' C colon cancer
      (3) Treatment of metastatic breast cancer

Leucovorin (folinic acid) potentiates the effects of 5-FU.

"Signature" adverse effects of fluorouracil are "hand and foot syndrome" and GI toxicity (mucositis).

Pyrimidine antimetabolites used to treat cancer include: fluorouracil, cytarabine, capecitabine, and gemcitabine.

4. Gemcitabine
   a. Mechanism similar to cytarabine
   b. Uses
      (1) Treatment of metastatic breast cancer
      (2) Locally-advanced or metastatic
         (a) Non-small cell lung cancer (NSCLC)
         (b) Pancreatic cancer
      (3) Advanced, relapsed ovarian cancer

D. Ribonucleotide Reductase Inhibitor
1. Hydroxyurea
2. Uses; treatment of:
   a. Melanoma
   b. Refractory chronic myelocytic leukemia (CML)
   c. Relapsed and refractory metastatic ovarian cancer
   d. Radiosensitizing agent in the treatment of squamous cell head and neck cancer
   e. Adjunct in the management of sickle cell patients

IV. Mitotic Inhibitors (Box 29-3)
A. Vinca alkaloids
1. Vinblastine
   a. Mechanism of action
      (1) Cell cycle-specific (CCS)
         • Active during the M phase; metaphase
      (2) Binds to tubulin (microtubular protein)
      (3) Prevents polymerization
   b. Uses
      (1) Hodgkin's and non-Hodgkin's lymphomas
      (2) Testicular carcinoma (in combination with cisplatin and bleomycin)
      (3) Mycosis fungoides
      (4) Kaposi's sarcoma
      (5) Histiocytosis (Letterer-Siwe disease)
      (6) Choriocarcinoma
2. Vincristine
   a. Mechanism similar to vinblastine
   b. Use to treat
      (1) Leukemias
      (2) Hodgkin's disease
      (3) Non-Hodgkin's lymphomas
      (4) Wilms' tumor
      (5) Neuroblastoma
      (6) Rhabdomyosarcoma
3. Vinorelbine
   a. Mechanism similar to vinblastine
   b. Uses
      (1) Treatment of NSCLC
      (2) Off label for treatment of:
         (a) Breast cancer
         (b) Cervical cancer
         (c) Ovarian cancer

B. Taxanes
1. Paclitaxel
   a. Mechanism of action

Hydroxyurea used to treat cancer and sickle cell patients.

Taxanes stabilize and vinca alkaloids inhibit formation of microtubular structure.

Vinblastine: BLASTs the bone marrow

"Signature" adverse effect of vincristine (dose-limiting): neurotoxicity, such as peripheral neuropathy

BOX 29-3 CHEMOTHERAPEUTIC DRUGS

Mitotic Inhibitors
Docetaxel
Ixabepilone
Paclitaxel
Vinblastine
Vincristine
Vinorelbine

(1) Cell cycle-specific (CCS)
  - Active during the G_2 and M phases
(2) Binds to tubulin
(3) Prevents depolymerization
  b. Used to treat
    (1) Refractory ovarian and breast cancers
    (2) Non-small cell lung cancer (NSCLC)
    (3) Treatment of AIDS-related Kaposi's sarcoma
2. Docetaxel
  a. Mechanism similar to paclitaxel
  b. Uses
    (1) Treatment of breast cancer
    (2) Locally-advanced or metastatic NSCLC
    (3) Hormone refractory, metastatic prostate cancer
    (4) Advanced gastric adenocarcinoma
    (5) Locally-advanced squamous cell head and neck cancer
3. Ixabepilone
  a. Mechanism related to the taxanes
    (1) Stabilizes microtubular function
    (2) Induces apoptosis
  b. Used to treat metastatic or locally-advanced breast cancer

V. **Podophyllotoxins** (Box 29-4)
  A. **Examples**
    1. Etoposide (VP-16)
    2. Teniposide
  B. **Mechanism of action**
    1. Cell cycle-specific (CCS)
      - Active during the G2 phase
    2. Inhibits topoisomerase II
  C. **Uses**
    1. Non-Hodgkin's lymphoma
    2. Testicular cancer
    3. Small cell lung cancer
    4. Acute lymphocytic leukemia (teniposide)
    5. Etoposide off label for many cancers

VI. **Camptothecins** (Box 29-5)
  A. **Irinotecan**
    1. Mechanism of action
      a. Converted by carboxylesterase enzymes to active metabolite (SN-38)
      b. SN-38 binds reversibly to topoisomerase I-DNA complex
      c. Prevents religation of the cleaved DNA strand
      d. SN-38 inactivated by UDP-glucuronosyl transferase 1A1 (UGT1A1) a polymorphic enzyme
    2. Uses
      a. Treatment of metastatic carcinoma of the colon or rectum
      b. Off label for treatment of
        (1) Lung cancer (small cell and non-small cell)
        (2) Cervical cancer
        (3) Gastric cancer
        (4) Pancreatic cancer

Taxanes stabilize and vinca alkaloids inhibit formation of microtubular structure.

Podophyllotoxins, topoisomerase II inhibitors cause double strand breaks in DNA.

Camptothecins, topoisomerase I inhibitors cause single strand breaks in DNA.

Irinotecan is used in the first-line treatment of metastatic colorectal cancer in combination with 5-FU and leucovorin.

BOX 29-4 CHEMOTHERAPEUTIC DRUGS

Podophyllotoxins
Etoposide
Teniposide

BOX 29-5 CHEMOTHERAPEUTIC DRUGS

Camptothecins
Irinotecan
Topotecan

(5) Leukemia

(6) Lymphoma

(7) Breast cancer

(8) Brain tumors

3. Boxed warning

a. Severe diarrhea may be dose-limiting and potentially fatal.

b. Two severe (life-threatening) forms of diarrhea may occur

    (1) Early diarrhea within 24 hours is characterized by cholinergic symptoms

        (a) Increased salivation

        (b) Increased diaphoresis

        (c) Increased abdominal cramping

          • Responsive to atropine

    (2) Late diarrhea after more than 24 hours leads to:

        (a) Dehydration

        (b) Electrolyte imbalance

        (c) Possible sepsis

          • Treated with loperamide

B. Topotecan

1. Mechanism of action

a. Binds to topoisomerase I

b. Religation of the cleaved DNA strand is blocked.

2. Used to treat:

a. Ovarian cancer

b. Small cell lung cancer

c. Cervical cancer (in combination with cisplatin)

VII. Hormones and Hormone Regulators (Box 29-6)

  A. Hormones

    1. Corticosteroids (see Chapter 23)

      • Prednisone

      a. Mechanism of antitumor effects

        (1) Inhibition of glucose transport

        (2) Inhibition of phosphorylation events

        (3) Induction of cell death in immature lymphocytes

      b. Uses

        • Often used in combination with other antineoplastic agents

          (1) Acute lymphoblastic leukemia (ALL) in children (with vincristine)

          (2) Chronic lymphocytic leukemia (CLL)

          (3) Multiple myeloma (with melphalan)

          (4) Hodgkin's and NHLs

  B. Modulation of hormone release and action (see Chapter 26)

    1. Aminoglutethimide

      a. Mechanism of action

        (1) Blocks first step in adrenal steroid synthesis

        (2) Inhibits estrogen synthesis (aromatase inhibitor)

> Early diarrhea from irinotecan is due to a cholinergic mechanism; blocked by atropine.

> Vincristine plus prednisone preferred induction therapy for children with ALL

BOX 29-6   CHEMOTHERAPEUTIC DRUGS

Hormones and Hormone Regulators

Hormones
  Prednisone

Modulators of Hormone Release and Action
  Anastrozole
  Aminoglutethimide
  Bicalutamide
  Exemestane
  Flutamide
  Fulvestrant
  Goserelin
  Letrozole
  Leuprolide
  Nilutamide
  Tamoxifen
  Toremifene

  b. Uses
    (1) Suppression of adrenal function in selected patients with Cushing's syndrome
    (2) Metastatic breast cancer
      • Must be administered with hydrocortisone
2. Aromatase inhibitors
  a. Examples
    (1) Anastrozole (reversible)
    (2) Letrozole (reversible)
    (3) Exemestane (irreversible)
  b. Mechanism of action
    (1) Inhibits aromatase
    (2) Enzyme that catalyzes the final step in estrogen synthesis
  c. Used to treat in postmenopausal women
    (1) Locally-advanced or metastatic breast cancer (estrogen receptor [ER]-positive or hormone receptor unknown)
    (2) Advanced breast cancer with disease progression following tamoxifen therapy
    (3) As an adjuvant of early ER-positive breast cancer
3. Estrogen antagonists
  a. Selective estrogen receptor modulators (SERM)
    (1) Examples
      (a) Tamoxifen
      (b) Toremifene
    (2) Mechanism of action
      (a) Blocks estrogen receptors in cancer cells that require estrogen for growth and development
      (b) Acts as a weak agonist at estrogen receptors in other tissues; examples—bone, uterus
    (3) Uses
      (a) Treat metastatic (female and male) breast cancer
      (b) Adjuvant treatment of breast cancer
      (c) Reduce risk of invasive breast cancer in women with ductal carcinoma *in situ* (DCIS)
      (d) Reduce the incidence of breast cancer in women at high risk
  b. Pure estrogen antagonist
    • Fulvestrant
    (1) Mechanism of action
      (a) Strong competitive binding to estrogen receptors
      (b) Produces a nuclear complex that binds to DNA; *but* inhibits estrogen effects
      (c) Has *no* estrogen-receptor agonist activity
      (d) Causes down-regulation of estrogen receptors and inhibits tumor growth
    (2) Uses
      (a) Treatment of hormone receptor positive metastatic breast cancer in postmenopausal women with disease progression following antiestrogen therapy
      (b) Off label uses; endometriosis; uterine bleeding
4. Androgen antagonists
  a. Examples
    (1) Flutamide
    (2) Bicalutamide
    (3) Nilutamide
  b. Mechanism of action
    • Inhibits the uptake and binding of testosterone and dihydrotestosterone by prostatic tissue
  c. Use
    • Treatment of metastatic prostatic carcinoma in combination with luteinizing hormone-releasing hormone (LHRH) agonists such as leuprolide
5. Gonadotropin-releasing hormone (GnRH) analogues (see Chapter 26)
  a. Examples
    (1) Leuprolide
    (2) Goserelin

Aminoglutethimide treatment must always be given in combination with hydrocortisone to prevent adrenal insufficiency.

Patients often complain of hot flashes.

Tamoxifen used both for the treatment and prevention of breast cancer.

Note the common ending -lutamide for the androgen antagonists.

b. Mechanism of action
   (1) GnRH agonist
   (2) A potent inhibitor of gonadotropin secretion when given continuously
   (3) Continuous administration results in suppression of ovarian and testicular steroidogenesis
   (4) Due to decreased levels of luteinizing hormone (LH) and follicle stimulating hormone (FSH)
   (5) Subsequent decrease in testosterone (male) and estrogen (female) levels
c. Uses
   (1) Advanced prostate or breast cancers (hormonal antagonist)
   (2) Endometriosis

VIII. **Monoclonal Antibodies** (Box 29-7)
   A. **General Information**
      1. Uses of currently available agents (Table 29-2)
      2. Brief discussion of key agents below
   B. **Alemtuzumab**
      1. Binds to CD52 antigen on normal and malignant β-lymphocytes
      2. CD52 antigen also found on:
         a. T lymphocytes
         b. Natural killer cells
         c. Macrophages
         d. Platelets
      3. Approved for CLL
   C. **Gemtuzumab ozogamicin**
      1. Directed toward the CD33 antigen that is expressed on:
         a. Leukemic cells
         b. Myelomonocytic cells

Continuous exposure GnRH agonists suppress LH and FSH secretion.

Alemtuzumab targets CD52 antigen on tumor cells.

BOX 29-7   CHEMOTHERAPEUTIC DRUGS

Antineoplastic Agent, Monoclonal Antibody
Alemtuzumab
Bevacizumab
Cetuximab
Gemtuzumab ozogamicin
Ibritumomab
Panitumumab
Rituximab
Tositumomab and iodine ^{131}I tositumomab
Trastuzumab

TABLE 29-2. Therapeutic Uses of Antitumor Monoclonal Antibodies

MONOCLONAL ANTIBODY	TARGET	TUMORS TREATED
Alemtuzumab	CD52	B-cell chronic lymphocytic leukemia Refractory T-cell prolymphocytic leukemia Multiple myeloma Treatment of autoimmune cytopenias
Bevacizumab	Vascular endothelial growth factor (VEGF)	Metastatic colorectal cancer Advanced nonsquamous, non-small cell lung cancer Metastatic HER-2 negative breast cancer
Cetuximab Panitumumab	Epidermal growth factor receptors (EGFR, HER1, c-ErbB-1)	Metastatic colorectal cancer Squamous cell cancer of the head and neck EGFR-expressing advanced non-small cell lung cancer (NSCLC)
Gemtuzumab ozogamicin	CD33	CD33 positive acute myeloid leukemia (AML) Salvage therapy for acute promyelocytic leukemia (APL)
Ibritumomab	Targets Indium-111 to CD20 positive tumors	Relapsed or refractory low-grade or follicular B-cell non-Hodgkin's lymphoma
Rituximab Tositumomab Iodine ^{131}I Tositumomab	CD20	Low-grade or follicular CD20-positive, B-cell non-Hodgkin's lymphoma (NHL); Large B-cell CD20-positive NHL Moderately- to severely-active rheumatoid arthritis (RA) in combination with methotrexate Rituximab has several off label uses
Trastuzumab	Human epidermal growth factor receptor 2 protein (HER-2)	HER-2 overexpressing breast cancer HER-2 overexpressing metastatic breast cancer

2. Coupled to calicheamicin, a cytotoxic molecule
3. Use
- Treatment of acute myelogenous leukemia (AML) in adults over 60 years of age in first relapse and have a CD33-positive tumor

   D. Rituximab
   1. Binds to CD20 antigen on B cells
   2. Used in B-cell non-Hodgkin's lymphoma

   E. Tositumomab
   1. Targets the CD20 antigen found on pre-B- and mature B-lymphocytes
   2. Used for treatment of CD20-positive follicular NHL whose disease is refractory to rituximab and has relapsed following chemotherapy

   F. Trastuzumab
   1. Binds to the HER2 protein on the surface of tumor cells
   2. Used for metastatic breast tumors that over express HER2 protein

IX. **Signal Transduction Inhibitors** (Box 29-8)
   A. General Information
   1. Uses of currently available agents (Table 29-3)
   2. Brief discussion of key agent below

   B. Imatinib
   1. Inhibits the Bcr-Abl tyrosine protein kinase found in CML
   2. Used for the treatment of:
      a. CML in patients who have failed alpha interferon therapy
      b. Metastatic and unresectable malignant gastrointestinal stromal tumors (GIST)

X. **Miscellaneous Antineoplastic Agents** (Box 29-9; see Table 29-4 for uses)

Gemtuzumab ozogamicin targets CD33 antigen on tumor cells.

Rituximab and tositumomab target CD20 antigen on tumor cells.

Trastuzumab targets HER2 antigen on tumor cells.

Imatinib treats CML and GIST.

BOX 29-8 CHEMOTHERAPEUTIC DRUGS

Antineoplastic Agent, Signal Transduction Inhibitor
Bortezomib
Dasatinib
Erlotinib
Gefitinib
Imatinib
Lapatinib
Nilotinib
Sorafenib
Sunitinib

TABLE 29-3. **Therapeutic Uses of Antitumor Signal Transduction Inhibitors**

AGENT	TARGET	TUMORS TREATED
Bortezomib	Inhibits proteasomes; leading to activation of signaling cascades, cell-cycle arrest, and apoptosis	Multiple myeloma Relapsed or refractory mantle cell lymphoma
Dasatinib Imatinib Nilotinib	BCR-ABL tyrosine kinase inhibitor	Gastrointestinal stromal tumors (GIST) kit-positive (Imatinib) Philadelphia chromosome-positive (Ph+) chronic myeloid leukemia (CML) Ph+ acute lymphoblastic leukemia (ALL)
Erlotinib	Epidermal growth factor receptor (HER1/EGFR)-tyrosine kinase	Locally advanced or metastatic non-small cell lung cancer (NSCLC) Locally advanced, unresectable or metastatic pancreatic cancer (first-line therapy in combination with gemcitabine)
Gefitinib	Tyrosine kinases (TK) associated with transmembrane cell surface receptors	Locally advanced or metastatic non-small cell lung cancer after failure of platinum-based and docetaxel therapies
Lapatinib	Tyrosine kinase (dual kinase) inhibitor	HER2/neu overexpressing advanced or metastatic breast cancer (in combination with capecitabine)
Sorafenib	Multikinase inhibitor	Advanced renal cell cancer (RCC) Unresectable hepatocellular cancer (HCC)
Sunitinib	Multikinase inhibitor	GIST resistant to imatinib Advanced renal cell cancer (RCC)

BOX 29-9 CHEMOTHERAPEUTIC DRUGS

Antineoplastic Agent, Miscellaneous
Aldesleukin
Alitretinoin
Altretamine
Arsenic trioxide
Asparaginase
Bexarotene
Denileukin diftitox
Mitotane
Pegaspargase
Porfimer
Tretinoin (Oral)

TABLE 29-4. **Therapeutic Uses of Miscellaneous Antitumor Agents**

AGENT	TARGET	TUMORS TREATED
Aldesleukin (IL-2)	Promotes proliferation, differentiation, and recruitment of T and B cells	Metastatic renal cell cancer Metastatic melanoma
Alitretinoin (gel)	Retinoid receptors	Cutaneous lesions in AIDS-related Kaposi's sarcoma
Altretamine	Alkylating- but has activity in alkylator-resistant patients	Palliative treatment of persistent or recurrent ovarian cancer
Arsenic trioxide	Damages DNA	Relapsed or refractory acute promyelocytic leukemia (APL)
Asparaginase Pegaspargase	Inhibit protein synthesis by hydrolyzing asparagine to aspartic acid and ammonia	Acute lymphocytic leukemia (ALL)
Bexarotene	Activates retinoid X receptor (RXR) subtypes	Cutaneous T-cell lymphoma (oral) Cutaneous lesions in patients with refractory cutaneous T-cell lymphoma (topical)
Denileukin diftitox	High-affinity for IL-2 receptor (CD25)	Cutaneous T-cell lymphoma (CTCL)
Mitotane	Affects mitochondria in adrenal cortical cells; ↓ cortisol	Inoperable adrenocortical carcinoma Treatment of Cushing's syndrome
Porfimer	Sensitizes tissues to light and oxygen, increasing production of free radicals	Obstructing esophageal cancer Microinvasive endobronchial non-small cell lung cancer (NSCLC) Ablation of high-grade dysplasia in Barrett's esophagus
Tretinoin (oral)	Nuclear receptors	Acute promyelocytic leukemia (APL)

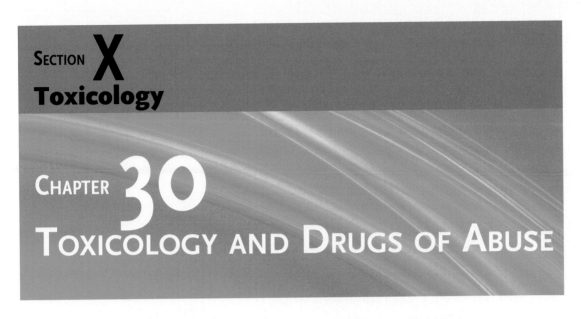

CHAPTER **30**
TOXICOLOGY AND DRUGS OF ABUSE

I. General Principles of Toxicology
A. Definitions
1. Toxicology is the study of the hazardous effects of chemicals, including drugs, on biologic systems.
2. Toxicity is a reflection of how much, how fast, and how long an individual is exposed to a poison.

B. Primary determinants of toxicity
1. Dose and dose rate
2. Duration of exposure
3. Route of exposure

C. Factors that affect toxicity
1. Biotransformation
   a. Methanol is transformed to formaldehyde and formic acid (toxic metabolites).
   b. Parathion is transformed to paraoxon (toxic cholinesterase inhibitor).
2. Genetic factors
   a. Polymorphic metabolism (toxicokinetics)
      • Individuals are *fast* or *slow* acetylators of isoniazid (slow acetylator have increased neurotoxicity).
   b. Polymorphic targets (toxicodynamics)
      • Increased risk of drug-induced torsades de pointes with mutations in ion channels leading to prolonged QT interval
3. Immune status (hypersensitivity)
   a. Penicillin allergies
   b. Sulfonamide allergies
4. Photosensitivity
   • Skin photosensitivity due to e.g., demeclocycline, sulfonamides, fluoroquinolones
5. Species differences
   • Malathion is rapidly inactivated by humans but *not* by insects
6. Age
   a. Toxicodynamics affected by age
      • Elderly more sensitive to benzodiazepines
   b. Toxicokinetic parameters vary with age
      (1) Decreased renal clearance in elderly
      (2) Decreased cytochrome P–450 activity in elderly
7. Gender
   • Hormonal status affects both toxicodynamic and toxicokinetic parameters.
8. Environmental factors
   • Aromatic hydrocarbons induce cytochrome P–450 activities
9. Nutritional status/protein binding

Paracelsus, the father of toxicology, wrote: "All things are poison and nothing is without poison, only the dose permits something not to be poisonous."

Large overdoses of chemicals often switch kinetics from first to zero-order because

Hypersensitivity to β-lactam antibiotics demonstrate cross-allergenicity including penicillins, cephalosporins, and carbapenems but *not* aztreonam.

Drugs with sulfonamide structures include: sulfonamide antimicrobials; sulfonylurea drugs used to treat diabetes, most diuretics, and celecoxib.

Elderly are often much more sensitive to drugs' adverse effects than young adults.

An example is tyramine in foods and drinks can cause a hypertensive action in patients taking monoamine oxidase inhibitors (e.g., phenelzine).

Drug-drug or drug-environmental chemical interactions can lead to marked enhancement of adverse effects.

Most poisons do *not* have a specific antidote.

10. Drug interactions
   • Interactions between drugs and between drugs and environmental chemicals may occur by both toxicokinetic and toxicodynamic mechanisms
11. Environmental Pathology (see Chapter 6; Rapid Review Pathology)

II. Symptoms and Treatment of Acute Poisoning (Table 30-1 and Table 30-2)
A. General Approach to the Poisoned Patient
1. Systematic
2. Treatment and diagnostic actions are in parallel
3. Basic goals
   a. Rapid stabilization of the patient
   b. Categorization of poison class
   c. Initiation of general treatment (supportive)
   d. Specific treatment when available
4. Remember that poisonings are often mixed, with multiple drugs/chemicals
5. Treatment often nonspecific
6. Prevent further toxin exposure
7. Enhance toxin elimination

TABLE 30-1. **Symptoms and Treatment of Poisoning**

AGENT	CLINICAL FEATURES	TREATMENT	COMMENTS
Acetaminophen	Elevated prothrombin time (PT), increased transaminase levels, hepatic necrosis	Acetylcysteine	Commonly used for suicide attempts
Alkalies (hydroxides in soaps, cleansers, drain cleaners)	GI irritation	Supportive care H$_2$O	No emesis or lavage More potent than strong acids
Bleach (sodium hypochlorite)	Irritation, delirium	Supportive care; milk, ice cream, or beaten eggs; antacids	No emesis
Carbon monoxide	Headaches, dizziness, metabolic acidosis, retinal hemorrhage	Supportive care, oxygen	Cherry-red blood
Corrosives	GI irritation, seizures, weakness	Milk, antacids, calcium gluconate (antidote for oxalates); milk of magnesia (antidote for mineral acids)	No emesis or lavage
Cyanide	Seizures, ECG changes	Amyl nitrite or sodium nitrite plus sodium thiosulfate Hydroxocobalamin	Rapid treatment necessary
Ethylene glycol	Renal failure; metabolic acidosis with anion gap	Ethanol IV or fomepizole (antidotes), sodium bicarbonate for acidosis, supportive care	Culprit: toxic metabolite (oxalic acid)
Heavy metals			
Arsenic	Vomiting, diarrhea, seizures, neuropathy, nephropathy	Chelation (dimercaprol or penicillamine); succimer for chronic exposure	Delayed reaction: white lines on fingernails (Mees' exposure lines)
Iron	GI irritation, blood loss, acidosis	Deferoxamine	Keep away from children
Lead	Abdominal pain, lead lines on gums, basophilic stippling, weakness, behavioral changes, peripheral neuropathy, encephalopathy	Chelation (dimercaprol, EDTA, succimer, or penicillamine)	In old paints and glazes
Mercury	Renal failure, GI irritation, behavioral changes	Chelation (dimercaprol); milk or eggs; succimer for chronic exposure	Delayed reaction: "mad as a hatter"
Hydrocarbons	Pulmonary infiltrates, CNS depression, seizures, tinnitus	Supportive care	No emesis or lavage Delayed reaction: pneumonitis
Methanol	Visual disturbance, metabolic acidosis, respiratory failure	Ethanol IV or fomepizole (antidotes), sodium bicarbonate for acidosis, supportive care	Culprit: toxic metabolite (formic acid)
Salicylates	Respiratory alkalosis, metabolic acidosis, increased temperature, tinnitus, respiratory failure, seizures	Supportive care, alkalinize urine, dialysis, cool down	Uncouple oxidative phosphorylation
Strychnine	Seizures, respiratory failure, rigidity	Supportive care, activated charcoal	Glycine antagonist in spinal cord, blocking nerve impulses

CNS, central nervous system; ECG, electrocardiogram; EDTA, ethylenediamine-tetraacetate; GI, gastrointestinal.

TABLE 30-2. **Specific Antidotes for Selected Drugs and Toxins**

ANTIDOTE	POISON
Drugs That Chelate Metals	
Calcium disodium edetate (CA^{2+},2Na$^+$EDTA)	Lead
Deferoxamine	Iron
Dimercaprol	Arsenic, gold, mercury, lead
Penicillamine	Lead, copper, arsenic, gold
Succimer	Lead; also used for chronic exposure to arsenic and mercury
Substances That Act Against Specific Drugs or Toxins	
Acetylcysteine	Acetaminophen
Amyl nitrite/sodium nitrate	Cyanide
Atropine	Cholinesterase inhibitor
Digoxin-specific FAB antibodies	Cardiac glycosides (e.g., digoxin)
Esmolol	Theophylline, caffeine, metaproterenol
Ethanol	Methanol or ethylene glycol
Flumazenil	Benzodiazepine
Fomepizole	Ethylene glycol, methanol
Glucagon	Beta blockers
Naloxone	Opioids
Oxygen	Carbon monoxide
Physostigmine	Anticholinergics
Pralidoxime (2-PAM)	Organophosphates; contraindicated for carbamates
Pyridoxine	Isoniazid
Sodium bicarbonate	Cardiac depressants (tricyclic antidepressants, quinidine)
Sodium thiosulfate	Cyanide

FAB, fragment antigen binding.

B. **ABCDTs of treatment**
1. **Airway** should be:
   a. Cleared of vomitus or any other obstruction
   b. An airway or endotracheal tube inserted
2. **Breathing** assessed by:
   a. Observation
   b. Measurements of arterial gases
   c. Pulse-oximetry
      • Intubate and mechanically ventilate if needed
3. **Circulation**
   a. Monitor
      (1) Pulse rate
      (2) Blood pressure
      (3) Urine output
   b. Start IV and draw blood for:
      (1) Glucose
      (2) Laboratory determination
4. **Drugs**
   a. Dextrose
      • Every patient with altered mental status
   b. Administer 100 mg of thiamine to alcoholic and malnourished patients
      • Prevents Wernicke-Korsakoff syndrome
   c. Naloxone
   d. Flumazenil
      • May cause seizures
   e. IV lorazepam or diazepam for seizure control
5. **Temperature** (cooling)
      • Tepid sponge bath or fan
C. **Remove stomach contents if indicated**
1. Gastric lavage
   a. *Not* recommended after 4 hours of poisoning
      • Usually *not* helpful after 1 hour

Treatment requires ABCDTs: Airway, Breathing, Circulation; Drugs, Temperature.

Thiamine prevents Wernicke-Korsakoff syndrome.

Remember multiple doses of naloxone may be required for opioid overdoses.

Flumazenil may cause seizures if used improperly.

Stop seizures with diazepam or lorazepam.

   b. Contraindications
      (1) After 30 minutes of ingestion of corrosive material
      (2) Ingestion of hydrocarbon solvents (aspiration pneumonia)
      (3) Coma, stupor, delirium, or seizures (present or imminent)
   c. Substances used to reduce absorption of poison
      (1) Charcoal
      (2) Cholestyramine (acidic compounds)
   d. Activated charcoal adsorbs many toxins if given immediately before or
      after lavage.
2. Induced emesis
   a. Same contraindications as for gastric lavage
   b. Makes use of syrup of ipecac (slow-acting oral emetic)
3. Current changes in emergency treatments
   a. Gastrointestinal (GI) decontamination
      (1) Ipecac now much less commonly used
      (2) Gastric lavage used much less
      (3) Whole bowel irrigation used more
      (4) Expanded use of activated charcoal

   b. Toxin elimination
      (1) Hemodialysis used much more than hemoperfusion
      (2) Expanded use of multiple doses of activated charcoal
D. History and physical examination provide clues to potential exposure.
   1. Oral statements may be unreliable.
   2. Always treat symptoms.
   3. Physical examination should focus on clues of intoxication.
   4. Vital signs should be checked

      • May lead to clues of intoxication
      a. Hypertension with tachycardia
         (1) Amphetamines
         (2) Cocaine
         (3) Antimuscarinics

      b. Hypotension and bradycardia
         (1) Beta blockers
         (2) Calcium channel blockers
         (3) Clonidine
         (4) Sedative-hypnotics

      c. Hypotension with tachycardia
         (1) Tricyclic antidepressants
         (2) Phenothiazines
         (3) Theophylline (acute)
         (4) β_2-agonists

      d. Rapid respiration
         (1) Salicylates
         (2) Carbon monoxide
         (3) Chemicals producing metabolic acidosis
         (4) Chemical producing cellular asphyxia (cyanide)

      e. Hyperthermia
         (1) Sympathomimetics
         (2) Anticholinergics
         (3) Salicylates
         (4) Uncouplers of oxidative phosphorylation (dinitrophenol)
         (5) Chemicals producing seizures or muscular rigidity

      f. Hypothermia
         (1) Phenothiazines
         (2) Ethanol
         (3) Other CNS depressants

      g. Eyes
         (1) Pupil constriction (miosis)
            (a) Opioids
            (b) Phenothiazines (α-blockade)
            (c) Cholinesterase inhibitors
            (d) Alpha receptor blockers

  (2) Pupil dilation (mydriasis)
   (a) Amphetamines
   (b) Cocaine
   (c) Lysergic acid diethylamide (LSD)
   (d) Phencyclidine (PCP)
   (e) Anticholinergics
 h. Skin
  (1) Flushed, hot, and dry
   (a) Atropine
   (b) Antimuscarinics
  (2) Excessive sweating
   (a) Cholinesterase inhibitors
   (b) Sympathomimetics
   (c) Parasympathomimetics
   (d) Nicotine
 i. Cyanosis
  (1) Hypoxemia
  (2) Methemoglobinemia (nitrites)
 j. Jaundice (liver toxicity)
  (1) Acetaminophen
  (2) Erythromycin estolate (cholestatic)
  (3) Carbon tetrachloride
  (4) Troglitazone
  (5) Valproic acid
 k. Abdomen
  (1) Ileus is typical of:
   (a) Antimuscarinics
   (b) Opioids
   (c) Sedatives
  (2) Hyperactive bowel sounds, cramping, and diarrhea; common with:
   (a) Organophosphates
   (b) Iron
   (c) Arsenic
   (d) Theophylline
   (e) Mushrooms
 l. Nervous system
  (1) Twitching and muscular hyperactivity
   (a) Anticholinergics
   (b) Sympathomimetics
   (c) Cocaine
  (2) Muscular rigidity
   (a) Antipsychotics (especially haloperidol)
   (b) Strychnine
  (3) Seizures (treat with intravenous diazepam or lorazepam)
  (4) Seizure producing agents
   (a) Theophylline
   (b) Isoniazid
   (c) Cocaine
   (d) Amphetamines
   (e) Tricyclic antidepressants
   (f) Diphenhydramine
   (g) Lidocaine
   (h) Meperidine
  (5) Flaccid paralysis and coma
   (a) Opioids
   (b) Sedative/hypnotics
   (c) Central nervous system depressants
E. Treatment for all poisons
 1. Symptomatic
 2. Supportive
 3. Antidotes when appropriate (see Table 30-2).

Margin notes: Open pupils: cocaine, sympathomimetics, parasympatholytics. High dose atropine flush; mechanism unknown. Excessive sweating; ganglionic stimulants parasympathomimetics and sympathomimetics. Liver toxins increase bilirubin accumulation leading to yellow color skin. Low bowel activity, parasympatholytics, opioids, sedatives. Hyperactive bowels; parasympathomimetics, iron, arsenic, mushrooms. Muscular rigidity produced by neuroleptics and convulsants. Treat seizures with diazepam or lorazepam. Pyridoxine best treats isoniazid-induced seizures. Flaccid paralysis and coma with marked CNS depression. For all poisons, always provide supportive treatment to minimize symptoms. For a few poisons, antidotes are available.

AT MUDPILES pneumonic for acidosis. **A**lcohol (chronic ethanol ketoacidosis), **T**oluene (renal tubular acidosis), **M**ethanol, **U**remia, **D**iabetic ketoacidosis, **P**araldehyde, **I**ron, **I**soniazid, **L**actic acid, **E**thylene glycol, **S**alicylates

Increased creatinine levels indicate renal toxicity; increased liver functional transaminases (LFTs) indicate hepatotoxicity.

Calculation of the osmolal gap is useful in evaluating causes of an increased anion gap metabolic acidosis. The plasma osmolality (POsm) is calculated— POsm = 2 (serum Na$^+$) + serum glucose/18 + serum blood urea nitrogen/2.8 + serum ethanol (mg/dL)/4.6 (if the patient is drinking ethanol) and is then subtracted from the measured POsm. A difference of less than 10 mOsm/kg is normal. A difference more than 10 mOsm/kg is highly suspicious for methanol and/or ethylene glycol poisoning.

Polyhydroxyl compounds produce an osmolar gap.

Results from toxicology screens are usually too late to help with treatment but are valuable in follow-up legal manifestations.

CT scans help rule out brain trauma.

Widening QRS caused by TCAs or quinidine is treated with sodium bicarbonate.

Potassium channel blockers prolong QT interval.

Treat torsades de pointes with magnesium sulfate.

Ammonium chloride acidifies the urine.

Acidification of the urine can lead to rhabdomyolysis.

F. **Laboratory and Procedures**
  1. Electrolyte analysis
    a. Anion gap = serum Na$^+$ − (serum HCO$_3^-$ + serum Cl$^-$)
      (1) Normal = 12 ± 2 mEq/L
      (2) Elevated by:
        (a) Renal failure
        (b) Diabetic ketoacidosis
        (c) Shock-induced lactic acidosis
        (d) Drug-induced metabolic acidosis
    b. Examples of toxins that elevate anion gap:
      (1) Salicylates
      (2) Methanol transforms to formic acid; also osmolar gap
      (3) Ethylene glycol transoforms to oxalic acid; also osmolar gap
      (4) Isoniazid
      (5) Iron
      (6) Metformin (lactic acidosis)
  2. Renal and liver functional tests
  3. Osmolar gap (solvents)
    a. Measured vs. calculated
      (1) 285 mOSmol (normal)
      (2) Calc. OS = $2\,Na^+ + \dfrac{glucose}{18} + \dfrac{BUN}{2.8}$
    b. Toxins that increase osmolar gap:
      (1) Ethanol
      (2) Methanol (also anion gap)
      (3) Ethylene glycol (also anion gap)
  4. Toxicology screens
  5. Computed tomography (CT) studies recommended if head trauma is suspected
  6. Electrocardiogram (ECG)
    a. Widening of QRS complex
      (1) Tricyclic antidepressants (TCAs)
      (2) Quinidine
    b. Torsades de pointes
      (1) Prolonged QT interval
      (2) Followed by ventricular tachycardia
      (3) A QRS that spirals around the *isoelectric line*
      (4) Caused by:
        (a) Quinidine (Class IA and III antiarrhythmics)
        (b) Tricyclic antidepressants (TCAs)
        (c) Phenothiazines
        (d) "Non-sedating" antihistamines (astemizole, terfenadine)
        (e) Cisapride
        (f) Fluoroquinolones
      (5) Prolonged QT caused by
        (a) β_1 Stimulation
        (b) Intense sympathetic activation
      (6) Factors that contribute to torsades de pointes
        (a) Hypokalemia
        (b) Hypomagnesemia
        (c) Hypocalcemia
        (d) Bradycardia
        (e) Ischemia
        (f) Tissue hypoxia
      (7) Treatment
        • Magnesium sulfate
G. **Increase the rate of excretion when appropriate.**
  1. Alteration of urine pH
    a. Acidification of urine
      (1) Use ammonium chloride
      (2) Increases excretion of weak organic bases
        (a) Phencyclidine
        (b) Amphetamines
      (3) *Not* often used today but often tested on Boards

   b. Alkalinization of urine
      (1) Use sodium bicarbonate or acetazolamide
      (2) Increases excretion of weak organic acids
         (a) Salicylates
         (b) Phenobarbital
   2. Cathartics
      a. Magnesium sulfate
      b. Osmotic diuretics
         (1) Mannitol
         (2) $MgSO_4$
         (3) Polyethylene glycol
   3. Whole bowel irrigation
      a. Body packers
         (1) Swallowed condoms filled with drugs of abuse
         (2) Used in drug trafficking
      b. Oral overdose with sustained release compounds
   4. Hemodialysis
   5. Peritoneal dialysis
   6. Hemoperfusion
III. **Teratogenic Effects of Specific Drugs:** (Table 30-3)
IV. **Dependence and Drugs of Abuse** (Table 30-4).
   • Repeated drug use may lead to dependence
   A. **Physical dependence**
      1. Examples
         a. Ethanol (Table 30-5)
         b. Barbiturates
         c. Opioids
      2. Symptoms
         a. Repeated administration produces
            (1) Altered or adaptive physiologic states
            (2) Signs and symptoms of withdrawal (abstinence syndrome)
         b. Withdrawal symptoms can last:
            (1) Days
            (2) Weeks
            (3) Months or occasionally longer
   B. **Psychological dependence**
      1. Examples
         a. Amphetamines
         b. Cocaine

Either acetazolamide or sodium bicarbonate can be used to alkalinize the urine.

Body packers are often used to smuggle drugs.

The smaller the volume of distribution (V_d), the more effective the hemodialysis.

Disulfiram discourages ethanol use.

Withdrawal symptoms occur when a physical dependent individual does not have substance in body.

TABLE 30-3. **Teratogenic Effects of Selected Drugs**

DRUG	ADVERSE EFFECTS
Alkylating agents and antimetabolites (anticancer drugs)	Cardiac defects; cleft palate; growth retardation; malformation of ears, eyes, fingers, nose, or skull; other anomalies
Carbamazepine	Abnormal facial features; neural tube defects such as spina bifida; reduced head size; other anomalies
Diethylstilbestrol (DES)	Effects in female offspring: clear cell vaginal or cervical adenocarcinoma; irregular menses and reproductive abnormalities, including decreased rate of pregnancy and increased rate of preterm deliveries Effects in male offspring: cryptorchism, epididymal cysts, hypogonadism
Ethanol	Fetal alcohol syndrome (growth retardation; hyperactivity; mental retardation; microcephaly and facial abnormalities; poor coordination; other anomalies)
Phenytoin	Fetal hydantoin syndrome (cardiac defects; malformation of ears, lips, palate, mouth, and nasal bridge; mental retardation; microcephaly, ptosis, strabismus; other anomalies)
Retinoids (systemic)	Spontaneous abortions; hydrocephaly; malformation of ears, face, heart, limbs, and liver; microcephaly; other anomalies
Tetracycline	Hypoplasia of tooth enamel, staining of teeth
Thalidomide	Deafness; heart defects; limb abnormalities (amelia or phocomelia); renal abnormalities; other anomalies
Valproate	Cardiac defects; central nervous system defects; lumbosacral spina bifida; microcephaly
Warfarin anticoagulants	Fetal warfarin syndrome (chondrodysplasia punctata; malformation of ears and eyes; mental retardation; nasal hypoplasia; optic atrophy; skeletal deformities; other anomalies)

Other substances known to be teratogenic: arsenic, cadmium, lead, lithium, methyl mercury, penicillamine, polychlorinated biphenyls, and trimethadione. Other drugs that should be avoided during the second and third trimesters of pregnancy: angiotensin-converting enzyme inhibitors, angiotensin receptor blockers, chloramphenicol, indomethacin, prostaglandins, sulfonamides, and sulfonylureas. Other drugs that should be used with great caution during pregnancy: antithyroid drugs, aspirin, barbiturates, benzodiazepines, corticosteroids, fluoroquinolones, heparin, opioids, and phenothiazines.

TABLE 30-4. **Drugs of Abuse**

DRUG	EFFECT	WITHDRAWAL	TREATMENT
Alcohol	Slurred speech, unsteady gait, nystagmus, lack of coordination, mood changes	Tremor, tachycardia, insomnia, seizures, delusions, hypertension	Clonidine, lorazepam, chlordiazepoxide, disulfiram
Amphetamines	Psychomotor agitation, pupil dilation, tachycardia, euphoria, hypertension, paranoia, seizures	Dysphoria, fatigue	Supportive care
Barbiturates	Same as alcohol	Anxiety, seizures, hypertension, irritability	Same as alcohol
Benzodiazepines	CNS depression, respiratory depression	Anxiety, hypertension, irritability	Supportive care, flumazenil
Caffeine	CNS stimulation, hypertension	Lethargy, headache, irritability	Supportive care
Cocaine	CNS stimulation, arrhythmias, psychomotor agitation, pupil dilation, tachycardia, euphoria, paranoia (similar to amphetamines)	Dysphoria, fatigue (same as amphetamines)	Supportive care
Lysergic acid diethylamide (LSD)	Anxiety, paranoia, pupil dilation, tremors, tachycardia, hallucinations Severe agitation may respond to diazepam	None	No specific treatment
Marijuana	Euphoria, dry mouth, increased appetite, conjunctival injection	Irritability, nausea	No specific treatment
Methylenedioxy-methamphetamine (MDMA, ecstasy)	Amphetamine-like hyperthermia, hypertension, jaw-clenching	Dysphoria, fatigue, brain damage	Reduce body temperature
Nicotine	CNS stimulation, increased GI motility	Anxiety, dysphoria, increased appetite	Bupropion, clonidine
Opioids	Pinpoint pupils, respiratory depression, hypotension	Dysphoria, nausea, diarrhea	Supportive care, naloxone, methadone, clonidine
Phencyclidine hydrochloride (PCP)	Aggressive behavior, horizontal-vertical nystagmus, ataxia, seizures, hallucinations	None	Life support, diazepam, haloperidol

CNS, central nervous system; GI, gastrointestinal.

TABLE 30-5. **Stages of Ethanol Poisoning***

DEGREE OF POISONING	BLOOD ALCOHOL LEVEL (mg/dL)	SYMPTOMS
Acute, mild	50–150	Decreased inhibitions, visual impairment, lack of muscular coordination, slowing of reaction time
Moderate	150–300	Major visual impairment, more pronounced symptoms of mild intoxication, slurred speech
Severe	300–500	Approaching stupor, severe hypoglycemia, seizures, death
Coma	>500	Unconsciousness, slowed respiration, complete loss of sensations, death (frequent)

*Disulfiram inhibits acetaldehyde dehydrogenase, which causes acetaldehyde to accumulate in the blood, resulting in nausea and vomiting if alcohol is consumed.

Psychological dependence promotes drug-seeking behaviors.

An addicted individual will continue to seek and use substances despite medical, financial, and social problems.

2. Affected individuals
   a. Use drug repeatedly for personal satisfaction
   b. Engage in compulsive drug-seeking behavior
C. Substance dependence (addiction)
  1. Chronic use results in a cluster of symptoms:
    a. Craving
    b. Withdrawal symptoms
    c. Drug-seeking behavior
  2. Continued use despite substance-related problems
    a. Medical
    b. Financial
    c. Social

COMMON LABORATORY VALUES

TEST	CONVENTIONAL UNITS	SI UNITS
Blood, Plasma, Serum		
Alanine aminotransferase (ALT, GPT at 30°C)	8–20 U/L	8–20 U/L
Amylase, serum	25–125 U/L	25–125 U/L
Aspartate aminotransferase (AST, GOT at 30° C)	8–20 U/L	8–20 U/L
Bilirubin, serum (adult): total; direct	0.1–1.0 mg/dL; 0.0–0.3 mg/dL	2–17 µmol/L; 0–5 µmol/L
Calcium, serum (Ca^{2+})	8.4–10.2 mg/dL	2.1–2.8mmol/L
Cholesterol, serum	Rec: <200 mg/dL	<5.2 mmol/L
Cortisol, serum	8:00 AM: 6–23 µg/dL; 4:00 PM: 3–15 µg/dL	170–630 nmol/L; 80–410 nmol/L
	8:00 PM: ≤50% of 8:00 AM	Fraction of 8:00 AM: ≤0.50
Creatine kinase, serum	Male: 25–90 U/L	25–90 U/L
	Female: 10–70 U/L	10–70 U/L
Creatinine, serum	0.6–1.2 mg/dL	53–106 µmol/L
Electrolytes, serum		
Sodium (Na^+)	136–145 mEq/L	135–145 mmol/L
Chloride (Cl^-)	95–105 mEq/L	95–105 mmol/L
Potassium (K^+)	3.5–5.0 mEq/L	3.5–5.0 mmol/L
Bicarbonate (HCO_3^-)	22–28 mEq/L	22–28 mmol/L
Magnesium (Mg^{2+})	1.5–2.0 mEq/L	1.5–2.0 mmol/L
Estriol, total, serum (in pregnancy)		
24–28 wk; 32–36 wk	30–170 ng/mL; 60–280 ng/mL	104–590 nmol/L; 208–970 nmol/L
28–32 wk; 36–40 wk	40–220 ng/mL; 80–350 ng/mL	140–760 nmol/L; 280–1210 nmol/L
Ferritin, serum	Male: 15–200 ng/mL	15–200 µg/L
	Female: 12–150 ng/mL	12–150 µg/L
Follicle-stimulating hormone, serum/plasma (FSH)	Male: 4–25 mIU/mL	4–25 U/L
	Female:	
	Premenopause, 4–30 mIU/mL	4–30 U/L
	Midcycle peak, 10–90 mIU/mL	10–90 U/L
	Postmenopause, 40–250 mIU/mL	40–250 U/L
Gases, arterial blood (room air)		
pH	7.35–7.45	[H^+] 36–44 nmol/L
P_{CO_2}	33–45 mmHg	4.4–5.9 kPa
P_{O_2}	75–105 mmHg	10.0–14.0 kPa
Glucose, serum	Fasting: 70–110 mg/dL	3.8–6.1 mmol/L
	2 hr postprandial: <120 mg/dL	<6.6 mmol/L
Growth hormone–arginine stimulation	Fasting: <5 ng/mL	<5 µg/L
	Provocative stimuli: >7 ng/mL	>7 µg/L
Immunoglobulins, serum		
IgA	76–390 mg/dL	0.76–3.90 g/L
IgE	0–380 IU/mL	0–380 kIU/L

(Continued)

TEST	CONVENTIONAL UNITS	SI UNITS
IgG	650–1500 mg/dL	6.5–15 g/L
IgM	40–345 mg/dL	0.4–3.45 g/L
Iron	50–170 µg/dL	9–30 µmol/L
Lactate dehydrogenase, serum	45–90 U/L	45–90 U/L
Luteinizing hormone, serum/plasma (LH)	Male: 6–23 mIU/mL	6–23 U/L
	Female:	
	Follicular phase, 5–30 mIU/mL	5–30 U/L
	Midcycle, 75–150 mIU/mL	75–150 U/L
	Postmenopause, 30–200 mIU/mL	30–200 U/L
Osmolality, serum	275–295 mOsm/kg	275–295 mOsm/kg
Parathyroid hormone, serum, N-terminal	230–630 pg/mL	230–630 ng/L
Phosphatase (alkaline), serum (p-NPP at 30° C)	20–70 U/L	20–70 U/L
Phosphorus (inorganic), serum	3.0–4.5 mg/dL	1.0–1.5 mmol/L
Prolactin, serum (hPRL)	<20 ng/mL	<20 µg/L
Proteins, serum		
Total (recumbent)	6.0–8.0 g/dL	60–80 g/L
Albumin	3.5–5.5 g/dL	35–55 g/L
Globulin	2.3–3.5 g/dL	23–35 g/L
Thyroid-stimulating hormone, serum or plasma (TSH)	0.5–5.0 µU/mL	0.5–5.0 mU/L
Thyroidal iodine (^{123}I) uptake	8–30% of administered dose/24hr	0.08–0.30/24hr
Thyroxine (T_4), serum	4.5–12 µg/dL	58–154 nmol/L
Triglycerides, serum	35–160 mg/dL	0.4–1.81 mmol/L
Triiodothyronine (T_3), serum, Radioimmune assay (RIA)	115–190 ng/dL	1.8–2.9 nmol/L
Triiodothyronine (T_3) resin uptake	25–38%	0.25–0.38
Urea nitrogen, serum (BUN)	7–18 mg/dL	1.2–3.0 mmol urea/L
Uric acid, serum	3.0–8.2 mg/dL	0.18–0.48 mmol/L
Cerebrospinal Fluid		
Cell count	0–5 cells/mm³	$0–5 \times 10^6$/L
Chloride	118–132 mEq/L	118–132 mmol/L
Gamma globulin	3–12% total proteins	0.03–0.12
Glucose	50–75 mg/dL	2.8–4.2 mmol/L
Pressure	70–180 mm H_2O	70–180 mm H_2O
Proteins, total	<40 mg/dL	<0.40 g/L
Hematology		
Bleeding time (template)	2–7 min	2–7 min
Erythrocyte count	Male: 4.3–5.9 million/mm³	$4.3–5.9 \times 10^{12}$/L
	Female: 3.5–5.5 million/mm³	$3.5–5.5 \times 10^{12}$/L
Erythrocyte sedimentation rate (Westergren)	Male: 0–15 mm/hr	0–15 mm/hr
	Female: 0–20 mm/hr	0–20 mm/hr
Hematocrit (Hct)	Male: 40–54%	0.40–0.54
	Female: 37–47%	0.37–0.47
Hemoglobin A_{IC}	≤6%	≤ 0.06%
Hemoglobin, blood (Hb)	Male: 13.5–17.5 g/dL	2.09–2.71 mmol/L
	Female: 12.0–16.0 g/dL	1.86–2.48 mmol/L
Hemoglobin, plasma	1–4 mg/dL	0.16–0.62 mmol/L
Leukocyte count and differential		
Leukocyte count	4500–11,000/mm³	$4.5–11.0 \times 10^9$/L
Segmented neutrophils	54–62%	0.54–0.62
Bands	3–5%	0.03–0.05
Eosinophils	1–3%	0.01–0.03
Basophils	0–0.75%	0–0.0075
Lymphocytes	25–33%	0.25–0.33
Monocytes	3–7%	0.03–0.07
Mean corpuscular hemoglobin (MCH)	25.4–34.6 pg/cell	0.39–0.54 fmol/cell
Mean corpuscular hemoglobin concentration (MCHC)	31–37% Hb/cell	4.81–5.74 mmol Hb/L

Mean corpuscular volume (MCV)	80–100 μm³	80–100 fl
Partial thromboplastin time (activated) (aPTT)	25–40 sec	25–40 sec
Platelet count	150,000–400,000/mm³	150–400 × 10⁹/L
Prothrombin time (PT)	12–14 sec	12–14 sec
Reticulocyte count	0.5–1.5% of red cells	0.005–0.015
Thrombin time	<2 sec deviation from control	<2 sec deviation from control
Volume		
Plasma	Male: 25–43 mL/kg	0.025–0.043 L/kg
	Female: 28–45 mL/kg	0.028–0.045 L/kg
Red cell	Male: 20–36 mL/kg	0.020–0.036 L/kg
	Female: 19–31 mL/kg	0.019–0.031 L/kg
Sweat		
Chloride	0–35 mmol/L	0–35 mmol/L
Urine		
Calcium	100–300 mg/24hr	2.5–7.5 mmol/24hr
Creatinine clearance	Male: 97–137 mL/min	
	Female: 88–128 mL/min	
Estriol, total (in pregnancy)		
30 wk	6–18 mg/24hr	21–62 μmol/24hr
35 wk	9–28 mg/24hr	31–97 μmol/24hr
40 wk	13–42 mg/24hr	45–146 μmol/24hr
17-Hydroxycorticosteroids	Male: 3.0–9.0 mg/24hr	8.2–25.0 μmol/24hr
	Female: 2.0–8.0 mg/24hr	5.5–22.0 μmol/24hr
17-Ketosteroids, total	Male: 8–22 mg/24hr	28–76 μmol/24hr
	Female: 6–15 mg/24hr	21–52 μmol/24hr
Osmolality	50–1400 mOsm/kg	
Oxalate	8–40 μg/mL	90–445 μmol/L
Proteins, total	<150 mg/24hr	<0.15 g/24hr

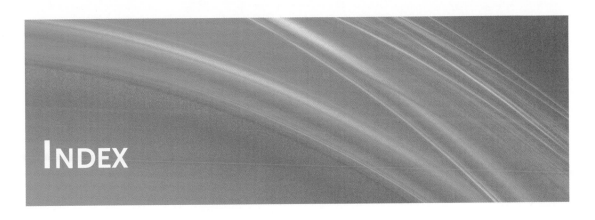

INDEX

Note: Page numbers followed by *b* indicate boxes, *f* indicate figures and *t* indicate tables.

A

Abacavir, 285*b*, 288, 291*t*, 292*t*
Abatacept, 192*b*, 192*t*, 194, 196*b*, 197, 199*t*
Abciximab, 138*f*, 139, 140*t*
Absence seizures, 71*t*, 72*b*, 74
Absorption, drug, 3, 4*f*
Abuse. *See* Drug abuse
Acarbose, 231
ACE inhibitors. *See* Angiotensin-converting enzyme
      inhibitors
Acebutolol, 44, 45*t*
Acetaminophen, 9, 9*b*, 21, 21*b*, 157, 158*t*, 159*t*
Acetazolamide, 9, 126*t*
Acetylation, 7, 8
Acetylcholine (ACh), 23, 23*b*, 24, 24*f*, 25*t*, 30*b*,
      32, 53
   as ganglionic stimulant, 32, 32*b*
   inhibitors, 181, 182*b*, 183*t*
   in motor end plate, 48, 48*f*
Acetylsalicylic acid. *See* Aspirin
ACh. *See* Acetylcholine
ACTH. *See* Adrenocorticotropin
Activity, drug, 20
Acyclovir, 7*b*, 285*b*, 287, 291*t*
Adalimumab, 188, 189*t*, 192*b*, 195, 196*b*, 198, 199*t*
Adefovir, 285*b*, 288, 291*t*
Adenosine, 101, 102*t*
ADH. *See* Antidiuretic hormone; Vasopressin
ADH antagonists, 134, 135*t*
ADHD. *See* Attention-deficit/hyperactivity disorder
Administration routes, 4, 5*t*
Adrenal medulla, ANS activity in, 27
Adrenergic drugs, 36–46, 45*t*
   adrenoreceptor agonists as, 36, 37*f*, 38*t*, 39*b*, 45*t*
   adrenoreceptor antagonists as, 41, 42*b*, 45*t*
   adrenergic pathways, 24*f*, 26, 26*t*
α₂-Adrenergic receptor agonists, 105*b*, 106, 111*t*
β₂-Adrenergic receptor agonists, 172, 173*b*,
      174, 176*t*
α₁-Adrenergic receptor antagonists, 105*b*, 107, 111*t*
β-Adrenergic receptor antagonists, 42, 42*b*, 105, 105*b*,
      111*t*, 114*b*, 114*f*
   as antianginal, 114*b*, 114*f*, 115, 116*t*
   as antiarrhythmic, 96*b*, 98, 102*t*
   for heart failure, 119, 120*b*, 122, 123*t*
Adrenocorticosteroids, 216, 217*b*, 218*f*, 218*t*,
      219*f*, 224*t*
Adrenocorticotropin (ACTH)-related preparations, 206*b*,
      208, 211*t*
Adrenoreceptor agonists, 36, 37*f*, 38*t*, 39*b*, 45*t*
β₂-Adrenoreceptor agonists, uterine effects of, 243*b*,
      244, 245*t*
Adrenoreceptor antagonists, 41, 42*b*, 45*t*
   α, 41, 42*b*
   β, 42, 42*b*
Adverse drug effects, 21
Affinity, 18
Agonist, 14
   full, 18
   inverse, 18
   partial, 14, 18

Albuterol, 5*t*, 20, 25*t*, 40, 45*t*, 172, 176*t*
Alcohol, 1, 5*t*, 8, 8*b*, 8*t*, 10, 21, 21*b*
   abuse of, 326*t*
   as CNS depressant, 11, 61
   poisoning, 325, 326*t*
Aldosterone, 217*b*, 222
Aldosterone antagonists, 130*f*, 131, 133*t*
Alemtuzumab, 316, 316*b*, 316*t*
Alendronate, 239
Alfuzosin, 41, 45*t*
Aliphatic phenothiazines, 80
Aliskiren, 110, 111*t*
Alkylating drugs, 305, 305*b*
Allergies, 21, 175, 176*b*, 177*t*
Allopurinol, 200*b*, 201
Allylamine antifungal drugs, 297*b*, 297*f*, 300, 301*t*
Alosetron, 184, 184*b*, 186*t*, 187, 187*t*, 188*t*
Aluminum hydroxide, 179*b*, 180, 182*t*
Amantadine, 92, 93*t*, 284, 285*b*, 291*t*
Amides, as local anesthetic, 67*b*, 68, 69
Amikacin, 269, 269*b*, 271, 276*t*, 282*b*, 283
Amiloride, 126*t*
γ-Aminobutyric acid (GABA), 56, 56*f*
γ-Aminobutyric acid (GABA) mimetics, 47,
      48*b*, 50*b*
Aminocaproic acid, 146
Aminoglutethimide, 217*b*, 223, 314*t*, 314*b*
Aminoglycosides, 5*t*, 21, 21*b*, 269, 269*b*
Aminophylline, 174, 176*t*
5-Aminosalicylic acid (5-ASA), 187, 189*t*
Amiodarone, 99, 102*t*
Amitriptyline, 82, 83*t*, 86*t*
Amlodipine, 109, 111*t*
Ammonium chloride, 9
Amoxapine, 84, 86*t*
Amoxicillin, 261, 262*b*, 264, 267*t*
Amphetamine, 4*f*, 9, 20, 25*t*, 40, 87, 88*t*, 326*t*
Amphotericin B, 297*b*, 297*f*, 298, 301*t*
Ampicillin, 260*t*, 262*b*, 264, 267*t*
Amprenavir, 285*b*, 288, 291*t*
Amyl nitrate, 5*t*
Amyl nitrite, 113
Amylinomimetic, 226*t*, 231, 233*t*
Anagrelide, 139, 140*t*
Anakinra, 196*b*, 197, 199*t*
Anastrozole, 314*b*, 315
Androgens, 246*b*, 252, 254*t*, 255*t*
Androgen antagonists, 314*b*, 315
Anemia, 147, 148*t*
Anesthetics, 64–69
   general, 64, 65*b*
   inhalation, 64, 65*b*, 65*t*
   local, 22, 67, 67*b*
   parenteral, 65*b*, 66
   preanesthetic medications, 67, 67*t*
Angiotensin receptor blockers (ARBs), 105*b*, 110, 111*t*,
      119, 120*b*, 122, 123*t*
Angiotensin-converting enzyme (ACE) inhibitors, 105*b*,
      109, 111*t*, 119, 120*b*, 122, 123*t*
Anidulafungin, 297*b*, 297*f*, 299, 301*t*
ANS. *See* Autonomic nervous system
Antacids, 179*b*, 180, 182*t*